The History and Compilation of Zhang Zhongjing's *Wu Zang Lun*

People who have studied acupuncture and Chinese medicine recognize Zhang Zhongjing as the author of two seminal texts that are among the most influential in Chinese medical history: the *Treatise on Cold Damage Disorders* (Shāng Hán Lùn, 伤寒论) and *Essential Prescriptions from the Golden Cabinet* (Jīn Guì Yào Lüè, 金匮要略). However, what is less well-known is that Zhang Zhongjing authored several other texts, all of which were lost over time, with the sole exception of the *Five Viscera Theory* (Wǔ Zàng Lùn, 五藏论). This was discovered in 1900 in a hidden library of China's Mogao Caves of Dunhuang by a Taoist priest named Wang Yuanlu.

***The History and Compilation of Zhang Zhongjing's* Wu Zang Lun** stands as the first comprehensive work in English detailing the history and compilation of Zhongjing's *Five Viscera Theory* (Wǔ Zàng Lùn, 五藏论). It uses storytelling to illuminate the historical context of the eight versions of this book that were discovered: five versions found in Dunhuang and three versions from Zhejiang China, Korea, and Japan respectively. By exploring the origin and development of these versions this book not only delves into traditional Chinese medicine but also intertwines fascinating elements of humanities, history, and geography. The reader is offered insight into the Dunhuang manuscripts' background and the significance of Zhongjing's contributions to medical literature.

The History and Compilation of Zhang Zhongjing's *Wu Zang Lun*

Five Viscera Theory

Qiang Cao and Yun Xiao

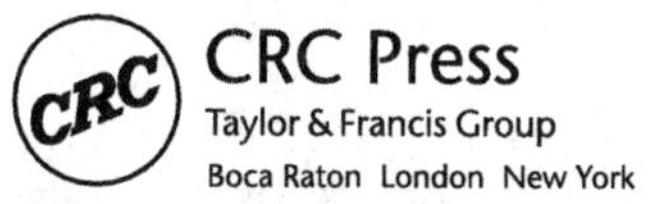
CRC Press
Taylor & Francis Group
Boca Raton London New York

CRC Press is an imprint of the
Taylor & Francis Group, an **informa** business

Cover Image Credit: Shutterstock.com.

In the Hidden Library, the colored statue of Wu Hongbian, dressed in monk's robes and emulating the Medicine Buddha, sits in full lotus position on a rectangular meditation platform.

First edition published 2025
by CRC Press
2385 NW Executive Center Drive, Suite 320, Boca Raton FL 33431

and by CRC Press
4 Park Square, Milton Park, Abingdon, Oxon, OX14 4RN

CRC Press is an imprint of Taylor & Francis Group, LLC

ISBN: 978-1-032-69819-9 (hbk)
ISBN: 978-1-032-69006-3 (pbk)
ISBN: 978-1-032-69820-5 (ebk)

DOI: 10.1201/9781032698205

Typeset in Times
by Apex CoVantage, LLC

Contents

Author Biographies

Qiang Cao, ND, L.Ac

Professor Cao has an impressive career spanning over 45 years, primarily teaching traditional Chinese medicine (TCM). He started his career at Shanghai University of TCM in China, where he taught from 1977 to 1987 before moving to the United States to study naturopathic medicine. He co-founded the acupuncture and oriental medicine program at Bastyr University, where he has been teaching Chinese medicine for 35 years.

In addition to his teaching, Prof. Cao's research has been published in peer-reviewed journals in China, focusing on clinical research on Qingpi extract injection to treat various conditions such as septic shock, cardiogenic shock, anaphylactic shock, neurogenic shock, and paroxysmal supraventricular tachycardia. Prof. Cao has also played a significant role in conducting research on the effectiveness of Qingpi injection for the treatment of paroxysmal supraventricular tachycardia, which was published in the *Journal of Integrated Traditional Chinese and Western Medicine.*

While Prof. Cao's primary focus has been on academic teaching and clinical acupuncture practice in the United States, he has also been a core faculty member teaching fundamental courses in acupuncture and Chinese herbal medicine. He has extensive expertise in Zhang Zhongjing's theories and has been teaching TCM medical classics since the 1990s. He taught Zhang Zhongjing's "Treatise on Cold Damage Disorders" for the doctoral program in the first decade of the 21st century.

In 2011, Prof. Cao's interest in Dunhuang medicine was piqued when he encountered Zhang Zhongjing's *Wu Zang Lun* at an academic conference at Gansu University of TCM in China. Since then, he has been studying this theory for over a decade and has conducted extensive research on this book. In 2012, he presented his paper on "Hypothesis on the Authorship and Collection of the Dunhuang Manuscript Fragments of Zhang Zhongjing's *Wu Zang Lun*" at the 20th Academic Symposium on Zhang Zhongjing's Theory, which was published in the symposium proceedings.

Yun Xiao, DAc, L.Ac.

Dr. Yun Xiao, as an adjunct faculty at Bastyr University and an experienced acupuncturist and herbalist at Wedgwood Acupuncture & Botanical Medicine, holds an impressive educational background with a doctorate in acupuncture and a master's in acupuncture and East Asian medicine from Bastyr University, alongside a bachelor's in herbal medicine from Shanghai University of TCM. Her deep passion for medical literature has driven her to explore ancient medical classics, firmly believing in their value to enhance our understanding of medicine's evolution and its application in innovative health solutions.

Her notable collaboration with Professor Cao on Zhang Zhongjing's *Wu Zang Lun* underscores her dedication to enriching medical theory and practice by reconnecting with historical insights. A recognized voice in TCM, Dr. Xiao's lectures deliver critical insights into TCM, embodying her commitment to integrating ancient wisdom with contemporary medical strategies.

Preface

Individuals studying acupuncture and traditional Chinese medicine (TCM) are well-acquainted with Zhang Zhongjing's two seminal texts, the *Treatise on Cold Damage Disorders* (Shāng Hán Lùn, 伤寒论) and the *Essential Prescriptions from the Golden Cabinet* (Jīn Guì Yào Lüè, 金匮要略), collectively referred to as the *Treatise on Cold Damage and Miscellaneous Disorders* (Shāng Hán Zá Bìng Lùn, 伤寒杂病论). These works are among the most influential in the history of Chinese medicine. The *Treatise on Cold Damage Disorders* delves into the treatment principles for diseases caused by external factors, while the *Essential Prescriptions from the Golden Cabinet* stands as the earliest extant monograph on the diagnosis and treatment of a variety of diseases. Together with the *Yellow Emperor's Classic of Internal Medicine* (Huáng Dì Nèi Jīng, 黄帝内经) and *Shennong's Classic of Materia Medica* (Shén Nóng Běn Cǎo Jīng, 神农本草经), these texts are celebrated as the "four great classics of traditional Chinese medicine." Within this esteemed quartet, Zhang Zhongjing's contributions are particularly distinguished and unparalleled.

In 2012, while serving as a professor of TCM at Bastyr University in the United States, I participated in a conference dedicated to the works of Zhang Zhongjing at the Gansu University of Chinese Medicine in China. It was during this time that I stumbled upon the *Five Viscera Theory* (Wǔ Zàng Lùn, 五藏论), and I also had the opportunity to explore the Mogao Caves in Dunhuang. This experience left me feeling quite humbled; despite my extensive knowledge and proficiency in Chinese medicine, capable of confidently addressing my students' myriad inquiries, I was utterly perplexed by the *Five Viscera Theory* (Wǔ Zàng Lùn, 五藏论). It raised the question: Did Zhang Zhongjing actually author this text? This encounter sparked a profound fascination with both the *Five Viscera Theory* (Wǔ Zàng Lùn, 五藏论) and the narratives surrounding the Mogao Caves, leading me to dedicate over ten years to researching Zhang Zhongjing's *Five Viscera Theory* (Wǔ Zàng Lùn, 五藏论).

In my research into the literature, I discovered that besides the *Treatise on Cold Damage Disorders*, Zhang Zhongjing also authored other works, including two volumes of *Zhang Zhongjing's formula for gynecological disorders* (Zhāng Zhòng Jǐng Liáo Fù Rén Fāng, 张仲景疗妇人方), 15 volumes of *Zhang Zhongjing's Formula* (Zhāng Zhòng Jǐng Fāng, 张仲景方), one volume of *Five Viscera Theory* (Wǔ Zàng Lùn, 五藏论), *Zhang Zhongjing's Treatise on treating the yellow* (Zhāng Zhòng Jǐng Liáo Huáng Jīng, 张仲景疗黄经), *Zhang Zhongjing's Theory of Mouth and Tooth* (Zhāng Zhòng Jǐng Kǒu Chǐ Lùn, 张仲景口齿论), and one volume of *Zhang Zhongjing's Discussion about Diseases and Essential Formula* (Zhāng Zhòng Jǐng Píng Bìng Yào Fāng, 张仲景评病要方). However, due to prolonged wars, ravages of conflict, and other such reasons, all these works, except *Five Viscera Theory* (Wǔ Zàng Lùn, 五藏论), have been lost to history, with only their titles remaining. Even the *Five Viscera Theory* (Wǔ Zàng Lùn, 五藏论), which has survived, exhibits variations among different versions.

Throughout the years, the Dunhuang manuscripts have emerged as a pivotal subject in cultural research, drawing interest from around the world. Among this extensive trove of over 50,000 documents, a seemingly modest number – about a hundred – are dedicated to medicine, representing a mere 0.2% of the entire collection. Yet it's remarkable that among these medical texts, *Five Viscera Theory* (Wǔ Zàng Lùn, 五藏论) stands out, with five distinct versions available.

Zhang Zhongjing's *Five Viscera Theory* (Wǔ Zàng Lùn, 五藏论) is represented by five manuscripts unearthed in Dunhuang, which are preserved in the British Library as S. 5614, in the National Library of France (Bibliothèque nationale de France), Paris, as P. 2115, P. 2755, and P. 2378, and in the Saint Petersburg branch of the Institute of Oriental Studies of the Russian Academy of Sciences as Дx. 01325V. In addition to these five manuscripts, there are three non-Dunhuang versions, including a version in the Korean *Categorized Collection of Medical Formulas* (Yī Fāng Lèi Jù, 医方类聚), a handwritten manuscript by the renowned physician Zhang Yicheng from North Zhejiang (with a preface by Zhang Yuansu), and the Gakkundō wooden-movable type edition from Japan.

Interestingly, while Zhang Zhongjing's *Five Viscera Theory* (Wǔ Zàng Lùn, 五藏论) was referenced in a 2005 publication titled *Medieval Chinese Medicine* (中世纪中国医学), which discussed four versions of the text, it did not include the original writings. Moreover, within English-language academic journals, there is scarcely any abstract, translation, or research article related to Zhang Zhongjing's *Five Viscera Theory* (Wǔ Zàng Lùn, 五藏论).

After dedicating six years to literature research and gathering insights, I had the honor of joining forces with Dr. Yun Xiao to embark on an in-depth exploration of this monumental TCM work, *Five Viscera Theory* (Wǔ Zàng Lùn, 五藏论). A decade of dedication allowed us to collaboratively complete an initial draft of nearly 1 million characters.

My journey began in the 1980s when I moved from Shanghai University of TCM to the United States to develop the acupuncture and Chinese herbal medicine program at Bastyr University. Over 35 years of teaching at Bastyr and a total of 45 years immersed in the teaching and clinical practice of TCM have provided me with a deep and broad foundation of knowledge. Leveraging my theoretical understanding and clinical experience, I aimed to elucidate the complex concepts within Zhang Zhongjing's *Five Viscera Theory* (Wǔ Zàng Lùn, 五藏论), covering the broad spectrums of astronomy, geography, the core principles of Chinese medicine, and the extensive pharmacology of medicinal plants, along with their clinical applications.

In the course of my research, I deeply realized that my interpretations may not accurately reflect the essence of Zhang Zhongjing's philosophy. It dawned on me that only by allowing students to first engage with the most authentic versions of *Five Viscera Theory* (Wǔ Zàng Lùn, 五藏论) can we spark a genuine comprehension of Zhang Zhongjing's insights. This revelation has led me to considerable reflection. What, then, is the correct way forward?

Going back to the Tang Dynasty, there's a story behind the idiom "throwing a brick to attract jade" that carries deep meaning. During this period, Zhao Gu and Chang Jian, two poets renowned for their extraordinary talent, deeply admired each other's work. When Chang Jian learned that Zhao Gu planned to visit Lingyan Temple, he penned the opening lines of a poem, hoping to spark inspiration in Zhao Gu. True to expectations, upon encountering these lines on the temple's wall, Zhao Gu seamlessly added his verses, elevating it to a complete and exquisite poem. This act of initiating a modest contribution to inspire greater excellence from others is what gave rise to the saying "throwing a brick to attract jade," symbolizing the use of one's humble input to draw out the brilliant contributions of others.

In an innovative approach, this book shines a light on *Five Viscera Theory* (Wǔ Zàng Lùn, 五藏论), encapsulating its significance within a concise 80,000 words. Through engaging storytelling, it explores the genesis and evolution of this seminal work, providing readers with a glimpse into its historical context, authorship, and the practical applications that underscore its value. The book meticulously presents eight pristine versions, offering a unique opportunity to appreciate the text's foundational role in Chinese medicine. What is it that elevates this document to the status of a classical masterpiece? How has it influenced the trajectory of Chinese medical history? And what implications might it hold for the vibrant fields of acupuncture and herbal medicine today?

For example, in Zhang Zhongjing's *Five Viscera Theory* (Wǔ Zàng Lùn, 五藏论), there's a treasure trove of knowledge with records of hundreds of herbs and a variety of prescriptions, such as using Ephedra for treating cold-induced fevers, the hallucinogenic effects of prolonged consumption of cannabis flowers, and the opium-laced Western medicine known as Theriac, renowned for its ability to cure all kinds of diseases. As we all know, the breakthrough discovery of artemisinin, a cornerstone in modern malaria treatment, owes its success to the meticulous study of ancient texts on TCM. Given this precedent, who can predict whether Zhang Zhongjing's writings might yield the next groundbreaking discovery akin to artemisinin?

Seattle, famously known as the city of rain, has recently seen its winters graced with a generous blanket of snow each year. The Burke-Gilman Trail, just steps from my home, is a beloved recreational pathway that welcomes a diverse crowd – walkers, runners, cyclists, inline skaters, and commuters. This trail was once an abandoned railway line running along Lake Washington's shores and through Seattle's east, now repurposed into one of Washington State's cherished routes. Whenever I face doubts or seek inspiration for my writing, a leisurely walk along the Burke-Gilman Trail invariably provides me with clarity and fresh ideas.

This winter has been extraordinarily cold, bringing with it another layer of snow. The Burke-Gilman Trail now wears a blanket of snow several inches thick. With early winter, moist snowflakes scatter across the forests lining the path, and the weight of the snow causes branches to snap and break, floating down through the air. These drifting snowflakes, like dandelion seeds caught in a breeze, are the muse for my writing, wafting with the wind. As they gently fall, they resemble the delicate petals of pear blossoms dancing in the sky, mirroring the mysteries in my writing that are soon to be unraveled by the warmth of the earth. The nearby lake and distant mountains fade into the snowy mist, their colors lost; further still, they merge with the hazy sky, enshrouded in a veil of mist. In such a vast and tranquil environment, one can truly sense the passage of time and awaken to deep insights. I envision a figure in the distance, a Taoist priest no taller than four feet, struggling to move forward. Could this be the figure of Wang, the humble Taoist? I yearn to ask him if he has ever encountered *Five Viscera Theory* (Wǔ Zàng Lùn, 五藏论). Following his footsteps, I pursue.

Qiang Cao

1 Wang Tao-shih, the Discoverer of the Hidden Library of Dunhuang

"After enduring countless hardships, he no longer harbors desires for fame and fortune."

– The Epitaph of Wang Tao-shih

In the closing chapter of the 19th century, the land was held captive by a fierce and unyielding winter. The Dang River, once a flowing serenade, lay imprisoned beneath a relentless siege of ice and snow. Its tranquil journey hidden, as if silenced by winter's stern hand. The valley, now a realm of desolation, echoed with the merciless howling of the wind. This gust, a ruthless maestro, orchestrated a symphony of snowflakes and sand, each note striking the burdened trees like a myriad of icy daggers. The river's surface, a battlefield scarred and fractured, bore witness to the season's unforgiving onslaught, each crack and crevice telling a tale of winter's harsh and unrelenting dominion.

On the opposite bank of the Dang River, a figure in the garb of a Taoist monk struggled amidst despair. He was of small stature, barely reaching four feet, his stooped and frail body topped by an incongruously large head. His Taoist robe, worn and tattered. His eyes, as small as a mouse's, did not seem to search for anything. Clouded with murkiness and streaked with red, they were windows to an inscrutable mind, perhaps devoid of any thoughts. His hair was cropped extremely short, seemingly to highlight his comical ears that had caught many a local tale in his travels. His forehead bore deep furrows, etched with the dust of his tumultuous and impoverished wanderings.

The piercing cold wind grew even more fierce here, cutting through his collar and sleeves. Beyond his Taoist robe, he had no protection against the relentless chill. Shivering incessantly, he tried to curl up to shield his neck from the icy gusts, but his efforts seemed in vain; his entire body was nearly frozen solid. He attempted to step forward, seeking warmth, but his legs betrayed him, trembling nonstop, refusing to move. The northwest wind, wild like an untamed stallion, carried a mix of sand, dust, and snowflakes, almost ready to sweep him up and whisk him away into the maelstrom.

Suddenly, from the northwest, a long howl pierced the vast wilderness, spreading in every direction and echoing back through the steep valleys. With his many years of wandering, he had accumulated a wealth of experience and instantly recognized the sound as the call of wolves. Before he could even think, one wolf, then two, ten,

DOI: 10.1201/9781032698205-1

hundreds, and thousands joined in the howling. Their cries rose and fell in waves, as if declaring war and simultaneously performing a ritual for their prey. The sound surged like a tide, wave after wave, relentless.

The howling grew closer and closer, enveloping him until he could barely breathe. Despair engulfed him when, on a snow-draped slope not a hundred steps away, he spotted a formidable pack of northwest wolves. With unwavering focus, their piercing eyes were locked squarely on him, intensifying the sense of imminent peril. They were too numerous to count; their silvery fur blended seamlessly with the snowy landscape. Only their eyes, emitting a haunting azure glow by the hundreds, shone like sharp iron nails, flickering in the fading twilight, revealing hunger and savage intent. The Daoist monk – their prey – stood frozen, unable to move.

The closest wolf to him was at least twice as robust, its body towering over half a person when standing. Its upright ears resembled two sharp arrows, sending shivers down one's spine.

Engulfed in profound terror, he drifted between clarity and delirium. The wolves before him were not ordinary beasts; they were white skeletons clad in wolf skins. Their sharp teeth dripped with fresh blood. In an instant, they could sever his head; within minutes, his flesh and bones would be torn to shreds, swallowed into their bellies. Their enormous jaws opened and closed, propelling the horde of skeletal specters towards him. Was this the White Bone Demon from *Journey to the West* (Xī Yóu Jì, 西游记), craving the flesh of Priest Tang-sen?

"I am not Priest Tang-sen! Even if you consume my flesh, it won't grant you eternal life!" His heart pleaded ceaselessly, beseeching any deity, any immortal, to come to his rescue. His body was covered in goosebumps, akin to the spines of a hedgehog. Cold sweat dripped down, following the raised hairs, soaking his Taoist robe. He turned hastily, fleeing with all his might, yet the footsteps behind him drew nearer. He could feel a pair of skeletal claws almost grasping his collar from behind.

He could no longer run, no longer escape. Dizzy and parched, he stood there in a daze, utterly defenseless. Like a lamb awaiting slaughter, he awaited his body to be torn asunder, to be devoured. He attempted to breathe, inhaling and exhaling, not knowing which breath would be his "final gasp."

Perhaps it was a hallucination born from extreme fear, or maybe it was the culmination of years of unwavering faith in the Buddha. At the very moment he believed he was on the verge of death, suddenly, all around him fell into a profound silence. In the distance, countless splendid rays of light began to ascend, so brilliant that he could hardly open his eyes. The radiance was so intense that he struggled to distinguish whether it originated from the heavens or the earthly realm. In that moment, all his fear dissolved into nothingness. The horde of white skeletons clad in wolf skins that had surrounded him vanished, unnoticed and unremembered.

He steadied himself, his hands still icy, his feet trembling uncontrollably. He pinched his own emaciated thigh, feeling the pain. Had he truly arrived in the legendary Western Pure Land? Was he in the process of becoming an immortal, or had he already attained enlightenment? His mind was clouded with confusion. His gaze followed the myriad threads of radiant light, stretching endlessly. At the culmination of that luminous spectacle, he perceived the destination guided by the Buddha himself. It was only later that he realized that place was the renowned Mogao Caves in Dunhuang.

The Dunhuang Oasis lies at the western end of the Hexi Corridor, surrounded by snow-capped mountains, with Yangguan to the front and Yumen Pass to the rear. Its centerpiece is the Crescent Lake, resembling a pool, encircled by the echoing sands of the desert, with the Dang River winding like a ribbon. The name "Dang River" originates from a Mongolian phrase, meaning the river of fertile grasslands. This name is not mere flattery. The Dang River is a stream of melted ice and snow from the Qilian Mountains, flowing into Dunhuang, and it is also the only underground river in China that flows from south to north. Under the nurturing flow of the Dang River, the once-barren desert has transformed into a lush oasis. For thousands of years, the Dang River has flowed serenely, moistening Dunhuang. It breathes new vitality and opportunities into the Mogao Caves while silently witnessing the rise and fall of generations in this land.

Legend has it that the Mogao Caves are a mysterious and magical place, believed to be a sacred site where numerous immortals manifest, as recorded in the murals within the caves. According to historical records, in the second year of Jianyuan during the former Qin dynasty (around 366 AD), an ascetic monk named Le Zun[1] stood at the edge of a cliff in the Dang River Valley, gazing at the distant Sanwei Mountain. He witnessed the peaks radiating countless golden lights under the glow of the evening sun, shining brilliantly and exceptionally pure. The scene was incredibly peculiar, even giving the illusion of a "thousand Buddhas." Inspired by this sight, monk Le Zun conceived a grand aspiration and decided to carve caves and construct temples here. After centuries of continuous construction, the Mogao Caves gradually developed into a Buddhist holy land with over a thousand grottoes, commonly known as the "Caves of a Thousand Buddhas."

In the same vein as monk Le Zun, who witnessed the radiant Buddha light, there walked a traveler in a Daoist robe named Wang Yuanlu.[2] Hailing from Macheng in Hubei, he was born around the year 1850 (the thirtieth year of the Daoguang reign). Came from a family of peasants, he acquired some knowledge of letters in his early years and had a modest understanding of the written word. However, during his youth, due to natural disasters and famine, he was compelled to flee to the northwestern region of Suzhou (present-day Jiuquan City, Gansu Province).[3]

During the early years of the Guangxu Emperor's reign in the Qing Dynasty, Wang Yuanlu, driven by financial hardships, found himself compelled to join the military. This decision, born out of necessity, provided him with a means to secure his basic livelihood. However, engaging daily in killings, robberies, and heinous crimes, including rape and pillage, became unbearable for this inherently simple-hearted farm boy. Despite his limited education, Wang Yuanlu was a devout soul. He had previously read *Journey to the West* (Xī Yóu Jì, 西游记), a novel that narrates the story of Xuanzang, also known as Tang-sen, a 29-year-old monk from the Tang Dynasty's Zhenguan era (628 AD), who embarked on a journey to retrieve the supreme scriptures and traveled to India, known as the Western Regions at that time. During this westward expedition, Xuanzang and his three disciples faced innumerable hardships, totaling 81 tribulations. Xuanzang swore, "Not until I attain the great teachings will

I take a single step back." They traversed an 800 mile desert devoid of any living creatures, a place where "no birds flew above, no beasts roamed below, all around was vast emptiness, devoid of humans and horses." Sometimes they endured hunger and starvation, while at other times, they faced threats from bandits and even pursued by ferocious wolves. Nevertheless, the Mogao Caves remained their sanctuary, allowing them to rest and recuperate.

Wang Yuanlu held profound admiration for Tang Xuanzang, respecting the monk's unwavering spirit dedicated to the Buddhist faith, regardless of personal gains or losses. He longed to venture to the Western Paradise just like Xuanzang, seeking the timeless scriptures that could bestow upon people a life of happiness. Some had told him that ancient people could see deities, but in the present age, human hearts had turned corrupt, and therefore, divine beings no longer revealed themselves to the world. Wang Yuanlu aspired to be a kind soul capable of glimpsing the divine. Thus, he laid down his weapons, bidding farewell to his life as a soldier, and returned to his homeland.

However, China at that time was engulfed in turmoil and calamity, making it nearly impossible for him to find a stable home. Years of wandering left him in a state of confusion; he didn't know where he could settle down or which path he should tread for his future. Only carried by the aspiration to attain enlightenment, he became a Taoist monk, embraced a life of seclusion in the local community. He adapted the monastic name "Fazhen." Interestingly, not many people referred to him as "Fazhen"; most simply called him "Wang Tao-shih."

That year, Wang Tao-shih had entered the latter half of his life's journey. Despite his monastic vows, life as a Taoist monk remained harsh. He endured scarcity in food and clothing, persevering through days of hardship. Reflecting on the decades that had slipped away, he lacked the audacious spirit of the Monkey King or the supernatural abilities of the White Dragon Horse. He remained destitute, his aspirations unfulfilled. Stagnating in place, he seemed resigned, believing that his life was destined to continue in this manner.

Yet perhaps due to an inner unwillingness to accept his fate or out of sheer necessity, he eventually made a firm decision. He resolved to follow in the footsteps of Tang Xuanzang, embarking on the journey alone. Carrying his alms bowl, he set forth along the eastern bank of the Dang River, beginning his solitary pilgrimage towards the west.

The wandering life of this peasant-turned-Taoist priest was never chronicled in the annals of Chinese official history. Whether he encountered the pursuit of the white skeletons clad in wolf skins, during his journey to the west, only to be saved by the divine radiance, remains a mystery lost to the sands of time. However, the epitaph on Wang Yuanlu's tomb does record that he not only faced demonic tribulations on his pilgrimage to the west, growing disenchanted with fame and fortune, but also stood atop the peak of Mount Sanwei. Like the venerable Monk Le Zun, he gazed into the distance at the ancient caves of a thousand Buddhas and exclaimed with boundless passion, "This is the Western Paradise!"[4]

In *Journey to the West* (Xī Yóu Jì, 西游记), Xuanzang is portrayed as a revered, almost divine figure, enduring 81 trials that would overwhelm any ordinary mortal.

Contrasting this, Wang Yuanlu recognized his own limitations as an ordinary man, far from the realm of immortality. Nevertheless, he found enlightenment in the divine radiance that seemed to guide him to the Mogao Caves of Dunhuang. For him, this place emerged as a sanctuary, possibly the very destination where the Buddha meant for him to spend his life. Despite the desolate terrain of the Mogao Caves, marked by sporadic offerings and incense, the site was still cared for by nearby villagers. The absence of luxury or lavish meals didn't diminish the tranquil and elegant atmosphere that brought peace to Wang Yuanlu's heart. Having spent years adrift without the comfort of family or friends, he chose to make this serene place his final abode, spending his remaining years in its quiet embrace. Despite being a Taoist in a Buddhist holy site, the people of Dunhuang embraced both Buddhism and Taoism. The coexistence of different beliefs did not hinder him from finding solace and a home in this place.

Initially, Wang Yuanlu's life was marked by poverty, frequently struggling to secure even three meals a day. At that time, the Mogao Caves were in a state of desolation, nearly engulfed by shifting sands and sparse grasslands, creating a landscape where foxes and wolves roamed freely, emphasizing its isolation from the outside world. Fortunately, Wang Yuanlu was gifted with a few valuable skills. His eloquence made him an effective preacher, and he had a basic knowledge of Taoist arts. This enabled him to read fortunes, perform divination, and even name newborns. More and more people seeking divination and guidance came to him, contributing to the prosperity of his Taoist temple. Despite his modest appearance, Wang Yuanlu succeeded in establishing a Taoist temple amidst the Buddhist sacred site, dedicating it to the worship of the three principal Daoist deities. He emerged as a prominent figure, representing the Daoist tradition within the Mogao Caves.

Every day, he diligently went out for alms, conducted Taoist rituals for people, and provided divination and fortune-telling services. Though his income wasn't abundant, it sufficed to sustain his basic needs. Wang Tao-shih remained a devout Daoist monk; even as his life became more comfortable, his thoughts didn't turn towards acquiring possessions or considering marriage. He invested his surplus money into clearing the sand from the Mogao Caves, repairing the cracked grottoes, and leveling the uneven dirt path in front of the entrance. He also employed workers to transcribe Buddhist scriptures from the caves and restore the Buddha statues eroded by time.

At the top of the sand dunes in the Mogao Caves, bathed in the lingering twilight, Wang Tao-shih sometimes wondered, "Would the group of ethereal blue-eyed white skeletons clad in wolf skins come back, just like in the past?" Of course, he hoped not. Now, he had become a local celebrity, confidently strolling with elegant steps, humming tunes, and enjoying the grace of the evening sun. Although he had never actually seen what Western gentlemen looked like, he felt he bore a certain resemblance to them. Perhaps the scenery of the Western Pure Land sought by Xuanzang was no different from this, he thought.

Soon after, Wang Tao-shih noticed a three-story cave several dozen meters north of his residence, which he deemed an ideal place for worship. Thus, he hired people to clean the area and invited a local scholar, Mr. Yang, to help receive worshippers and assist in transcribing Taoist scriptures. These caves were later designated as Cave 16 of the Mogao Caves. However, the story had only just begun.

Mr. Yang, a dedicated scholar, primarily spent his days immersed in books, having few other interests. His one notable indulgence was enjoying the occasional smoke from his dry pipe, yet at that specific time and place, one unintended action sparked a series of poignant events. Both glory and adversity were woven into the tapestry of history, beginning on May 26, 1900, when Mr. Yang lit his cigarette. From that moment onward, Wang Yuanlu's world underwent a transformation, and his name would forever be intertwined with the Mogao Caves of Dunhuang.[5]

Mr. Yang's pipe was quite long; he couldn't reach it with his own arm to light it. Unlike the wealthy who had others to light their pipes, Mr. Yang lacked such luxury. Ingeniously, he used a long reed to light his pipe, skillfully igniting and drawing on it with a rhythmic puff, bringing the tobacco to life. This clever method served him well. Reluctant to part with the reed after his smoke, knowing he'd need it again, Mr. Yang resourcefully preserved it by tucking it into a crevice in the wall behind him.

Mr. Yang's approach to smoking stood in stark contrast to that of the farmers on the village outskirts, who would typically squat in a corner against a wall for a quick puff. In comparison, Mr. Yang's method was far more refined. After a busy day, Mr. Yang would sit at his desk, brew a pot of tea, then relax with a pipe of tobacco. When in good spirits, he could even blow out a few elegant smoke rings. Once he finished smoking, he would rhythmically tap the bowl of the pipe against the wall beside him, "thud, thud, thud," to clear out the ashes, preparing it for his next use.

That day was no different from the usual. Mr. Yang lit his tobacco with a reed and casually stuck the reed into the wall behind him. This time, however, he noticed that the reed penetrated the wall without any obstruction, leading him to suspect a hollow space behind it. Curious, he gently tapped the wall with his pipe and, indeed, heard a hollow echo resonating from within. Upon discovering this, Mr. Yang quickly informed Wang Tao-shih of his findings. At the time, Wang Tao-shih was preoccupied with thoughts of acquiring furniture for the Daoist temple, so he only gave cursory attention to Mr. Yang's report, casually acknowledging it before suggesting that Mr. Yang take a rest.

After dinner, Wang Tao-shih's thoughts returned to Mr. Yang's earlier words, sparking a growing conviction that a mystery lay hidden behind the wall. He mulled over the possibilities: Could there be chests brimming with treasures, a hidden Buddha hall adorned with statues, or was it merely an empty room? This intrigue intensified his curiosity, leaving him restless in bed, unable to find sleep. Finally, in the stillness of the night, he roused Mr. Yang, resolved to explore the mystery shrouded in darkness.

The night in the northwest bore a stark contrast to the serene nights of Jiangnan. It was a realm of howling winds, interlaced with gusts of sandstorms, all enveloped in an endless expanse of darkness. Wang Tao-shih, armed with a pickaxe, and Mr. Yang, holding an oil lamp, made their way cautiously towards Mr. Yang's desk. In the pitch darkness, only the wavering glow of the oil lamp cast their shadows, lending them an almost ghostly appearance. As the dim light flickered, Wang Tao-shih could discern deep cracks veining the wall.

Over the years, Wang Yuanlu had endured many difficult days, having been a soldier, a wanderer, and faced numerous challenges. He didn't consider himself a fortunate person. The tranquility of his current life had already brought him contentment. He didn't seek fame or wealth; he simply wished for a peaceful and stable existence, to repair temples, and spend the latter part of his life in peace. He had accepted this fate. In this lifetime, he was just an insignificant individual, a common peasant. However, somehow, he recalled Sun Wukong from *Journey to the West* (Xī Yóu Jì, 西游记), the Great Sage who subdued demons and vanquished evil. On this night, he felt as though he had transformed into Sun Wukong, his pickaxe akin to the Sea-Calming Needle and the Golden Cudgel, ready to dispel all difficulties and obstacles.

He spat on both of his hands, raised the pickaxe high, and with a resounding thud, smashed a huge hole into the wall in an instant. Looking inside, he could hardly see anything. Swiftly, he took the oil lamp from Mr. Yang and projected its light deep into the cave. He was rooted to the spot in disbelief, eyes widening at the sight that unfolded before him. His mind seemed to buzz, echoing with astonishment, as if it had been jolted by an unseen force. In the confines of the small, airtight cave, a staggering collection of books and scrolls of various sizes and types was packed tightly, occupying every inch of space. Overwhelmed, he found it hard to grasp the reality of the incredible scene within this compact cave. The Daoist was unable to fathom that, from that moment on, his life's trajectory would be completely rewritten. This momentous strike, like a thunderbolt from a clear sky, marked the beginning of one of the most significant archaeological discoveries in both China and the world. From that point onward, the Daoist monk's name became inextricably linked with the Hidden Library.

Of course, at that moment, Wang Yuanlu couldn't have foreseen the impact of his discovery. He refocused his attention, his first thought being to examine these scrolls and books. Carefully, he stepped across the hole of the cave. Inside, scrolls and books filled the entire room. Moving around in the limited space was challenging; he had to be mindful of the oil lamp, fearing it might get knocked over. Particles of dust hung in the air, carrying a subtle sweet aroma, as if mixed with the scent of earth. These books appeared ancient, most were yellowed, some even had mottled spots. The Daoist monk carefully picked up the nearest scroll and delicately brushed away the surface dust. As he slowly unrolled it, a sweet, earthy scent drifted up to him – the unmistakable aroma of ancient books. Involuntarily, the Daoist monk took a few more breaths, as if in an instant, he had transformed into a scholar, experiencing the refined pleasure of learning. He read line by line, though unsure how much he truly understood. Nevertheless, he immersed himself completely, losing track of time. Amidst this collection of ancient texts, the Daoist monk felt a sense of purpose for the first time, as if the mission Xuanzang felt on his journey to the Western Paradise for the scriptures. He had a basic literacy, enough to understand that these ancient texts were indeed treasures, predominantly consisting of Buddhist scriptures and similar works. The radiant light that guided him to this place seemed like a divine revelation from the Buddha himself. He felt both honored and overwhelmed, finding it hard to believe that the Buddha had chosen an ordinary peasant like him. The Daoist monk certainly did not dare to take this lightly. The room was filled with countless treasures; how should he handle them? The only thought that came to mind was to hand them to the imperial court.

Early the next morning, under the rising sun, Wang Tao-shih carefully selected a few scrolls and scriptures, neatly placing them in his rough cloth bag. Determined, he made his way to the county town, intending to deliver these treasures to the then Dunhuang county magistrate, Yan Ze. Despite the county yamen being difficult to access, with guards bearing stern faces and harsh words, he ultimately managed to deliver these treasures inside. He hoped the imperial court would swiftly transport the ancient books from that room to a secure storage place in the national treasury. The presence of so many valuable treasures in his possession made him feel uneasy and anxious.

And so Wang Tao-shih made repeated trips to the county town and provincial capital, carrying as many finely copied scriptures and Buddhist paintings as he could. He offered them as tributes to the higher-ranking officials, hoping the court would recognize the significance of this remarkable discovery. Even the newly appointed Dunhuang county magistrate, Wang Zonghan, and the then Gansu provincial scholar, Ye Changchi, received Wang Tao-shih's offerings to varying degrees.

One year, two years, then three passed by. Over the span of three years, Wang Tao-shih's dedication to these ancient books intensified, wearing down numerous pairs of shoes in his persistent efforts to draw the imperial court's attention to their significance. He pondered whether this might be a test deliberately set by the Buddha, akin to the 81 trials faced by Tang Xuanzang on his journey. Wang Tao-shih even hired a local artist to paint scenes from Tang Xuanzang's stories on the walls. The murals depicted the legends along Tang Xuanzang's pilgrimage route. In one mural, Tang Xuanzang stood by a turbulent river, his faithful steed, the White Dragon Horse, laden with scrolls. A giant tortoise was swimming towards him, ready to help him cross this "trial." Clearly, the mural portrayed the moment when Tang Xuanzang, bringing 20 bundles of Buddhist scriptures, prepared to return from India to China. Illiterate Wang Tao-shih speculated that the scrolls in the cave might be the scriptures Tang Xuanzang had brought back from India. Therefore, he steadfastly held onto his faith, believing that with one more attempt, with a little more effort, his mission could be accomplished.

Who would have imagined that all of this would take more than three years? Finally, in the year 1904 (the thirtieth year of Emperor Guangxu's reign), he received a letter from the provincial government of Gansu, informing him that due to budget constraints, they could not afford to transport the relics to Lanzhou. Therefore, they ordered these artifacts to be kept on-site, under the personal supervision of Wang Yuanlu. Of course, no funds were provided for the safekeeping. Despite the setback, Wang Tao-shih was unwilling to give up easily. He chose two boxes of scriptures, rented a mule, and embarked on a journey by foot, heading to report the situation to higher authorities. However, every time he recalled the experience of being chased by the white skeletons clad in wolf skins in the past, fear gripped his heart, making him shiver with dread.

Nevertheless, he pressed on without rest, traversing the distance of over 800 miles day and night, eventually arriving in Jiuquan. There, he found his former superior, Ting Dong, who had been promoted to a higher rank. After skimming through a few scrolls of scriptures, Ting Dong gave his final verdict: "The writing here is not even as good as what I can produce." With disdain, he dismissed Wang Tao-shih. From that moment on, no one cared about these matters anymore.

Wang Tao-shih even risked his life by writing a letter to the Empress Dowager Cixi, pleading for attention to his discovery. In his letter, he wrote:

> Suddenly, there was a thunderous explosion in the sky, and at the same time, a crack appeared in the mountain. I, along with fellow workers, eagerly dug with hoes and unexpectedly revealed a Buddhist cave, containing ten thousand ancient scriptures.[6]

Clearly, he deliberately mystified the discovery process of the Hidden Library, attempting to convey that it was a divine arrangement, hoping to gain the attention it deserved.

However, during that time, the Qing Dynasty had already entered a period of irreversible decline. The capital had just experienced the chaos of the Boxer Rebellion, leaving the city in ruins. Even major homicide cases went unresolved, let alone the concerns of a Daoist priest in the distant desert of the northwest. He didn't know how many times he had knocked on the doors of the officials nor how many times he had been met with indifferent gazes. Every time, he wore the exhaustion of his journeys, his face covered in dust and weariness. Meanwhile, the Dang River continued its tranquil flow, seemingly oblivious to the worldly vicissitudes unfolding around it.

After all, the artifacts were sent, the letters were written, but all he ever received was rejection, and he couldn't fathom how much bitterness he had endured. After years of persistence, this was the result he had obtained. Doubt began to creep into his mind. Were these scriptures truly precious treasures, or just a pile of useless waste paper? If they were treasures, why was there no one caring for them, not even attempting to steal a few? If they were mere scraps, then what meaning did his years of effort hold? The room was evidently filled with ancient artifacts, where each paper bore such an elegant script and the paintings were of exquisite beauty – how could they not be considered treasures?

At the break of each day, Wang Tao-shih would step into the tranquil Hidden Library, gazing at the dense array of scrolls and ancient texts. With each visit, his heart felt heavier, as the once-inspiring treasures now represented helplessness and disillusionment. They are just like tasteless chicken ribs – unsatisfying to savor yet regrettable to cast aside.

Wang Tao-shih gradually came to the somber realization that the scriptures were merely valueless sheets of paper. His journey had seen him evolve from an inexperienced, youthful farmer to a young solder and ultimately to a Taoist monk deeply marked by life's many ups and downs. Regardless of his devout chanting and spiritual practices, the fate of humanity continued to be painted with strokes of suffering, the shadows of illness and anguish ever-present, like unyielding companions.

Thus, he began in an almost desperate manner to collect the tattered scriptures, burning them into ashes, mixing them with water, and proclaiming it a healing remedy, selling it to the local populace. This act was perhaps a solace for the soul or a silent protest against a life of resignation. The harsh reality of the world may scorn such actions, yet in that era, who could claim to be free from their own struggles and moments of helplessness?

Fate did not grant Wang Yuanlu the opportunity to become a renowned practitioner of traditional Chinese medicine. While Wang Yuanlu's limited literacy allowed him to appreciate the elegance of the murals and the value of the scriptures, had he been able to read a few more characters like Mr. Yang, he would have certainly discovered some medical-related scrolls concealed in the Hidden Library. Among them was a long-lost medical text by the famous Han Dynasty physician Zhang Zhongjing. Had Wang Yuanlu devoted himself to the study of these medical classics, he might have achieved renown in the medical field, becoming known and respected as "Doctor Wang" and leaving a profound legacy in the annals of medical history.

REFERENCES

1. 李正宇，"乐傅史事纂诂 [J]." *敦煌研究*，No. 2 (1985): 149–156.
2. 方广锠, "王道士名称考 [J]." *敦煌研究,* No. 4 (2016): 111–118.
3. 荣新江, *敦煌学十八讲 [M]: 第三讲 王道士其人*. (北京: 北京大学出版社, 2001), 52.
4. 刘进宝, *藏经洞之谜 [M]: 敦煌文物流散记* (兰州: 甘肃人民出版社, 2000), 4.
5. 荣新江, "王道士—敦煌藏经洞的发现者 [J]." *敦煌研究*, No. 2 (2000): 23–28.
6. 陈双印, "莫高窟王道士《催募经款草丹》再考 [J]." *史料研究*, No. 9 (2022): 31–37.

2 Aurel Stein, a Love Story from Budapest

"Tang Xuanzang has always been my guardian deity of China."

– Sir. Aurel Stein

Day after day, year after year, Wang Tao-shih steadfastly guarded the ancient treasure trove of scriptures, a place seldom sought after by others. Sometimes, he stood on the cliffs of the Dang River valley, reminiscent of Monk Le Zun from bygone days. However, the splendid rays of light that once graced these heights were no longer visible to him. Amidst howling winds, gathering storm clouds, and the jagged slashes of lightning, Wang stood under the vast sky, his presence seemingly as inconsequential as a speck of dust, vulnerable to being swept away by the merest gust.

Over five years had elapsed since the momentous discovery of the Dunhuang Hidden Library. During this time, Wang Tao-shih led a serene and contented life, practicing with a few disciples and occasionally conducting Taoist rituals or divinations for the villagers nearby. In October 1905, word reached Wang of several foreign visitors with distinctive appearances in Dunhuang, seeking information about the Mogao Caves. This news was soon followed by the arrival of the 42-year-old Russian geologist and geographer Vladimir Obruchev, along with his assistant. Fresh from a successful expedition in Northern Xinjiang, where they had unearthed numerous valuable relics, Obruchev's thirst for discovery was unquenched. Driven by this zeal, he set his sights on the Mogao Caves, eager to uncover more historical treasures. At the dawn of the 20th century, Central Asia was akin to an untapped frontier, enigmatic and irresistibly inviting. It drew adventurers and explorers from around the world, each enthralled by the region's mysterious allure, repeatedly braving its uncharted terrains in search of the fabled treasures.

What exactly draws these explorers with such eagerness? And what constitutes the "fabled treasures" they seek? To understand this, we must delve into a manuscript known as the *Bower Manuscript*.[1]

Rewinding to April 8, 1888, Andrew Dalgleish, a British Scottish merchant, was attacked and killed by Dad Mahomed, a Pashtun from Quetta, at the Karakoram Pass while en route to Xinjiang. The local Qing Dynasty officials refused to intervene in the case on the grounds that the perpetrator was not a subject of the Qing Empire, resulting in Mahomed evading justice and his whereabouts becoming unknown.

In June 1889, Lieutenant Hamilton Bower (1858–1940) of the 17th Bengal Cavalry and Major W. B. Cumberland of the British Indian Army took advantage of a leave to embark on a hunting and exploration expedition to the Pamir Plateau within Chinese territory. On November 13, 1889, Bower received a secret order from a messenger

DOI: 10.1201/9781032698205-2

dispatched by Captain Ramsay, the British Joint-Commissioner of Ladak, instructing him to take charge of the investigation into the case and to capture the perpetrator. Bower immediately led his team eastward, eventually reaching Kucha.

Shortly after Bower's arrival in Kucha, a local Afghan merchant named Ghulam Qadir Khan visited him, claiming to have found some manuscripts inside an ancient Buddhist stupa near the Qumtura caves.[2] Bower recalled:

> The man proposed a nocturnal visit to the underground city, fearing trouble if anyone knew he was leading a European there. I readily agreed, and we set out at midnight. He showed me a bundle of manuscripts written on birch bark, eager to sell them.

The manuscript consisted of 51 leaves of birch bark. Although Bower could not understand the content, he happily purchased the text at a low price. Later, Bower had the man guide him to the ruins where the documents were excavated. There, amidst numerous architectural remnants and a collapsed cave, Bower found no other treasures.

After acquiring the ancient documents, with the capture and subsequent death of the perpetrator Mahomed, Bower returned to Leh on April 1, 1890, bringing back to Shimla in British India the birch bark manuscripts and other artifacts he had purchased in Kucha.

On September 30, 1890, Bower sent the manuscript to Colonel James Waterhouse, who was about to step down as the president of the Asiatic Society of Bengal, hoping that he could find a scholar capable of discerning the true meaning and value of the manuscript. However, the content of these documents remained undeciphered for a long time. It wasn't until the beginning of 1891 that the distinguished German-born British scholar Augustus Rudolf Hoernle learned about the birch bark manuscript. After obtaining the original document, Hoernle began an in-depth study and quickly uncovered many significant clues. He discovered that these ancient texts were written in Sanskrit using the Brahmi script of the Gupta period, around the 4th to 6th centuries CE, which was prevalent in India and Central Asia. The manuscript comprised seven sections, with the first three being parts of ancient Indian traditional medicine, Ayurveda, which had been long lost and never before discovered. The fourth and fifth sections were the earliest known texts on divination by dice, while the sixth and seventh sections are on incantations (Dharani) against snake bites. These findings proved that the manuscript was among the world's oldest Sanskrit and Brahmi script documents, later named the "Bower Manuscript." It was subsequently acquired by Edward Nicholson, the head of the Bodleian Library at the University of Oxford, for the modest sum of 50 pounds and is preserved in the Bodleian Library to this day, remaining one of its most treasured items.[3]

It was the *Bower Manuscript* that sparked an international frenzy for Central Asian archaeology. Numerous countries, including the United Kingdom, France, Russia, and Japan, dispatched expeditions to the region, including Xinjiang, in hopes of uncovering more precious ancient documents during their explorations.[4]

Let's return to the arrival of the 42-year-old Russian geologist and geographer Vladimir Obruchev,[5] who can be considered one of the earliest foreigners to arrive in Dunhuang. After concluding his expedition in Northern Xinjiang, he set his sights on Dunhuang, faced with a choice between two distinct paths. The more traveled route ran along the southern foothills of the Tian Shan mountains, well-equipped with stations for changing horses and favored by officials and merchants. Alternatively, a shorter yet far more ominous path lay along the southern edge of the Kumtag Desert. This route, infamously known as the "Valley of Demons," was shrouded in tales of supernatural occurrences and had long been abandoned.

Despite the daunting reputation of the Valley of Demons, Obruchev chose this path, driven by his adventurous spirit. He sent his assistant and the caravan along the safer southern road, while he, accompanied by a local guide, embarked on the perilous journey through the Valley of Demons. This barren landscape, with its scarcity of vegetation and peculiar terrain, was scattered with the intact skeletons of camels and other animals. The area was notorious for fierce winds that could swiftly erode the protruding red rock layers. In such conditions, travelers were forced to crawl, lest they be swept away by the gusts.

Nighttime in the valley brought its own set of terrors for Obruchev. Eerie shadows flickered in the darkness, and the desert air carried the sounds of camel bells, horse neighs, and donkey brays, sometimes even echoing with ethereal music. His guide cautioned him against pursuing these mysterious sounds, warning that they could lead them astray into the depths of the desert. Although a lover of adventure, Obruchev had no intention of perishing in this forsaken place. With careful steps and heightened alertness, he navigated through the Valley of Demons. After a tense and arduous month, he finally emerged from its chilling grasp, reaching the destination of his journey – the Mogao Caves of Dunhuang.

Prior to his arrival in Dunhuang, Obruchev had learned of the monks' impoverished lifestyle there. Hence, he brought a considerable array of items, including cloth for making robes, incense and candles for religious rituals, lamp oil, incense burners, and various everyday essentials. Indeed, the monks at the temple greeted these contributions with great appreciation and, in return, were eager to share valuable local insights with him.

Obruchev got excited by the tales he heard from the monks about the Hidden Library, which was brimming with ancient scrolls and manuscripts. He became deeply interested in visiting the Hidden Library. The library's preservation was attributed to its stable environment, free from sunlight, preventing mold, pests, and rodents from damaging the texts. In light of a decree issued by the Gansu provincial governor a year earlier, entrusting Wang Yuanlu with the relics, access was highly restricted, even to the monks.

The protocol for entering the Hidden Library was meticulous: visitors first entered an antechamber, pausing briefly for prayer, then moved to a second chamber, waiting again before finally entering the innermost chamber. Here, they would pause once more before touching the manuscripts. A lantern, crafted from oiled paper and inscribed with prayers for each room, was used to deter any malevolent spirits from infiltrating the trove. The monks explained to Obruchev that these practices served two purposes: first, to allow the body's moisture to evaporate and, second, to dispel any evil thoughts. However, Obruchev couldn't care less about these customs. For him, he just wanted the treasures within.

Obruchev, a geologist with little knowledge of Sinology or archaeology, was more captivated by the prospect of monetary profit rather than the academic value of the ancient texts. He intended to have experts well-versed in Central Asian history evaluate these potential treasures upon his return to determine their true value. Keeping expenses minimal was a key consideration for him. He was well aware that Wang Tao-shih's long-standing efforts had yielded little more than unresolved outcomes, and he also knew that there was little interest in purchasing these ancient manuscripts. Skillfully navigating this situation, Obruchev managed to secure a favorable deal. For the modest price of six packs containing about 50 stearic wax candles each, he acquired over 600 ancient scrolls and Buddhist scriptures from the Hidden Library.

After leaving the Mogao Caves, Obruchev didn't head to Dunhuang City but instead proceeded directly northwest to evade inspection and questioning by the Chinese government. At that time, the political situation in Central Asia was in utter chaos. Mongolia, China, and various British and Russian forces each held sway over their respective territories. Who would bother about those old books that didn't gleam like gold?

Later, Obruchev transported these artifacts back to Russia. The exact amount he earned from selling these relics is unknown nor did they reportedly make any significant impact in Russia. It's possible that Obruchev later regretted bringing such a seemingly useless and burdensome haul across such a vast distance. Perhaps only Wang Tao-shih remained dedicated to finding a more deserving resting place for these ancient scriptures.

In 1907, seven years after the discovery of the Hidden Library, Wang Tao-shih's hair had turned grey and his dream of emulating Xuanzang had faded. Yet he remained fondly attached to Wu Cheng'en's *Journey to the West* (Xī Yóu Jì, 西游记). Interestingly, the story of Xuanzang's pilgrimage is extensively documented in the Dunhuang Mogao Caves. There are no fewer than six murals depicting the arduous 17-year journey of Xuanzang and Sun Wukong. For instance, in Cave 3 of the Yulin Caves on the north side of the western wall, there's a mural. In it, Tang Xuanzang and Sun Wukong, dressed in monk's robes, stand on the bank of a raging river, hands joined in prayer, paying homage to Guanyin. Sun Wukong and the White Dragon Horse stand side by side, the horse bearing large lotus flowers and scriptures wrapped in fine silk, glowing with Buddha's light. Dressed for a long voyage, in short jackets and hemp shoes, with their trouser legs tied up, they appear ready for the challenges of their journey. Sun Wukong, with his signature golden headband and flowing hair, stands prominently. Perhaps at that time, the Taoist priest Wang would occasionally take the time to admire the *Journey to the West* (Xī Yóu Jì, 西游记) murals. Later on, he even commissioned someone to paint another mural depicting Xuanzang's journey to the Western Regions in the front corridor of the cave temples. However, this time, he was no longer alone in his admiration.

In the spring of 1907, the British-Hungarian archaeologist Aurel Stein arrived at the remote desert oasis of Dunhuang in northwest China. After Hoernle deciphered the *Bower Manuscript* in 1891, Stein shifted his research focus from Kashmir to China's Tarim Basin. Stein stated,

> In 1891, the famous birch bark manuscript obtained by Colonel Bower from Kucha became known to Indologists. Since then, I have set my sights on southern Xinjiang, convinced that this was the place to pursue archaeological endeavors.

Stein was deeply enamored with Central Asian culture. Born in Budapest, Hungary, he was considered an eccentric prodigy from a young age, often dismissed as a dreamer by his family. He studied ancient scripts and was proficient in seven languages. At the age of 22, he moved to England to specialize in Oriental languages and archaeology. Later, he served as a principal at several schools in India. Since learning about Eastern languages, Stein had been captivated by the stories of Xuanzang. From then on, this Tang Dynasty monk became his most admired figure. Stein's admiration for Xuanzang stemmed from his childhood yearning to explore and travel across Central Asia, and historically, the greatest traveler of the Asian interior was undoubtedly Xuanzang. Without Xuanzang's accounts, the history of 7th-century India and Central Asia might have remained obscure. Xuanzang's precise recording of his journey's mileage greatly impressed Stein. After reading *The Great Tang Dynasty Records on the Western Regions* (Dà Táng Xī Yù Jì, 大唐西域记), Stein became obsessed with the book. All previously unsolved mysteries seemed to be answered in its pages. He decided to venture to the great Gobi Desert, in search of the prosperous civilizations described by Xuanzang in his writings.[6]

In 1900, Sir Aurel Stein embarked on his inaugural journey to China, driven not by wealth or fame but by a salaried profession. Supported by funding from the British and Indian governments, Stein realized his dream of retracing the steps of the ancient monks. With Xuanzang's *The Great Tang Dynasty Records on the Western Regions* (Dà Táng Xī Yù Jì, 大唐西域记) in hand, he journeyed from India, steadily making his way eastward, until he finally arrived in China.

During his expedition from India through the vast, uninhabited expanse of the Gobi Desert between 1900 and 1901, Sir Aurel Stein often found himself precariously balanced between life and death. Yet he steadfastly believed that Xuanzang, the revered Buddhist monk whose journey he sought to emulate, was watching over him as a guardian deity. Drawing inspiration and guidance from Xuanzang's *The Great Tang Dynasty Records on the Western Regions* (Dà Táng Xī Yù Jì, 大唐西域记), Stein unearthed the Dandan Oilik site, a significant Buddhist site dating back to the Tang Dynasty, hidden deep within the desert. In this remote site, Stein uncovered a series of vibrant murals. Among them was a painted panel portraying a legendary king of sacred rats and another mural depicting a mythical scene. Stein named this latter mural "Guardian of the North." These artistic treasures were later hailed as "masterpieces of ancient oriental painting art." Remarkably, it was the depiction of the "Guardian of the North" that seemed to bridge time and space, connecting Stein to Xuanzang in a mystical and timeless encounter.

This was Stein's description of this mural:

> It shows a woman standing in an oblong tank of water, enclosed by a tessellated pavement and filled with lotuses. The figure, 18 inches high as far as seen above the water, is nude except for a large red headdress resembling an Indian pagri and profuse ornaments around the neck, arms and wrists, and is drawn with remarkable verve, in simple but graceful outlines of true flesh-colour. The right hand, with its shapely fingers, rests against the breasts, while the left arm is curved down towards the middle of the waist. Fourfold strings of small bells (or beads?) are shown hanging in elegant curves around the hips, just as in representations of dancing-girls and other female attendants

> in early Indian sculpture, while, curiously enough, an elaborate vine-leaf appears where post-classical convention would place its fig-leaf. The woman's face is turned to her proper right, down towards a small figure of a male, also nude, who is shown as if trying to rise from the water by holding to her side. Further to the left appear the head and shoulders of another small male figure, just rising above the water as if in the act of swimming. In the foreground, and in front of the tank, the foot of the fresco showed in faint but unmistakable outlines a small riderless horse, closely resembling, in its dappled colours.[7]

Stein held a deep appreciation for this painting. In describing its artistry and significance, he expressed his admiration with thoughtful and eloquent remarks:

> The delineation of the lotus-flowers rising from the tank in a variety of forms, closed or half open, as well as their colours, ranging from dark blue to deep purple, seemed quite true to nature, and distinctly suggested that these sacred flowers were familiar to the painter from personal observation. The pool is also painted with a riderless horse and a bathing girl facing her own right and looking down at the little boy. It is reminiscent of its theme may be a love myth, that is, Xuanzang recorded in *The Great Tang Dynasty Records on the Western Regions* (Dà Táng Xī Yù Jì, 大唐西域记), about a story took place in the river South of Xinjiang, a dragon girl who is a celestial maiden seeking for a lover from the earth.

Stein drew upon a narrative from Xuanzang's *The Great Tang Dynasty Records on the Western Regions* (Dà Táng Xī Yù Jì, 大唐西域记), the enchanting tale of "The Dragon Maiden's Quest for a Husband." This ancient story unfolds southeast of Yutian City, where a vital river, once the lifeblood of local agriculture, mysteriously dried up. Legend attributed this calamity to a dragon's influence. In response, the king erected a temple alongside the river, invoking the dragon's favor. It was there that the dragon maiden gracefully emerged upon the waves. Mourning her deceased husband and feeling adrift, she proposed a deal to the king: find her a new spouse, and the river would regain its flow. The king selected a minister, who, clad in white and mounted on a white horse, ventured into the underwater Dragon Palace. With this union, the river's waters began to flow again, ensuring the land's prosperity and the well-being of its people.

If Stein's analysis was correct, then the nude woman in the mural represented the dragon maiden, with the boy beside her likely symbolizing her new husband who entered the Dragon Palace on a white horse. This interpretation aligns with the ancient Buddhist art practice where divine figures are depicted larger and humans smaller, making the relationship between the characters in the painting quite plausible. It seems almost like a twist of fate that Stein, after 1,300 years, followed the steps of Xuanzang, the man he deeply admired, and encountered the dragon maiden from Xuanzang's tales in the vast desert. The joy and satisfaction Stein experienced upon this discovery were indescribable. The mural had silently adorned the temple for over a thousand years, maintaining its pristine beauty. Out of respect for its integrity, Stein chose not to remove it but instead photographed it. Unfortunately, the original mural has long since disappeared from its site, and the whereabouts of Stein's photograph's negative are unknown. Today, only studies based on the photograph developed by

Stein are possible. This encounter might symbolize the intertwined destinies of Stein and Xuanzang, crossing time and space. Xuanzang's legacy inspired Stein, and in turn, Stein validated the historical accounts in Xuanzang's *The Great Tang Dynasty Records on the Western Regions* (Dà Táng Xī Yù Jì, 大唐西域记).

It was this very follower of Xuanzang who returned to China in 1906 and arrived in Dunhuang on March 12, 1907. Here, he was destined to encounter another follower of Xuanzang. One of these individuals, born in Budapest, was an archaeology expert, while the other, raised in the rural countryside of China, was an ordinary citizen. Although seemingly unlikely to have any connection on the surface, these two individuals were brought together in the same narrative, united by their shared reverence for Xuanzang.

Certainly, the narrative wasn't always straightforward. Before arriving in Dunhuang, Stein had only heard of the Mogao Grottoes, also known as the Thousand Buddha Caves, and was unaware of the existence of the Hidden Library. Thus, he planned to stay in Dunhuang for just two weeks, briefly surveying the caves and replenishing supplies and food before heading to the Lop Nur Desert for archaeological excavations. However, shortly after arriving in Dunhuang, he learned from a Xinjiang merchant settled in the area about the Hidden Library discovered by Wang Tao-shih a few years earlier. Stein, with his profound fascination for Eastern culture, naturally became intrigued by the Hidden Library and decided to investigate further.

On March 16, Stein reached the Mogao Grottoes. In a twist of fate, Wang Tao-shih was away, raising funds for the upkeep of the caves.[8] A novice monk from the upper temple at the Grottoes presented Stein with an exquisitely penned scripture. Stein, despite not understanding Chinese characters, instantly recognized the manuscript's antiquity from its appearance. This prompted him to patiently await Wang Tao-shih's return before proceeding with his explorations.

Certainly, Stein didn't just wait idly. During Wang Tao-shih's absence for alms collection, he ventured to the westernmost end of the Great Wall of China and discovered a collection of Han Dynasty bamboo slips and documents. Based on these documents, Stein identified the long-debated site of Yumen Pass, confirming the existence of the Han Dynasty Great Wall. Among the bamboo slips he found, there were more than ten medical texts, one of which described:

> For treating chronic cough, chest pain, paralysis, diarrhea, chronic abdominal distension, and typhoid fever: take one fen of Ren Shen, Zi Wan, Chang Pu, Xi Xin, Gui Zhi, and Shu Jiao, and ten fen of Wu Tou. Mix them together and take the mixture, the person should have diarrhea at the hour of Shenshi (3–5 pm). If it doesn't work, take the medicine again. A major bowel movement will bring immediate relief. Truly effective.

Stein probably couldn't understand the Chinese characters on these slips. Fortunately, he didn't discard them as useless, allowing scholars nowadays the opportunity to study these ancient texts.

The discovery of these bamboo slips, although fragmented, provides a vibrant snapshot of medical practices from two millennia ago. These artifacts are a treasure trove for medical research. Stein's find reveals that in the remote outposts near the Great Wall's beacon towers during the Han Dynasty, soldiers were treated for typhoid fever using traditional Chinese herbal medicine. Fascinatingly, these slips indicate that the Han Dynasty favored purgative methods for treating typhoid, in stark contrast to the renowned medical sage Zhang Zhongjing's approach of inducing sweating with ephedra. This intriguing detail not only adds a new dimension to the understanding of ancient Chinese medical practices but also unexpectedly connects Stein's discovery to the academic study of Zhang Zhongjing's medical philosophies.

Over a span of more than two months, Stein finally met Wang Tao-shih. Initially, the Taoist monk paid little attention to the foreigner with eyes as blue as the northwest wolves. He had never seen such clear, strikingly blue eyes, reminiscent of the autumn waters of the Dang River. Wang Tao-shih couldn't fathom the thoughts of this foreigner with his piercingly blue eyes. But perhaps by coincidence or fate, Stein discovered that Wang Tao-shih, like himself, deeply revered Tang Xuanzang, the monk who journeyed to the Western Paradise. This revelation brought an immediate connection between these two seemingly unrelated individuals, instilling a sense of belated camaraderie. Stein, with his limited Chinese, expressed his admiration for Xuanzang to Wang Tao-shih, recounting his journey across mountains and deserts from India, following in Xuanzang's footsteps. When the conversation turned to Xuanzang, Wang Tao-shih couldn't hide his excitement. He was amazed that this distant foreigner was also an admirer of Xuanzang. Could Stein be the emissary sent by Xuanzang to retrieve the scriptures that had ceased to exist in India? Wang Tao-shih then showed Stein the murals he had commissioned, depicting stories from *Journey to the West* (Xī Yóu Jì, 西游记). Stein was bewildered by these paintings, which narrated tales of Xuanzang's western journey, including characters like the Monkey King and Pigsy, stories he was completely unfamiliar with. He had not encountered any records in Xuanzang's *The Great Tang Dynasty Records on the Western Regions* (Dà Táng Xī Yù Jì, 大唐西域记) about the holy monk being coveted by countless demons, occasionally abducted, and then rescued by his peculiar-looking disciples. But what did that matter? To Wang Tao-shih, Stein was someone who truly understood him. His years of perseverance were finally not in vain.

Finally, as night fell, Wang Tao-shih led Stein to the Hidden Library. Just like Obruchev before him, Stein first entered the antechamber, pausing there momentarily for a prayer, before moving on to the next room. This progression continued from one chamber to the next. Outside, the wind continued to howl with the sound of swirling sand, but inside, there was utter silence. Gradually, Stein's breathing became rapid, his excitement palpable. The dim light from Wang Tao-shih's oil lamp faintly revealed Stein's flushed face, glistening with sweat on his forehead. Wang Tao-shih's hand, holding the lamp, trembled noticeably. Though unable to communicate verbally with Stein, Wang Tao-shih sensed a deep significance in this moment. He felt as though he was escorting a divine emissary, coming to review his years of guardianship and to take charge of his mission. With each step further into the cave, Wang Tao-shih's heart raced faster; with each room they entered, his trembling hand grew more unsteady, almost extinguishing the lamp.

Throughout his years of spiritual practice, Wang Tao-shih believed he had atoned for his past sins as a soldier. He had become a good person, one who could see deities. Finally, he brought Stein into the Hidden Library. Confronted with an entire room filled with ancient scrolls, Stein was utterly dumbstruck. That night, Wang Tao-shih opened the doors of the Dunhuang Hidden Library to Stein, revealing a treasure trove of history and knowledge.

People later speculated that there were three main reasons why Wang Tao-shih sold the scriptures to Stein. First, after seven long years of seeking assistance from officials at various levels, his efforts were consistently ignored, leading to his disillusionment. Second, he had a grand vision of cleaning the caves, constructing a three-story building, and installing wooden bridges, for which he needed funds. Third, their shared admiration for Tang Xuanzang served as a bridge transcending national and language barrier.

As for Stein, he is considered one of the greatest explorers of the 20th century. During his four Central Asian expeditions, he brought back valuable artifacts that he donated to British and Indian museums. Stein was not only an outstanding scholar and expert in his academic field but he was also highly praised for his personal character, sense of responsibility, and dedication. His contributions received high acclaim from both the Chinese and international academic communities. His exploratory journeys spanned from the Hindu Kush mountains to the Pamir Plateau, from the Kunlun Mountains to the Lop Nur Desert, and from the abandoned routes of the ancient Silk Road to the Great Wall fortresses buried under sand. Stein saw every step of his journey as following in the footsteps of Xuanzang.

Stein's adventurous life was marked by extraordinary challenges. He once lost several toes to frostbite in the snowy mountains and nearly didn't survive an ordeal in the Lop Nur Desert. In Turpan, he even faced confrontations with armed bandits. A life dedicated to exploration meant that he remained unmarried, with the legendary Tang Dynasty monk Xuanzang serving as his spiritual guardian throughout his journeys. In 1943, at the age of 81, Stein finally received permission to conduct archaeological explorations in Afghanistan, a dream he had long cherished. Unfortunately, he caught a cold that developed into bronchitis and ultimately suffered a stroke, passing away in Kabul. In accordance with his wishes, Stein's remains were buried in a Kabul cemetery. Reflecting on Stein's legendary life, his years of exploration in Dunhuang stand out as the most brilliant peak of his career.

Wang Tao-shih, the unassuming Taoist monk who safeguarded the Dunhuang treasures, never had the chance to attend Stein's funeral nor learned if the treasured scriptures were taken back to India. In his later years, he often lingered by the Dang River, his thoughts filled with memories of the foreigner who, like him, revered Xuanzang. With his sunken, toothless lips gently moving, it seemed he still had words left unsaid for Stein. As time passed, his concern for the scattered scrolls in the Hidden Library only grew deeper, harboring a persistent hope in his heart that they would eventually find a tranquil and rightful home.

In his heart, Wang Tao-shih silently said to Stein:

> Stein, do you remember the story of "The Dragon Maiden's Quest for a Husband" you once told? Perhaps all of this was destined, for the discovery of the Hidden Library has tied a bond that spans a thousand years. The scrolls within this cave are like the mythic dragon maiden, and you, the white-clad knight. I entrust these scrolls to you, as a king entrusts the dragon maiden to her groom. Stein, you must not let everyone down;

provide your beloved dragon maiden a wonderful home. May the waters of the Dang River flow endlessly, nourishing the earth and benefiting the people.

REFERENCES

1. 任曜新，"新疆库木吐喇佛塔出土鲍威尔写本研究 [D]." 博士论文，兰州大学 (2012): 18–25.
2. 林梅村，"鲍威尔写本的发现地 [J]." *读书*, No. 8 (2023): 56–60.
3. 王冀青，"库车文书的发现与英国大规模搜集中亚文物的开始[J]." *敦煌学辑刊*，No. 2 (1991): 64–73.
4. 范振宇,王兴伊，"《鲍威尔写本》的研究进展 [J]." *中医药文化*, Vol. 13, No. 8 (2018): 36–43.
5. [俄] 费·阿·奥勃鲁切夫，*荒漠寻宝[M]*：*敦煌千佛寺院的宝藏*，王沛译 (乌鲁木齐：新疆人民出版社, 2010), 188.
6. Annabel Walker, *Aurel Stein Pioneer of the Silk Road* (London: John Murray Ltd, 1995), 36.
7. Sir. Aurel Stein, *On Ancient Central Asian Tracks: First Exploration at a Sand-Buried Site*. CH IV. (London: Macmillan and Co., Limited, 1933), 61
8. Sir. Aurel Stein, *Serindia: Detailed Report of Explorations in Central Asia and Westernmost China Vol.2: Chapter XXL – The Caves of Thousand Buddhas, Section III. Wang Tao-shin and His Restored Temple* (Oxford: The Clarendon Press, 1921), 801.

3 Paul Pelliot, a Dear Friend of Dunhuang

"Without him, Sinology would wander as a parentless child."

– One of Pelliot's French colleagues

On a dusky evening in late spring of 1945, the Mogao Caves of Dunhuang in Gansu Province were enveloped in a peaceful and solemn silence. Spring had gently arrived, but the chill of Dunhuang's climate lingered, leaving traces of snowflakes and a thin layer of ice on the Dang River, reminiscent of winter's past. The setting sun bestowed its final tender glow upon the peaks of the Mogao Grottoes, bathing the ancient golden-hued structures in a divine radiance. Nearby, on the vast expanse of the Gobi Desert, a man, lost in thought, rode a chestnut-colored horse. He sped towards Anxi, over a hundred kilometers from Dunhuang, as if in desperate pursuit of some unattainable dream.

The man was Chang Shuhong,[1] director of the China National Research Institute of Dunhuang Art. Revered as the guardian of Dunhuang's art, his name was closely associated with the splendor of Dunhuang. Four days earlier, his wife, Chen Zhixiu, left Dunhuang under the guise of seeking medical treatment. In reality, she had eloped with someone else, leaving Chang Shuhong with their young children.

Chen Zhixiu, who had studied in France with Chang Shuhong, journeyed from Chongqing to Dunhuang with her daughter two years prior to reunite with him. The mother and daughter braved numerous hardships and challenges, enduring a grueling journey that lasted a month before they finally reached Dunhuang. On the day of their arrival in Dunhuang, the first meal that greeted them consisted only of a bowl of coarse salt, a bowl of vinegar, and a bowl of plain noodles.

Back then, Dunhuang was a landscape dominated by endless yellow sand, with vast stretches of the Gobi Desert surrounding the dwellings, with desolation all around and not a single village in sight. Packs of wolves would often roam these barren lands. In this harsh environment, every step taken depended on one's steadfast feet, and every conversation required loud shouting to be heard over the barriers of wind and sand. Inside the houses, the cold was piercing, devoid of even the slightest warming equipment.

The departure of Chen Zhixiu placed Chang Shuhong in the solitary position of caring for their young children, plunging his life into deeper hardship and challenge. Yet this did not diminish his profound fascination with Dunhuang. From a young, handsome man to a white-haired, elderly figure, he remained a devoted guardian of the Dunhuang art, tirelessly studying and preserving it across the thousands of miles of vast Gobi Desert. Once, the renowned Japanese writer Daisaku Ikeda asked

DOI: 10.1201/9781032698205-3

him, "If you were to be reborn, what profession would you choose?" Chang Shuhong replied, "I am not a Buddhist and do not believe in reincarnation. However, if I were to be reborn as a human again, I would still be 'Chang Shuhong.' I would want to finish the work I have yet to complete."

Chang Shuhong, who could have enjoyed a brilliant future in the French art world, surprisingly chose an unusual path. He abandoned the easily attainable fame and fortune, dedicating the rest of his life selflessly to the protection and in-depth study of the remote Dunhuang. His life's trajectory shifted dramatically on a cold winter night in 1935. At that time, he was just a Chinese youth studying in France. During an aimless stroll along the Seine in Paris, his attention was captivated by a book at an old bookstore. This six-volume set titled *The Dunhuang Grottoes Illustrated* (Les Grottes de Touen-Houang) introduced the mystically charged name "Dunhuang" into his world for the first time. The murals and sculptures of the Thousand Buddha Caves in Gansu's Dunhuang, with their dazzling colors and profound historical depth, struck a chord in his heart, igniting his curiosity and reverence for this enigmatic land. This forgotten album, found on a bookstall, acted like a key unlocking the door to destiny, leading Chang Shuhong into an unknown and vast new world. It not only completely altered his life course but also transformed this descendant of the Manchu nobility into a guardian of Dunhuang's art, renowned in China and across the world.

The author of this book was Paul Pelliot. Who was he, and why did a Frenchman write a book about China's Dunhuang? We seem to find some answers in Philippe Flandrin's biography, *The Seven Lives of the French Mandarin: Paul Pelliot or the Passion of the Orient* (Les Sept Vies du mandarin français: Paul Pelliot ou la Passion de l'Orient).[2] In 1984, Flandrin embarked on a journey seeking Eastern wisdom. Arriving in Dunhuang, China, a key stop on the ancient Silk Road and a land full of legends, he encountered an information panel at the entrance of the Thousand Buddha Caves. It prominently featured the name "Paul Pelliot," a Frenchman, along with a list of his alleged "heinous crimes" against the Dunhuang Hidden Library. Pelliot was accused of plundering numerous artifacts from the library through bribery of Wang Tao-shih.

Flandrin wondered if this man, labeled a "robber," ended his life in some dark prison. Curious, Flandrin returned to France and delved into Pelliot's history. He discovered they were both alumni of the Sorbonne University. To his surprise, Pelliot's life in France was quite illustrious. Through interviews with Pelliot's colleagues and students, Flandrin learned that Pelliot was not only a top-tier Sinologist in France but also revered as the founding father of Sinology among Western experts. He was considered an authority and pioneer in Sinology throughout the Western world. It was said that without Pelliot, Sinology would be like an orphan without parents, lacking foundation and support.

Interestingly, Pelliot was not just a scholar. His life was like a colorful tapestry, intertwined with multiple identities: perceived as a robber, colonialist, soldier, explorer, politician, and even a spy. Was Paul Pelliot a thief or a great figure? What exactly did he do in Dunhuang?

In June 1906, Paul Pelliot, a French Sinologist and explorer proficient in 13 languages, formed an expedition team with Louis Vaillant, a military doctor, and Charles Nouette, a naturalist and photographer.[3]

During the preparation phase of this expedition, Pelliot, true to his habit, studied Xuanzang's *Great Tang Dynasty Records on the Western Regions* (Dà Táng Xī Yù Jì, 大唐西域记). In the blank spaces of the book, he penciled in dense annotations and profound insights, each stroke reflecting his thirst for knowledge and passion for exploration. By then, Stein had already become a renowned figure. Pelliot decided to follow in the footsteps of Xuanzang and compete with Stein, a formidable rival, in this unparalleled contest of exploration.

Pelliot's team set off from Paris, journeying eastward. Traversing through layers of history, they passed through the ancient and majestic Saint Petersburg. Overcoming mountains and rivers, the expedition team finally arrived in the mysterious and legendary lands of Central Asia.

In Urumqi, Pelliot learned about Wang Tao-shih's unexpected discovery of the Hidden Library, which piqued his curiosity for this expedition. Coincidentally or perhaps by fate, he unexpectedly reunited there with Aisin Gioro Zailan, his former enemy.[4] Zailan, a cousin of the Emperor, had represented the Qing government in joining forces with the Boxers to resist foreign powers. During the Boxer Rebellion, when the French Embassy was besieged by the Boxers, Pelliot was inside the embassy. He tried to confront the Boxers outside the embassy but was captured and personally interrogated by Zailan. This history indeed made them enemies. After the defeat, Zailan was demoted and sent to Xinjiang due to his involvement with the Boxers.

As time passed, these former adversaries, now in distant Xinjiang, transformed their enmity into friendship. Zailan invited Pelliot to a banquet at his home. During their conversation, Pelliot inquired about the Hidden Library. Zailan recalled that during his journey through Dunhuang, a Taoist monk had given him an ancient scroll. To demonstrate goodwill, he decided to present the scroll as a gift to Pelliot. When Pelliot returned to his accommodation and examined the manuscript closely, he quickly recognized it as a precious 7th-century manuscript. This unexpected gift greatly intrigued Pelliot, prompting him to immediately lead his expedition team from Urumqi straight to Dunhuang.

In January 1908, Paul Pelliot and his team arrived in Hami, the site of the ancient and prosperous Kingdom of Gaochang, referred to as "Yiwu" by the great Master Xuanzang in *Great Tang Dynasty Records on the Western Regions* (Dà Táng Xī Yù Jì, 大唐西域记). In the heart of winter, Paul Pelliot and his team embarked on a month-long journey across the frozen landscape of Hami. Bracing against the harsh elements – wind, frost, snow, and rain – they persevered. In February 1908, exactly a year following Stein's pioneering exploration of the Dunhuang Hidden Library, Pelliot, at the helm of his small but determined party, made their way into the hallowed halls of the legendary Mogao Caves of Dunhuang. Although Xuanzang did not mention Dunhuang extensively in *Great Tang Dynasty Records on the Western Regions* (Dà Táng Xī Yù Jì, 大唐西域记), it was a regular stop on his journeys to and from the Western Regions.

Paul Pelliot once stated that Dunhuang, during the era of Xuanzang, was not only a crucial outpost for the westward dissemination of Chinese culture but also served as a bridge linking ancient Asian civilizations with the Far East. On that ancient land, every step was imprinted with historical traces, and every glance offered a reflection of bygone eras. In this silent expanse, Pelliot and his team members seemed to traverse through time and space, walking alongside Xuanzang, jointly witnessing the millennia of changes and heritage in Dunhuang.

Wang Tao-shih, once a mere Taoist monk, had now become the custodian of the Hidden Library, appointed by the county government. He was well-versed in hosting Chinese officials, understanding that their visits typically involved offering scriptures free of charge. Drawing on his successful interaction with the foreign friend Stein, Wang Tao-shih realized that he needed to present himself to foreigners as the guardian of the scriptures brought back by the great master Xuanzang from the Western Regions, rather than speaking fancifully of the Monkey King and Pigsy. Despite his short stature and wearing a Tang monk-style Taoist robe that didn't quite fit, topped with a lotus-shaped Pilu crown reminiscent of Xuanzang in *Journey to the West* (Xī Yóu Jì, 西游记), he greeted Pelliot with great decorum and performed solemn Taoist rituals. With a thin mustache on his chin and a constant amiable smile on his face, his demeanor was humble, frequently bowing with clasped hands and devoutly offering incense and prayers. He confided to Pelliot that it was divine guidance in a dream that led him to discover the Hidden Library. Thus, Wang Tao-shih bore the solitary responsibility of protecting this sacred cave. He informed Pelliot that Stein had previously surveyed the cave for three days and had paid a considerable sum for some of the manuscripts. Pelliot understood his implication and quietly contemplated his approach.

Pelliot, known for his remarkable social acumen and keen intellect, adeptly maneuvered through complex social interactions. The specifics of how he gained Wang Tao-shih's trust remain unclear, but it's likely that his fluent Chinese, characterized by a distinct Beijing accent, resonated with the Taoist monk. Demonstrating a desire to purchase some of the manuscripts, Pelliot was met with even warmer hospitality than Stein had experienced. This preferential treatment might have been influenced by Wang Tao-shih's financial struggles in refurbishing the Mogao Caves, leading to Pelliot being allowed personal access to the Hidden Library to handpick documents.

Wang Tao-shih informed Pelliot that the key to the Hidden Library was kept in Dunhuang county town and needed to be retrieved from there. Consequently, Pelliot waited patiently in Dunhuang, despite his internal anxiety about the potential mishaps Wang Tao-shih might encounter on the way. During this waiting period, he meticulously numbered, measured, and photographed the Mogao Caves, becoming the first scholar to conduct such a comprehensive study of the Dunhuang Mogao Caves.[5]

When the heavy doors of the Hidden Library finally opened for Pelliot, he stood in astonishment. He recorded this heart-racing moment in his diary:

> At last, we held the mysterious key in our hands. On a day of penitential worship, I stepped into this sacred domain. The impact on my heart was indescribable! I had thought that the collection here had greatly diminished due to the loss of documents eight years ago. However, as I entered this small cave, merely two and a half meters squared, the sight before me was astonishing. Three walls were stacked with scrolls as high as a person, each wall bearing two or three layers of thick manuscripts. Many Tibetan manuscripts were carefully sandwiched between wooden boards, tightly bound with ropes, lying quietly in the corners. Among those bundled scrolls, I could faintly make out characters in both Chinese and Tibetan.

Pelliot was surprised and exhilarated by these treasures, previously unstudied in depth by Chinese scholars.

He began to peruse these scrolls and found many were incomplete, some with only titles remaining. However, Pelliot didn't overlook any item. Faced with these vast collections of scrolls, Pelliot set for himself a few selection criteria: prioritize those marked with dates, then choose various documents outside the common Buddhist canon, and finally, select manuscripts in languages other than Chinese, representing different ethnic texts.

Relying on his extensive Sinological background and rich archaeological knowledge, Pelliot astonishingly sifted through over 15,000 manuscripts to select the most valuable texts at an astonishing pace. He proudly stated, "It is absolutely impossible that there are any scrolls in this cave that I haven't examined." A photograph showing Pelliot himself records his time crouched in the cave, facing the mountainous piles of scriptures, inspecting each item and page by the dim light of a candle. In Pelliot's own words, he proceeded at a speed "reserved for philologists," examining 1,000 scrolls a day, opening 100 per hour, thus reviewing all the documents in the Hidden Library.

We must realize that Pelliot was not reading in his native French nor in the widely spoken languages of English or Russian in Europe. The manuscripts in the Hidden Library formed a cultural Tower of Babel, encompassing texts written in Chinese, Sanskrit, Tibetan, Uighur, Turkic, Sogdian, and various other Eastern Iranian scripts. If there was anyone in the world who could thoroughly understand these ancient languages, it was undoubtedly Pelliot alone.

In the mysterious Hidden Library, shrouded by the deep sands of the desert, Pelliot spent three weeks fully immersed in the in-depth study of the ancient texts. Mundane needs like food and sleep became trivial to him. Even Wang Tao-shih, who typically liked to give orders, was rendered speechless by Pelliot's intense focus. In this solitary and sacred space, Pelliot's soul seemed captivated by the endless charm of the manuscripts, his body nearly collapsing several times in this vast ocean of knowledge. Now, let us glimpse into Pelliot's precious experiences in the Hidden Library through his diary entries.[6]

On the first day, March 3, 1908, he wrote:

> On this Tuesday before Lent, I spent a full ten hours in the Hidden Library. That shrine, adorned with Buddha statues and divine tablets, about 10 feet long on each side, had its three walls piled high with scrolls. I was almost crawling on the ground to sort through and organize these manuscripts. Despite the soreness in my back, the day's discoveries left me immensely satisfied.

On the third day, March 5, 1908, he recorded:

> Around 2:30 in the afternoon, I began to feel shortness of breath and experienced some discomfort in my heart. Clearly, this was due to the lack of sufficient oxygen while working in the cramped shrine for an extended period. However, after half an hour of fresh air, these discomforts disappeared. Despite this, I knew that my body was not accustomed to working in such confined spaces for long durations.

During this time, despite being in a challenging environment, Pelliot maintained his thirst for knowledge and dedication to discovery. In his writings, the Hidden Library was not just a repository of documents but also a sacred place for his spiritual exploration and historical discoveries.

In the Hidden Library buried deep in the desert, Pelliot's days were filled with the joy of discovery and academic passion. For him, each dawn heralded a new harvest of knowledge and wisdom. He was immersed in his world, enthralled by the precious documents covering fields such as religion, literature, art, and politics. With his extraordinary stamina and profound understanding of Sinology and various languages, Pelliot perused every scroll in the library. He wrote in his notes: "I did not miss any precious item. I not only reviewed every manuscript but also carefully examined every piece of paper." During this process, he even discovered and selected some treasures from traditional Chinese medical manuscripts, which are often difficult to understand from a Western cultural perspective.

On the 12th day, March 14, 1908, Pelliot recorded a historical coincidence that he found a manuscript named *On Exhaustive Deceit, Argumentation, and Bewilderment – Part Two: A Response to Essays on Alerting the Deluded* (Qióng Zhà Biàn Huò Lùn • Dá Jǐng Mí Lùn, 穷诈辩惑论卷下·答警迷论). The manuscript of Zhang Zhongjing's *Five Viscera Theory* (Wǔ Zàng Lùn, 五藏论) was unexpectedly found on the back of this document. This was later cataloged as P. 2115v.

On the 13th day, March 15, 1908, he discovered "an anonymous medical manuscript." Although he couldn't ascertain the identity of the author, given the rarity of medical-related manuscripts in the Hidden Library, we can speculate that this might be the famous, incomplete *Verses on Medicinal Properties* (Yào Xìng Gē Jué, 药性歌诀), cataloged as P. 2755.

Until the evening of March 25, after three weeks of relentless effort, Pelliot finally completed his meticulous selection of manuscripts from the Hidden Library. He chose about 2,000 of the most valuable documents from the thousands of scrolls, considering them to be treasures of incalculable historical value. Pelliot then engaged in a crucial negotiation with Wang Tao-shih, which ultimately determined the fate of these ancient texts. On May 12, Pelliot noted in his diary this epoch-making moment: "Tonight, the matter of purchasing the ancient manuscripts has finally been settled. I have acquired the Chinese and Tibetan manuscripts I meticulously selected, as well as the treasures from the Tibetan clapboards, although I could not obtain everything."

In this transaction, Pelliot's fluent Chinese and exceptional social skills played a decisive role. Wang Tao-shih eventually agreed to sell these invaluable treasures to Pelliot for 500 taels of official silver (approximately 90 British pounds). Compared to Stein, who knew nothing of Chinese, Pelliot, proficient in 13 languages, including Chinese, selected each manuscript as a unique treasure. This included obscure traditional Chinese medical texts like Zhang Zhongjing's *Five Viscera Theory* (Wǔ Zàng Lùn, 五藏论), a rarity at the time. At the young age of 30, Pelliot had become a knowledge seeker transcending cultural boundaries. His achievements were not only a personal glory but also set a standard for future scholars in the field of Sinology.

After acquiring a large collection of artifacts from Dunhuang, Pelliot shipped most of them back to France. He then traveled from Hanoi by sea to China, planning to purchase Chinese books in Beijing for the National Library of France, before taking the train through Russia to return to Paris. Upon his arrival in Beijing, the academic and collecting circles were shocked to hear about Pelliot's substantial discovery of precious manuscripts in Dunhuang. Pelliot even showed some of the Dunhuang manuscripts he carried with him to Chinese officials in Beijing. The scholar Yun Yuding wrote in his diary:

> Local officials and scholars never inquired about these texts, and now they have been handed over to the French, transported thousands of miles across the ocean to Paris. Isn't this a matter of great regret and shame? Do we still have people who care about our heritage in China? The local officials of Anxi are not to blame; what about Chen Su-sheng, the Educational Commissioner? Did he never hear of these matters? How shameful!

Consequently, the Beijing political and academic circles decided to host a grand banquet at the Grand Hôtel des Wagons-Lits for Pelliot not only to express their admiration for this Sinology prodigy but also in the hope that Pelliot, upon returning to France, would photograph the Dunhuang manuscripts onto the then-popular glass plate photographs and send them back to China. The idea was to compile and print these photographs into books in China, with the costs covered by contributions from the banquet attendees.[7]

Pelliot attended the banquet, where he spoke fluently in Chinese about his exploratory experiences in the Western Regions and displayed several precious Dunhuang manuscripts. The attendees included prominent figures from the political and academic circles of the time. During that splendid evening, Yun Yu-ding, representing the guests, stood up to toast Pelliot, expressing deep admiration and envy for his relentless academic pursuits and exceptional talent.

Pelliot responded with evident emotion, saying:

> I was dispatched by my country for research purposes; discovering these treasures was a fortunate accident. Although these collections now belong to the French government, knowledge and learning are the commonwealth of all humanity. Should there be any need for photographic transcription and the like, I will spare no effort to support it.

After returning to France, Pelliot remained true to his promise, maintaining close and deep connections with Chinese scholars. He continually sent copies of the Dunhuang manuscripts to Luo Zhenyu, Wang Guowei, and other Chinese academic giants, providing them with many valuable document replicas and photographs. Luo Zhenyu and Wang Guowei were both excited but slightly regretful that these historical materials were first discovered by a foreigner. Luo Zhenyu delved deeply into these documents, writing the milestone work *Bibliography of Dunhuang Grotto Scriptures and the Origin of Their Discovery* (Dūn Huáng Shí Shì Shū Mù Jí Fā Jiàn Zhī Yuán Shǐ, 敦煌石室书目及发见之原始), which quickly garnered widespread attention in the academic world. Pelliot also published *New Perspectives on Chinese Art and Archaeology* (中国艺术和考古新视野), promoting the research achievements of Luo Zhenyu and Wang Guowei in European academic circles.

The Chinese academic world began its formal exploration of Dunhuang studies thanks to the critical discoveries of the late 19th and early 20th centuries. These discoveries are inseparably connected to the pivotal roles played by Wang Tao-shih, Stein, and Pelliot. Pelliot, with his deep Sinological knowledge, conducted thorough analyses and research on the Dunhuang manuscripts, earning him recognition as the "Father of Dunhuang Studies." His work first brought the world's attention to Dunhuang's invaluable heritage. The initial interactions between Luo Zhenyu, Wang Guowei, and Pelliot laid the groundwork for the field. Their efforts led to the gradual growth and eventual global recognition of Dunhuang studies.

Over the subsequent decades, numerous Chinese scholars, driven by their passion for Dunhuang studies, embarked on journeys to France, where Pelliot generously offered his assistance and support. In 1912, Dong Kang introduced the Japanese scholar Naoki Kano to Pelliot in Paris; Kano was the first Japanese scholar to study the Dunhuang manuscripts in Europe. On March 2, 1921, Cai Yuanpei, during his visit to Europe and America, made a special trip to meet Pelliot in Paris. In 1925, Wang Guowei and Chen Yinke had the opportunity to personally see the precious Dunhuang scrolls. In August 1926, Hu Shi visited Pelliot during his trip to Europe. Guided and introduced personally by Pelliot, Hu Shi was granted access to the manuscript room of the library to view the Dunhuang scrolls. Hu Shi highly praised Pelliot in his diary, describing him as "the leading Western scholar of Chinese studies, with the greatest achievements and the widest influence."

Subsequently, scholars like Liang Sicheng, Chen Yinke, and Pu Jiangqing also journeyed to Paris to study the Dunhuang manuscripts. Between 1934 and 1939, Wang Zhongmin conducted an in-depth study of all the Dunhuang documents and took thousands of photographs. Regrettably, a portion of these valuable research achievements was destroyed in China during World War II.

Chinese scholars held Paul Pelliot in high regard not only for his exceptional academic achievements but also for his respect and unwavering support for Chinese scholars. Consequently, the Institute of History and Philology of the Academia Sinica in China specially appointed him as a Corresponding Research Fellow, acknowledging his significant status in the academic community. It was due to Pelliot's recommendation that in 1932, the Institute of History and Philology, represented by Li Ji, received the prestigious Prix Stanislas Julien from the French Academy. This award, highly esteemed in Sinology, signified the extraordinary achievements and international recognition of Chinese scholars in the field of archaeology. Pelliot's relentless support and advocacy played a crucial role in gaining international academic recognition for Chinese scholars, particularly in confirming the existence of the Shang Dynasty in China.

Paul Pelliot was highly respected and welcomed in China, but in France, many doubted him, considering him a boastful show-off, almost like a reincarnation of Marco Polo. He was fiercely criticized by colleagues at the Ecole Française d'Extrême-Orient, accused of wasting public funds and bringing back forged documents, which made it difficult for him to secure funding for the organization and publication of the Dunhuang manuscripts. They even believed that the British explorer Aurel Stein had already taken all the manuscripts from Dunhuang. Facing such scorn, Pelliot endured for months. However, during a banquet, a heated argument over the Dunhuang manuscripts led him to lose control and slap the other party. This impulsive act resulted in a court case, and Pelliot was fined 5 francs, earning him the nickname "The Noseglass Smasher."[8] It wasn't until 1912, after Stein published the *Ruins of Desert Cathay* and confirmed the existence of numerous undiscovered manuscripts in Dunhuang, that the public skepticism towards Pelliot began to fade.

Paul Pelliot was an erudite scholar, proficient in both ancient and modern Eastern and Western knowledge. His achievements were remarkable in every field he explored, making pioneering contributions in multiple domains. He had a great fondness for densely annotating his own collection of books, with notes filling almost every page. Regrettably, after his passing, his widow, Marianna, did not donate these valuable collections to institutions as other academic masters had done. Instead, she dispersed and sold them to various research institutions, booksellers, and scholars in Europe and America.

Marianna had a special fondness for Russian carved glassware. Among her cherished items was a three-legged candy dish, intricately engraved with a pair of closely linked hearts and the image of two people embracing under a tree. Beside them was the inscription: "Was hier in treuer liebe brennt, bleibt auch un tode ungetrennt" (What burns here in true love, remains inseparable even in death).[9] She meticulously cleaned these glass pieces every day, perhaps believing that love should not be tainted by even a grain of sand. Her approach to her husband's books was similar; the dense annotations that Pelliot had written in his lifetime seemed to irk her like a thorn in the eye. Unsentimentally, she erased the handwritten notes of the Sinologist, effectively removing the countless hours of effort and dedication Pelliot had invested in them.

Returning to early 20th-century China, the impassioned appeals of scholars like Luo Zhenyu finally garnered official attention. The government ordered the resealing of the Dunhuang scripture caves and prohibited outsiders from entering. However, the tragedy behind this decision lay in the mystery of funding for the maintenance and protection of these invaluable artifacts. Despite their vocal support at academic conferences, none of those scholars who had spoken out actually ventured into the desolate desert to personally inspect the conditions at Dunhuang. In the ensuing years, Japanese and Russian exploration teams continued their activities under the guise of archaeology in Dunhuang, relentlessly transporting away a vast number of precious documents.

In 1910, the Qing government made a significant decision to transfer all remaining manuscripts from Dunhuang to Beijing for safekeeping. It was estimated that there were about 8,000 documents at that time. The governor of Xinjiang oversaw this transfer, assigning the duty to the Dunhuang county magistrate to inventory these documents before transporting them to Lanzhou and then onward to Beijing. Regrettably, these officials did not handle these precious artifacts with the care they deserved. They merely covered the ancient texts with straw mats and hastily sent them to the capital. Throughout the lengthy journey of over 5,000 li, these documents not only suffered damage from natural elements but also faced theft and destruction from various sources.

It is even more disheartening that the theft and destruction of these manuscripts were primarily perpetrated by some officials and celebrities. Some of these officials even brought the invaluable manuscripts to their homes, allowing their family members to select and keep the most precious scrolls for themselves. To cover up their actions, they cut some of the longer scrolls into multiple pieces, ensuring they had the required count of 8,000 items. Subsequently, the stolen manuscripts were either handed over to the National Central Library in Nanjing or sold to Japanese collectors. To this day, it remains unknown how many manuscripts were lost or damaged during the long transportation process.

For Wang Tao-shih, who was in distant Dunhuang, these events were undoubtedly a severe blow. As the one who initially discovered and protected these artifacts, he underwent profound inner conflict and anguish. In 1914, when Stein visited the Mogao Caves for the second time, Wang Tao-shih candidly shared his inner turmoil with this "foreigner" from afar. According to Stein's *On Ancient Central Asian Tracks* (西域考古记), Wang Tao-shih expressed his regret for not having had enough courage and insight at the time to entrust all the scriptures to Stein for safekeeping.

According to records, over 10,000 Dunhuang manuscripts eventually arrived in Beijing, where they are now preserved in the Beijing Library. There are more than 40,000 Dunhuang manuscripts scattered abroad, most of which are housed in national libraries and museums around the world, where they receive proper protection and maintenance, including restoration of damaged and incomplete sections. Of these, Stein took away approximately over 10,000 scrolls and manuscripts, as well as more than 500 Buddha statues and silk paintings. Pelliot brought back more than 5,000 manuscripts, along with an unspecified number of silk and paper paintings. In addition, there are over 6,000 manuscripts scattered across Russia, Japan, and other places. These artifacts, now overseas, continue to be valuable resources for scholars and researchers.

If it weren't for the pivotal roles of Wang Tao-shih's initial discovery, Aurel Stein's diligent archaeological efforts, and Paul Pelliot's fervent academic passion, the fate of the Mogao Caves and their treasures would likely have been drastically different. These individuals collectively ensured Dunhuang's significant position within Chinese scholarly circles. Pelliot's contribution went beyond the mere rescue of imperiled artifacts; he also facilitated the provision of invaluable document replicas to China. Regrettably, the artifacts that remained in China suffered substantial damage due to a variety of reasons, resulting in a troubled and unfortunate trajectory for these cultural treasures.

Since the discovery of the Hidden Library by Wang Tao-shih in 1900, his life became entangled in a whirlwind of controversy. He faced relentless slander but also received defense and support from many. Wang Tao-shih, a devout Taoist, led an extremely austere life devoid of indulgences. He abstained from smoking and drinking, steered clear of gambling, and shunned any romantic involvements. His diet was simple, consisting of plain tea and bland meals, with water often serving as his soup. His lifestyle was akin to that of an ascetic monk.

Wang Tao-shih received over 1,500 taels of silver from individuals like Stein and Pelliot. However, he viewed these funds not as personal income but as donations. He maintained a detailed ledger, meticulously recording all income and expenditures. The money he acquired from foreigners was entirely allocated to the management, maintenance, and restoration of the Mogao Caves, as well as for hiring people to transcribe scriptures.

The unfortunate Wang Tao-shih was driven to madness in his later years. It's possible he truly lost his sanity, or perhaps he had to feign insanity to live in peace. In a 1926 letter to Stein, Werner mentioned:

> I once gave Wang Tao-shih a small sum of silver, only 75 taels. However, this amount was exaggerated to 100,000 silver yuan. Consequently, villagers approached Wang, demanding a share of this exaggerated fortune. Naturally, Wang couldn't produce such an amount, so when faced with threats to his life, he resorted to feigning madness to escape this calamity.

His later years were indeed challenging. He spent his days trying to avoid those who harbored resentment towards him or those who sought money from him. The place he devoted most of his life to conserving and repairing had become his shackles, a place that labeled him a sinner for eternity. He longed to follow Buddha, to let his spirit transcend. However, his physical being was as if pressed under heavy rocks on the east bank of the Dang River, unable to move. Thirty-one years after the momentous discovery of the Hidden Library, Wang Tao-shih, at the venerable age of 81, passed away. His departure marked the end of an era and his release from the burdens of a lifetime. At last, he could leave behind the place he had so diligently guarded, a world where survival had meant resorting to the guise of insanity. His commitment to protecting a treasure trove of history, despite the personal cost, remains a poignant testament to his dedication.

In a humble cave, just a stone's throw from the Hidden Library, stands a statue of a high monk, serenely positioned. This cave, so small it could be deemed pitiable, would make even visitors a millennium later feel claustrophobic for the statue. However, the monk's demeanor is one of detached tranquility, seemingly indifferent to the confinements surrounding him. Silently observing the unfolding tales, his face bears a faint smile, tempered by time, mirroring the quietude of a contemplative sage.

It's as if he silently imparts a revelation:

> Look, the Dang River has flowed quietly for a thousand years. It didn't choose the conventional path from west to east towards the sea, but instead, it veered from south to north, silently seeping underground, generously nurturing this once barren desert, transforming Dunhuang into a verdant oasis. Just as the Frenchman Pelliot said, "Knowledge is universal." At that pivotal moment in history, whether it was Wang Tao-shih, Stein, or Pelliot, they were like the waters of the Dang River, unswayed by the allure of wealth, not chasing after greed and opulence. Thanks to them, these precious scriptures have been preserved in various forms. Alas, even the beloved *Five Viscera Theory* (Wǔ Zàng Lùn, 五藏论) by Zhang Zhongjing survived, continuing to illuminate human health with its wisdom.

REFERENCES

1. 袁芳霞, "魂系敦煌—记常书鸿的艺术人生[D]." 硕士论文. 西北师范大学 (2005), 16.
2. [法] 菲利普·弗朗德兰, *伯希和传[M]*，一梧译（桂林: 广西师范大学出版社, 2017), i–iii.
3. [法] 保罗·伯希和，*伯希和西域探险记[M]*，耿昇译 (昆明：云南人民出版社，2011), 4.
4. 法] 保罗·伯希和，*伯希和敦煌石窟笔记[M]*，耿昇译 (兰州: 年甘肃人民出版社, 2007), 13.
5. Peter Hopkirk，*Foreign Devils on the Silk Road: The Search for the Lost Treasures of Central Asia* (London: John Murray, 1988), 183.
6. [法] 保罗·伯希和，*伯希和西域探险日记（1906–1908）[M]*，耿昇译 (北京: 中国藏学出版社，2014), 481.
7. 王冀青，"清宣统元年 (1909年) 北京学界公宴伯希和事件再探讨[J]." *敦煌学辑刊*, No. 2 (2014): 130–142.
8. [法] 菲利普·弗朗德兰, *伯希和传[M]*，一梧译 (桂林：广西师范大学出版社, 2017), 31.
9. [法] 菲利普·弗朗德兰, *伯希和传[M]*，一梧译 (桂林: 广西师范大学出版社, 2017), 271.

4 Dang River, Where the Water Brought Out Zhang Zhongjing's *Wu Zang Lun*

Dunhuang Studies represent the new trend in today's global academia.

– Chen Yinke

The water of the Dang River not only cleanses the dust of the natural world but also purifies the souls of people, injecting vitality into this land. Outside the Yumen Pass, the clear springs of the Dang River resemble a melodious song from heaven, flowing amidst the sparkling waves of lakes and mountains, where birdsong and the fragrance of flowers compose a hymn of spring. The water continues to flow, while the trees grow lusher and the flowers bloom in competition, becoming even more dazzling and eye-catching.

In past times, to capture the beauty of the scenery permanently, people could only rely on painting and writing. Over thousands of years, numerous skilled monks and artists embarked on journeys to Dunhuang. They devoted their lifetime skills to meticulously replicate the appearance of the Dang River, the Thousand Buddha Caves, the murals, and the scriptures without any discrepancy. However, each artist's brushstrokes and style were inevitably unique, leading to distinctly characterized works. Painting and writing, these two forms of art, have played an indispensable role in the history of human civilization. Through them, people have witnessed the transmission and transformation of civilizations. However, it is challenging to determine how much of this passed-down civilization is accurate and how much is vague and unclear. Just like the revered medical sage Zhang Zhongjing, to this day, no one can precisely describe his appearance nor does anyone know exactly how many medical masterpieces he wrote.

Fortunately, in the 19th-century wave of innovation in Europe, a revolutionary invention completely transformed the way humans record and disseminate civilization – the camera. August 19, 1839, marks a significant date when the Frenchman Daguerre introduced the world's first true camera. Since then, the art of photography gradually began to replace painting as a new method for documenting significant historical moments and everyday life scenes. A splendid photograph not only carries the transmission of information and public education but also becomes

DOI: 10.1201/9781032698205-4

a part of historical testimony. It impacts our descendants and propels the continuous progress of social civilization.

Especially after Wang Tao-shih discovered the Dunhuang Hidden Library, it was the advent of this emerging photographic technology that enabled Stein to introduce the wonders of Dunhuang to the world. The thousands of photographs of Dunhuang taken by Pelliot and his team not only captured the unique charm of Dunhuang but also gave birth to the academic field of Dunhuang studies. Subsequently, Chinese scholars, utilizing photographs of Dunhuang artifacts, conducted in-depth research, leading to the flourishing development of Dunhuang studies. Therefore, photographs undoubtedly became an important tool for preserving the true appearance of historical documents, providing invaluable and detailed reference materials for the research in Dunhuang studies.

With the rise of photographic technology in the early 20th century, a door to new knowledge gradually opened, providing an opportunity for scholars from China and Japan to embark on unprecedented research endeavors. In this academic adventure, Chinese scholars such as Luo Zhenyu, Wang Guowei, Chen Yinke, Yuan Tongli, Luo Fuyi, and Ma Jixing, with their profound knowledge and relentless efforts, emerged as leading figures in this field. Similarly, in Japan, scholars like Naoki Kano, Genji Kuroda, Sakae Miki, and Saburō Miyashita also made outstanding contributions, adding brilliance to the burgeoning academic landscape of Dunhuang studies.

Talking about the origins of Dunhuang studies, it's essential to mention Luo Zhenyu. This master of Sinology made significant contributions to agronomy, archaeology, and oracle bone studies in China. He is revered as the foremost expert in ancient Chinese studies in modern Chinese history and is universally recognized as the founder of Dunhuang studies.[1]

Let's go back to the historical banquet with Paul Pelliot mentioned in the previous chapter. On an autumn night in 1909, Pelliot brought several precious manuscripts from the Dunhuang Hidden Library to the Grand Hôtel des Wagons-Lits in Beijing, stunning the scholars of the capital. Luo Zhenyu, the pioneer of Dunhuang studies, was most eager and personally planned this meeting with Pelliot. However, fate seemed to play a trick, as Luo fell ill and couldn't attend on the scheduled day. Fortunately, in China, it seems no problem can't be solved over a meal. After some discussion, both parties reached a consensus: Chinese scholars would pool funds, and Pelliot would provide the access to the artifacts for joint photographic reproduction of the documents from the Dunhuang Hidden Library. Eager and deeply invested in the collaboration, Luo Zhenyu swiftly transformed the outcomes of his meeting with Paul Pelliot into a seminal article titled *The Initial Discovery of the Catalogue of the Dunhuang Stone Chamber* (Dūn Huáng Shí Shì Shū Mù Jí Fā Jiàn Zhī Yuán Shǐ, 敦煌石室书目发见之原始). This groundbreaking piece was published in the *Eastern Miscellany* (Dōng Fāng Zá Zhì, 东方杂志) on November 7, 1909, marking a pivotal moment in the annals of Dunhuang studies. This article detailed 12 types of Dunhuang manuscripts and a list of 31 documents, with brief introductions to some of the manuscripts. From then on, China began systematic organization and cataloging research of the Dunhuang manuscripts. This article was not only the first academic paper on the artifacts unearthed from the Hidden Library of Dunhuang in

China but also in the world, marking the beginning of China's historical research on Dunhuang relics. Thus, November 7, 1909, is widely regarded as the birth date of "Dunhuang studies" in China.

Following his meeting with Paul Pelliot, Luo Zhenyu initially photographed 15 artifacts unearthed from Dunhuang, including "five volumes of manuscripts, two wooden carved sculptures, three stone carvings, and five mural paintings." These photographs, which can be considered among the earliest images of Dunhuang manuscripts and murals possessed by the Chinese academic community, were later stored in the library of the Imperial University of Peking. Luo Zhenyu even wrote a postscript for these photographs, reflecting the high regard in which he held them. At that time, the essence of the Dunhuang relics had already been taken to Europe by Aurel Stein and Paul Pelliot, leaving Chinese scholars with only photographs for their research. In December of the same year, Luo Zhenyu's compilation, *The Lost Scriptures of the Dunhuang Stone Chamber* (Dūn Huáng Shí Shì Yí Shū, 敦煌石室遗书), was published by the publisher Songfeng Shi (诵芬室).

Wang Guowei, a Sinology master born in Zhejiang,[2] showcased his exceptional talents early, passing the prestigious imperial examination at just 15. In the twilight years of the Qing Dynasty, he worked alongside Luo Zhenyu in the Ministry of Education, witnessing the decline of an era. Following the Xinhai Revolution, both scholars embarked on an in-depth study of Sinology. Their significant contributions, especially in the realms of oracle bone script and Dunhuang studies, cemented their reputations as eminent Sinologists.

Luo Zhenyu, with his insightful wisdom and astuteness, became a wealthy and capable social activist. Wang Guowei, on the other hand, was a melancholic and pessimistic individual, deeply immersed in academic research and indifferent to fame and fortune, earning the reputation of being "as honest as ham." After the Xinhai Revolution, Wang Guowei was appointed by Emperor Puyi to teach at the South Study Room, serving as Puyi's Chinese literature teacher. In 1924, following Feng Yuxiang's coup in Beijing which forced Puyi to leave his palace – the Forbidden City – Wang Guowei saw this as a great humiliation and was engulfed in despair as a loyal servant of the fallen dynasty.

On the eve of the Dragon Boat Festival in 1927, Wang Guowei found himself at Kunming Lake in the Summer Palace, his thoughts entwined with the ancient poet Qu Yuan. Qu Yuan, a loyal minister exiled and unable to serve his country, tragically drowned himself, a tale echoing across two millennia. His death stirred profound grief in the people of Chu, leading to the birth of the Dragon Boat Festival traditions – beating drums on the riverbanks, racing dragon boats, and casting rice-filled zongzi into the waters, all to honor and remember him.

Centuries later, Wang Guowei, burdened by his own deep sorrow and unwavering loyalty in a rapidly changing world, sought solace and release at the same lake. In his poignant final note, he wrote: "At fifty, death is all that remains. Witnessing the upheaval of my world, I refuse to be dishonored further." These words resonated with the pain of witnessing an era's end and a steadfast commitment to his ideals. In his last act, mirroring Qu Yuan's, Wang Guowei sought to escape the turmoil of his time, choosing a dignified end over a world he could no longer reconcile with.

Wang Guowei's passing, a towering figure in the academic world, deeply grieved countless people, all of whom felt a profound sense of loss at his departure. His work, *Poetic Remarks in the Human World* (Rén Jiān Cí Huà, 人间词话), especially the concept of "Three ching-chieh (states) of scholarship"[3] he described therein, continues to be widely cited, a testament to the depth of his thought. He described:

> Throughout the ages all those who have been highly successful in great ventures and in the pursuit of learning must of necessity have [successively] experienced three kinds of ching-chieh.
>
> "Last night the west wind shriveled the green-clad trees,
> Alone I climb the high tower
> To gaze my fill along the road to the horizon."
> Expresses the first state (ching).
> "My clothes grow daily more loose, yet care I not.
> For you am I thus wasting away in sorrow and pain."
> Expresses the second state.
> "I sought her in the crowd a hundred, a thousand times.
> Suddenly with a turn of the head [I saw her],
> That one there where the lamplight was fading."
> Expresses the third state.
>
> (Translated by Adele Austin Richett)

Perhaps only a master of Sinology like Wang Guowei could describe these three realms with such vivid and exhaustive detail.

Wang Guowei, a towering figure in the academic world, dedicated his life to researching a vast array of fields including philosophy, literature, the history of drama, oracle bone script, ancient artifacts, the history of the Shang and Zhou dynasties, Han and Jin dynasty bamboo slips, Han and Wei dynasty steles, Mongolian history, northwestern Chinese history, and Dunhuang manuscripts. Wang Guowei's journey in the academic realm was nothing short of extraordinary. His scholarship, deeply respected across various disciplines, ranged from philosophy and literature to the intricate studies of ancient artifacts and Dunhuang manuscripts. More than just a pioneer, he is celebrated as one of the foundational figures in Dunhuang studies. Throughout his illustrious career, he wove a rich tapestry of historical and cultural insights, leaving behind a legacy that continues to enlighten and inspire future generations. His profound contributions not only shaped his fields of study but also enriched our understanding of the past, making his work an invaluable treasure for those who follow.

Wang Guowei's research on Dunhuang was remarkable for its interdisciplinary approach. He creatively utilized a wide range of knowledge and skills, pioneering investigations into significant, unresolved, or previously overlooked issues spanning various academic fields. Particularly noteworthy was his introduction of the "dual evidence method"[4] as an academic principle, a significant innovation in 20th-century Chinese archaeology and textual research. This groundbreaking method, which synergized newly unearthed archaeological materials with existing literary documents, offered fresh perspectives for historical examination and interpretation. It paved new paths in the study of Chinese culture, demonstrating Wang Guowei's ingenuity and his lasting impact on academic research.

The so-called "dual evidence method" involves corroborating newly unearthed materials with traditional textual materials to verify the authenticity of ancient history. This approach emerged at a time when Eastern and Western academic thoughts intersected and a wealth of new historical materials were discovered. This methodology revolutionized historical research, which was no longer confined to relying solely on textual descriptions or narratives from predecessors. Instead, it involved verifying the authenticity of textual materials through physical artifacts excavated from the ground and vice versa. In this process, Wang Guowei played the role of a skilled detective, unraveling numerous historical mysteries that had remained unsolved. For instance, *Five Viscera Theory* (Wǔ Zàng Lùn, 五藏论) unearthed in Dunhuang serves as an outstanding complement and correction to ancient documentary records. Although this work was mentioned in ancient Chinese texts, it was relatively unknown; the discovery in Dunhuang essentially validated the historical accuracy of these records.

Wang Guowei and Luo Zhenyu, two towering figures in the academic world, met in Shanghai in 1898 and journeyed together through nearly three decades of challenges. Despite their contrasting personalities – Wang being deep and melancholic and Luo being astute and insightful – they demonstrated remarkable understanding and cooperation in their academic and professional lives. The intricacies of their friendship and collaboration, filled with complexities and nuances, perhaps remain fully understood only by themselves. Although their friendship ended in 1926, it did not diminish their individual and collective monumental contributions to Dunhuang studies. Both scholars are universally acknowledged and respected for their efforts and achievements in researching, excavating, and preserving the cultural heritage of Dunhuang. Their profound impact on Dunhuang studies extends beyond academia, leaving an indelible mark on both Chinese and global cultural history.

In our discussion, the term "Dunhuang studies"[5] has been mentioned multiple times. The academic community generally agrees that the origin of Chinese "Dunhuang studies" can be traced back to November 7, 1909, the day Luo Zhenyu published *The Initial Discovery of the Catalogue of the Dunhuang Stone Chamber* (Dūn Huáng Shí Shì Shū Mù Jí Fā Jiàn Zhī Yuán Shǐ, 敦煌石室书目发见之原始) in the *Eastern Miscellany* (Dōng Fāng Zá Zhì, 东方杂志). However, the coinage of the term "Dunhuang studies" came much later. It is widely believed that the term was first used by the Japanese scholar Ishihama Juntaro (1888–1968) in a lecture at the Kaitokudo in Osaka in 1925. Another view holds that the concept of "Dunhuang studies" was first introduced by the renowned Chinese Sinologist Chen Yinke in 1930 when he wrote the preface for Chen Yuan's book *An Analytical List of the Tun-huang Manuscripts in the National Library of Peiping* (Dūn Huáng Jié Yú Lù, 敦煌劫余录). Despite differing opinions on the origin of the term, it is undeniable that "Dunhuang studies" emerged as a natural result of the development of research on Dunhuang relics.[6]

Chen Yinke, in the preface to *An Analytical List of the Tun-huang Manuscripts in the National Library of Peiping* (Dūn Huáng Jié Yú Lù, 敦煌劫余录), wrote: "The scholarship of an era necessarily involves new materials and new questions. The use of these materials to investigate these questions signifies the new trend in the scholarship of that era." This publication became indispensable for researchers across various disciplines, including those focusing on Dunhuang studies and Buddhism. As the concept of "Dunhuang studies" gradually gained international recognition, Chen Yinke's role in shaping this field became increasingly evident. His research significantly influenced the development and understanding of this specialized area of study.

Chen Yinke, a legendary figure in the annals of Chinese academia,[7] was revered for his exceptional scholarly talent and distinctive personality, earning the accolade of being the "most promising scholarly seed" in the Chinese cultural sphere. Demonstrating remarkable memory and extensive knowledge from a young age, Chen studied in countries like Japan, Germany, France, and the United States. He mastered eight languages, including Sanskrit, Pali, Persian, Turkic, Tangut, English, French, and German, particularly excelling in Sanskrit and Pali. Intriguingly, despite his 23 years of study abroad, Chen chose not to obtain any academic degrees. Perhaps, in his view, degrees were merely symbolic papers, unable to measure the true essence of knowledge and wisdom.

The year 1925 held special significance for Chen Yinke. After spending over two decades studying abroad, he finally embarked on his journey back to China. Upon his return, he joined Tsinghua School, serving alongside luminaries such as Wang Guowei, Liang Qichao, and Zhao Yuanren as a professor at the Institute of Chinese Studies. Despite being only 36 years old at the time, Chen's extensive knowledge and multifaceted talents garnered immense respect from both students and faculty. His lectures spanned a wide array of topics from both Eastern and Western fields, attracting even Tsinghua's professors to attend his lectures. Revered as the "the professors' professor," this title aptly reflected his esteemed status in the academic world.

Chen Yinke's extensive overseas education and teaching experiences endowed him with a unique perspective in his academic pursuits. He employed a method combining Eastern and Western comparative textual analysis, achieving significant breakthroughs in the field of Chinese historical textual research. Throughout his life, he authored numerous works encompassing history, literature, religion, and more. Remarkably, even in his later years when he almost lost his eyesight, he continued to produce important manuscripts and monographs with the assistance of his aides.

Chen Yinke's connection to Dunhuang studies can also be traced back to another individual we mentioned earlier: Wang Guowei. At that time, China's cultural circle was remarkably interconnected. It was through Wang Guowei that Chen Yinke was introduced to Paul Pelliot in Paris. While the exact time and details of their meeting are not uniformly recorded, it is certain that the encounter between Chen Yinke, a rising Sinologist proficient in eight languages, and Pelliot, a Western scholar fluent in 13 languages and adept in Beijing dialect, must have been a moment of profound mutual recognition and admiration. This meeting inspired Chen Yinke to delve deeply into the study of Dunhuang manuscripts.

In the realm of Dunhuang studies, Chen Yinke made significant contributions as well. His efforts in rescuing, organizing, and establishing the Dunhuang manuscripts were instrumental. Chen's work played a vital role in the development and recognition of Dunhuang studies, leaving an indelible mark on this academic field.

Dunhuang studies, a discipline centered around the exploration of Dunhuang manuscripts, the art of the Dunhuang Caves, and their associated theories, also encompasses the history and geography of Dunhuang. Over a century has passed since the discovery of the scripture caves. Current statistics indicate that over 50,000 Dunhuang relics have been published, the majority being Buddhist scriptures. These also include historical records, local gazetteers, works of various schools of thought, contracts, and documents covering language, literature, art, and technology.

According to Ma Jixing's *Annotations on the Ancient Medical Texts from the Dunhuang Cave Library* (Dūn Huáng Gǔ Yī Jí Kǎo Shì, 敦煌古医籍考释),[8] Most of the relatively well-preserved Dunhuang manuscripts are currently housed in Europe. As of August 1991, the British Library boasted a collection of over 7,000 Dunhuang documents. Initially, these documents were roughly categorized based on language and the site of excavation, compiled under the general series Or.8210 to Or.8212. Or.8210 mainly includes Chinese manuscripts and printed works unearthed from the Dunhuang scripture caves; Or.8211 comprises documents obtained during Aurel Stein's first expedition, as well as Chinese slips from his second expedition to Dunhuang; and Or.8212 consists of documents in ethnic languages or mixed scripts. Subsequently, the British Library reclassified these documents, assigning them a numbering system based on Stein's surname, abbreviated as "S."

The National Library of Paris in France, following the British Library, holds the second-largest collection of Dunhuang manuscripts, with approximately 2,500 documents obtained by Paul Pelliot. These documents are cataloged with a numbering system that begins with Pelliot's surname, commonly abbreviated as "P."

The Saint Petersburg branch of the Institute of Oriental Studies at the Russian Academy of Sciences, as reported in *Russian Collection of Dunhuang Manuscripts* (É Cáng Dūn Huáng Wén Xiàn, 俄藏敦煌文献), houses over 19,000 cataloged Dunhuang documents. In Japan, institutions like Ryukoku University, Tenri University, Otani University libraries, and the Tokyo National Museum, along with some private collections, also preserve Dunhuang manuscripts, with a total of approximately over a thousand volumes.

In China, the Beijing Library (now the National Library of China) holds the largest collection of Dunhuang fragments, totaling over 16,000 scrolls. This includes more than 8,000 scrolls that have been cataloged and organized, as mentioned in Chen Yuan's *An Analytical List of the Tun-huang Manuscripts in the National Library of Peiping* (Dūn Huáng Jié Yú Lù, 敦煌劫余录), and additional scrolls that are yet to be sorted. Moreover, the Dunhuang Research Institute, the National Museum of Chinese History, the Palace Museum, the Gansu Provincial Museum, and the Peking University Library also house collections of Dunhuang manuscripts. Some Dunhuang manuscripts are also preserved in libraries in Taiwan.

The richness and historical significance of the Dunhuang manuscripts have gradually become a focal point in global cultural research over the past century. Among these is a branch that has continually attracted the attention of many medical scholars, namely, Dunhuang medicine. Despite being a relatively obscure field of study for most people, the Dunhuang manuscripts related to medicine are of great importance. Among the more than 50,000 Dunhuang manuscripts, there are just over a hundred related to medicine. While this might seem insignificant, these texts provide a crucial theoretical foundation and documentary resources for the study of the history of Chinese medicine and the development of modern medicine.

The creation of Dunhuang medical texts dates back to the pre-Qin period, with the majority originating from before the Sui and Tang dynasties. Most of these texts were transcribed during the Tang Dynasty and preserved as manuscripts. In terms of content, Dunhuang medical literature can be categorized into various fields: medical theory, diagnostic methods, acupuncture and moxibustion, materia medica, medical prescriptions, Buddhist and Taoist medical texts, and miscellaneous medical discussions. These categories represent the most abundant collection among the known unearthed medical documents in China.

The initial focus of research on Dunhuang medical documents was primarily on their collection and collation, with less emphasis on an in-depth study of their academic essence, such as ideas, concepts, techniques, and methodologies, as well as their scholarly value. In the preface to *An Analytical List of the Tun-huang Manuscripts in the National Library of Peiping* (Dūn Huáng Jié Yú Lù 敦煌劫余录), Chen Yinke stressed the importance of "effectively using materials to explore questions." He advocated for Dunhuang studies to move beyond mere material collection and to focus more on raising and investigating new questions, thereby advancing academic renewal and development. Contemporary Dunhuang scholars have started to recognize this, and they are now comprehensively, systematically, and deeply studying the academic essence and value of Dunhuang medical documents, making this a new trend in the field.

In the meanwhile, the study of Dunhuang medical manuscripts faces numerous challenges, including the fragmented and incomplete nature of the documents, and the difficulty in identifying colloquial characters, homophones, and errors within the texts. These issues have limited the number of scholars able to conduct in-depth research. Fortunately, several scholars have already undertaken extensive work in these areas, laying a solid foundation for the future utilization and study of these materials.

The Dunhuang medical manuscripts are dispersed globally, with the British Library and the National Library of France each housing over 30 types of Dunhuang medical documents. Additionally, libraries in Japan and various locations in China also hold a collection of these Dunhuang medical manuscripts.

A notable example is the manuscript of *Materia Medica with Collected Commentaries – Preface and Records* (Běn Cǎo Jīng Jí Zhù · Xù Lù, 本草经集注·序录), acquired in 1908 by Japanese scholars Tachibana Zuicho (1890–1968) and Kikkawa Koichiro. This manuscript was later obtained by the Chinese scholar Luo Zhenyu and included in his 1916 publication *Ji Shi Xian's Collected Works* (Jí Shí Ān Cóng Shū, 吉石盦丛书) titled *Kaiyuan Manuscript of Materia Medica with Collected Commentaries Preface and Example Fragments* (Kāi Yuán Xiě Běn Cǎo Jīng Jí Zhù Xù Lì Cán Juàn, 开元写本草经集注序例残卷). The original document is currently housed in the Ryukoku University in Japan.

In China, some Dunhuang medical manuscripts have been preserved in private collections. For instance, Luo Zhenyu once owned a fragment of *Remedies and Formulas of Mineral Medicine* (Liáo Fú Shí Fāng, 疗服石方), which he purchased from a bookstore in Tianjin. He later included its photo in his collection *Zhensong Hall Collection of Secret Books from the Western Frontier* (Zhēn Sōng Táng Cáng Xī Chuí Mì Jí Cóng Cán, 贞松堂藏西陲秘籍丛残), originally titled *Remnant Scrolls of Remedies and Formulas of Mineral Medicine* (Liáo Fú Shí Yī Fāng Cán Juàn, 疗服石医方残卷).

Additionally, another significant traditional Chinese medical text, *Key Methods of Medicine Administration for Organs and Viscera* (Fǔ Xíng Jué Zàng Fǔ Yòng Yào Fǎ Yào, 辅行诀脏腑用药法要), originally from Dunhuang, was once a treasured family heirloom of Zhang Wuonan. Regrettably, the original scroll was destroyed during the Cultural Revolution. Later on, Zhang Wuonan's grandson, Zhang Dachang, donated a copied version of this manuscript to the China Academy of Chinese Medical Sciences. Wang Xuetai undertook the task of organizing and annotating this work, and it was eventually included in the *Annotations on the Ancient Medical Texts from the Dunhuang Cave Library* (Dūn Huáng Gǔ Yī Jí Kǎo Shì, 敦煌古医籍考释), published in 1988 under the editorship of Ma Jixing.

It is noteworthy that the sum of Dunhuang's medical manuscripts amounts to just over 100 varieties,[9] which constitutes less than 0.2% of the total number of Dunhuang manuscripts. However, within this relatively small collection of medical texts, the presence of Zhang Zhongjing's *Five Viscera Theory* (Wǔ Zàng Lùn, 五藏论) in five different versions stands out significantly. This work is notable not only for its wide distribution among the countries that house these collections but also for the intense debate surrounding its authenticity. In recent years, significant progress has been made in verifying, editing, annotating, supplementing, and conducting related research on the Dunhuang versions of Zhang Zhongjing's *Five Viscera Theory* (Wǔ Zàng Lùn, 五藏论). This advancement in the study of these documents has been a major step forward in understanding the historical and medical value of this ancient text.

Up to the present, five distinct manuscript versions of Zhang Zhongjing's *Five Viscera Theory* (Wǔ Zàng Lùn, 五藏论) unearthed from Dunhuang have been discovered. They are as follows: the S. 5614 copy at the British Library, three copies at the National Library of France – P. 2115, P. 2755, and P. 2378 – and the Дx. 01325V copy currently preserved at the Saint Petersburg branch of the Institute of Oriental Studies of the Russian Academy of Sciences. Each of these copies offers a unique perspective on this ancient medical text, contributing to the broader understanding of its historical and medical significance.

Apart from the five Dunhuang manuscript versions of Zhang Zhongjing's *Five Viscera Theory* (Wǔ Zàng Lùn, 五藏论), there are also three well-known non-Dunhuang versions: the *Categorized Collection of Medical Formulas* (Yī Fāng Lèi Jù, 医方类聚) version from Korea; a hand-copied version by Zhang Yicheng, a renowned physician from North Zhejiang (with a preface by Zhang Yuansu); and the Japanese Gakkundō wooden-movable type edition of *Five Viscera Theory* (Wǔ Zàng Lùn, 五藏论). This last version was created by the Japanese scholar Taki Motokata, who extracted it from the extensive Korean medical work *Categorized Collection of Medical Formulas* (Yī Fāng Lèi Jù, 医方类聚). Each of these eight versions will be explored in detail in this book, highlighting their unique aspects and their importance in the history of Dunhuang medical studies.

Two thousand years ago, both Dunhuang and Loulan were places of splendor. However, the drying up of the Kongque River, a tributary of the Tarim River, deprived Loulan of its nourishment, leading to the ancient city's eventual submergence into the depths of the Taklamakan Desert, where it became a forgotten memory in the annals of history. In contrast, Dunhuang, blessed by the enduring flow of the Dang River, not only escaped the encroachment of the desert but also flourished over time, retaining its dazzling glory to this day. The Dang River's continuous water supply nourished the surrounding forests and grasslands, forming a natural barrier against the advancing desert, allowing Dunhuang to be preserved as a vibrant and beautiful oasis.

On April 18th, 1931, in the lunar calendar, Wang Tao-shih, a diligent and unassuming guardian, closed his eyes of wisdom, concluding his ordinary yet extraordinary life journey at the age of 81. His passing did not cause a sensation, but on the hundredth day after his departure, his devoted disciples erected a significant pagoda across from the Mogao Caves in his memory and honor. This pagoda, inscribed with an epitaph for Wang Tao-shih, faces the vast southern sky and stands 174 centimeters tall and 75 centimeters wide. The seal script at the top of the monument reads "His Virtue Extends Across a Hundred Generations," and it is flanked by two carved dragons on either side, symbolizing reverence and remembrance for Wang Tao-shih. Affectionately, it is known as the "Daoist Tower."

In the historical tapestry of Dunhuang, Wang Tao-shih resembles the king from the legend of "The Dragon Maiden's Quest for a Husband." His existence not only facilitated the legendary love story between Stein and the "Dragon Maiden" but also ensured the continuous flow of the Dang River, benefiting generations to come. His role in Dunhuang's history is like a mythical guardian, weaving his own legend into the fabric of time, much like the enduring and nourishing waters of the Dang River itself.

By the banks of the Dang River, the spirit of Wang Tao-shih seems to still wander, his steps marked by grace and composure. His eyes, once filled with worry and fear, now exude a sense of tranquility. He seems to whisper softly, with pride:

> I, Wang Tao-shih, am the true guardian of the Dunhuang Hidden Library. Without me, the legendary love story of Stein and the "Dragon Maiden" would cease to exist, and how then would the globally revered field of Dunhuang studies shine its light?

REFERENCES

1. 李晓林，"略论罗振玉对近代学术的贡献[D]." 硕士论文 东北师范大学 (2008), 17.
2. 魏友壮，"王国维的漫漫天涯路[J].'民间传奇故事'(A卷), No. 6 (2022): 63–65.
3. 李学利，"解读王国维'治学三境界'[J]."*太原理工大学学报*(社会科学版), No.1(2007): 43–45.
4. 彭汶，"试论王国维的'二重证据法'及其逻辑 – 方法论意义[J]." 江淮论坛, No. 4 (1990): 49–56.
5. 王冀青，"论'敦煌学'一词的词源 [J]." *敦煌学辑刊*，Vol. 38, No. 2 (2000): 110–132.
6. 屈小强, "陈寅恪与敦煌学 [J]." *文史杂谈*, No. 5 (2016): 98–103.
7. 任重, "陈寅恪先生传略 [J]." *石油大学学报（社会科学版）*, No. 4 (1998): 72–74.
8. 马继兴，*敦煌古医籍考释[M]*, (南昌: 江西科学技术出版社, 1988), 2.
9. 李应存, *实用敦煌医学[M]* (兰州: 甘肃科学技术出版社, 2007), 8.

5 The Truncated *Verses on Medicinal Properties* – P. 2755V Collected in France

"Despite the historical abundance of 'Wu Zang Lun' texts, . . . most have vanished into obscurity."

– Fan Xingzhun

Within the rich archives of the National Library of France in Paris, there is a fragment from Pelliot's Dunhuang collection, designated as Pel.chin.2755V (or simply P. 2755V).[1] Measuring 25.5 cm in height and approximately 80 cm in length, this fragment is meticulously written on both sides with a brush. Unfortunately, both the beginning and end are missing, casting it as an enigmatic piece without a clear start or finish. The front side displays a fragment of a Taoist text, neatly inscribed in regular script with clear, unaltered handwriting, identified as a part of the *Supreme Subtle Dharma Sutra on Fundamental Nature* (Tài Shàng Miào Fǎ Běn Xiàng Jīng, 太上妙法本相经). The reverse side presents a different scene with 58 lines of cursive script. The first half follows basic rules of line and character spacing, with occasional corrections, while the latter half, starting from the 36 line, features smaller writing and narrower spacing, resulting in blurred characters. This side, lacking both a title and author's name, primarily focuses on the properties of Chinese medicinal herbs and their clinical applications. Given Paul Pelliot's unlikely choice of an unknown Taoist scripture, this fragment is likely the "an anonymous medical manuscript" he discovered on March 15, 1908.[2]

However, this precious medicine related manuscript has often been misunderstood by scholars. Yuan Tongli referred to it as the *Verses on Medicinal Properties* in his work *Complete Catalog of Overseas Dunhuang Manuscript Photographs in the National Library of Peiping* (国立北平图书馆现藏海外敦煌遗籍照片总目).[3] In contrast, Huang Yongwu described it as *Experiential Medical Prescriptions* in his book *Treasures of Dunhuang* (Dūn Huáng Bǎo Zàng, 敦煌宝藏).[4] Another scholar, Fan Xingzhun, believed it to be the *Jivaka's Five Viscera Theory* (Qí Pó Wǔ Zàng Lùn, 耆婆五□脏论).[5]

The first person to bring P. 2775 into the academic field was Yuan Tongli. A distinguished alumnus of the Department of Foreign Languages at Peking University, Yuan polished his academic skills at the Tsinghua University Library and later pursued further studies across the ocean in the History Department at Columbia

DOI: 10.1201/9781032698205-5

University and at the New York State Library School. He returned to China in 1924, with all the knowledge he learned abroad.[6] As a pioneer of modern library science in China, he seemed predestined to be deeply connected with books. In 1929, he was invited to lead the National Library of Peiping, adopting the mission of preserving ancient texts and enlightening with new knowledge, thus beginning his quest to collect valuable academic materials from within China and abroad. Yuan's overseas educational experience expanded his perspective, allowing him to establish a broad network in the academic circles of Europe and America.

In 1934, destiny shifted its course. Yuan Tongli helped Wang Zhongmin and Xiang Da to set off on separate journeys to France and Britain, embarking on a historic quest to uncover Dunhuang manuscripts.[7] Once in Paris, Wang Zhongmin, aided by scholars like Paul Pelliot and Lionel Giles, not only witnessed the splendor of all the Dunhuang fragments in the National Library of Paris but also replicated nearly 10,000 invaluable manuscript photos for the National Library of Peiping and Tsinghua University. Meanwhile, Xiang Da's journey in England was laden with challenges. Faced with the British Museum's vast and unsorted collection of Dunhuang Chinese documents, he found it difficult to start his research. Amidst these vast piles of documents, his only option was to go through them one at a time. Restricted by the library's service rules, he was only able to review a fraction of the manuscripts, totaling just over 500 volumes.

The saying "trouble breeds success" was vividly exemplified in the life of Wang Zhongmin. With the outbreak of World War II, Europe was shrouded in the smoke of war, and China, too, suffered greatly from the turmoil. Against this backdrop of unrest, Wang faced immense challenges. Especially after the Marco Polo Bridge Incident, the necessity of relocating the National Library of Peiping southwards added complexity and danger to both domestic and international situations. In such circumstances, Wang diligently registered each of the precious photographs he had taken and compiled them into a catalog. Given the significance of these photos and the unstable conditions of the time, he decided to keep the photographs with him for safekeeping and only sent the catalog back to China.

In the autumn of 1939, Wang Zhongmin, with nearly 10,000 photographs in tow, made his way to the United States and temporarily stored them in Washington, D.C. After years of waiting and relentless effort, he finally managed to return to his homeland in early 1947. Safely bringing back these valuable photos to the National Library of Peiping, he reunited them with the catalog that had been sent back earlier. Wang Zhongmin's steadfast commitment ensured the preservation of these precious Dunhuang manuscript photographs, a contribution that profoundly influenced future scholarly research.

After Wang Zhongmin sent the catalog back to China, Yuan Tongli promptly organized it into the *Complete Catalog of Overseas Dunhuang Manuscript Photographs in the National Library of Peiping* (国立北平图书馆现藏海外敦煌遗籍照片总目), which included ten medical manuscript fragments classified under the category of medical texts. This was the first time that Dunhuang medical literature was independently categorized under medicine and officially published. This catalog was published in the *Quarterly Bulletin of Chinese Bibliography* (Tú Shū Jì Kān, 图书

季刊) new volume 2, issue 4, by the Peiping Library before 1940. Upon its release, it quickly garnered the attention of scholars and became a valuable resource for their research. Due to the P. 2755V fragment missing both its beginning and end, and having no visible title, with content mostly about medicinal properties and applications, Yuan Tongli mistakenly identified the *Five Viscera Theory* (Wǔ Zàng Lùn, 五藏论) as the *Verses on Medicinal Properties* (Yào Xìng Gē Jué, 药性歌诀) in this catalog, which led to the subsequent unfolding of events.

Fan Xingzhun,[8] a renowned medical historian revered as "the foremost collector of traditional Chinese medical texts in China," happened upon the book *Complete Catalog of Overseas Dunhuang Manuscript Photographs in the National Library of Peiping* (国立北平图书馆现藏海外敦煌遗籍照片总目). Within it, one entry particularly caught his eye: "Ming Tang Wu Zang Lun, one volume, four pages of enlarged photographs." Although this was just a part of the catalog and did not include the actual photos, these few words were enough to spark Fan's intense interest in the *Five Viscera Theory* (Wǔ Zàng Lùn, 五藏论). This curiosity marked the beginning of his deep dive into the exploration of this ancient medical text.

Since his youth, Fan Xingzhun had shown an extraordinary passion for ancient medical texts. He lived a frugal life, often scrimping and saving to collect precious medical books from various dynasties, even going so far as to use all his family's savings. By 1942, it was recorded that his personal collection had grown to an astonishing "over twenty thousand volumes," and it continued to expand over time. Fan lived in a rented small house, where, apart from essential furniture like chairs and desks, almost every space was occupied by books. Yet it was in this ocean of books that he found his greatest joy. His collection was not only vast but also immensely valuable, including original works from the Song and Yuan dynasties, manuscripts of medical experts from the Ming and Qing dynasties, and even extremely rare and unique editions.

Notably, despite his deep affection for his books, Fan always believed that books were "public assets of the world." He named his library the "Xifen Room" (栖芬室), symbolizing that these books were merely resting there temporarily. He once said, "If I do not use them, it is fitting to quickly disperse them to the world." This statement reflected his selfless attitude towards the dissemination of knowledge and his magnanimous spirit.

For Fan Xingzhun, a scholar who had perused thousands of books, the discovery that he had never come across the *Five Viscera Theory* (Wǔ Zàng Lùn, 五藏论) was indeed surprising. He recalled the *Five Viscera Theory* (Wǔ Zàng Lùn, 五藏论) mentioned in the Korean *Categorized Collection of Medical Formulas* (Yī Fāng Lèi Jù, 医方类聚) but realized that this text was not widely circulated in China at the time. This prompted him to reach out to Kim Tae-Dou in North Korea, through whom he borrowed the Korean edition of *Categorized Collection of Medical Formulas* (Yī Fāng Lèi Jù, 医方类聚) from the renowned medical expert Hong Choju. This version of *Categorized Collection of Medical Formulas* (Yī Fāng Lèi Jù, 医方类聚) was a cultural treasure in itself, produced in 1852 during Japan's Edo period by the medical family Kita. It was printed using the most advanced movable type technology of the time on high-quality "Hon Mino paper" from Mino City, Gifu Prefecture, and was eventually gifted by the Japanese government to the Korean government. After the fall of Korea, this set of books became a cherished possession of the Hong family.

Fan, having borrowed this precious collection, planned to compare the *Five Viscera Theory* (Wǔ Zàng Lùn, 五藏论) in it with the *Mingtang's Five Viscera Theory* (Míng Táng Wǔ Zàng Lùn, 明堂五脏论) mentioned by Yuan Tongli in the *Complete Catalog of Overseas Dunhuang Manuscript Photographs in the National Library of Peiping* (国立北平图书馆现藏海外敦煌遗籍照片总目). However, due to the lack of photographs, this plan was temporarily put on hold.

In 1943, Fan joined the Chinese and Western Medicine Research Institute, taking up work in the documentation department. His mind, however, continually lingered on the Dunhuang manuscripts related to the *Five Viscera Theory* (Wǔ Zàng Lùn, 五藏论). He suggested photocopying the medical book photos from the Dunhuang collection at the Peiping Library, a task eventually completed with the help of his colleagues. When he finally got the photos of the *Mingtang's Five Viscera Theory* (Míng Táng Wǔ Zàng Lùn, 明堂五脏论) and compared them with the *Five Viscera Theory* (Wǔ Zàng Lùn, 五藏论) from *Categorized Collection of Medical Formulas* (Yī Fāng Lèi Jù, 医方类聚), he found no similarities, a discovery that was undoubtedly a huge disappointment for him. But amidst this disappointment, fate seemed to offer a glimmer of hope. Fan unexpectedly discovered that the *Verses on Medicinal Properties* (Yào Xìng Gē Jué, 药性歌诀) (P. 2755V) listed by Yuan Tongli in the catalog astonishingly resembled the *Five Viscera Theory* (Wǔ Zàng Lùn, 五藏论) in *Categorized Collection of Medical Formulas* (Yī Fāng Lèi Jù, 医方类聚). Surprisingly, what Yuan had listed was not the *Verses on Medicinal Properties* (Yào Xìng Gē Jué, 药性歌诀) but the *Five Viscera Theory* (Wǔ Zàng Lùn, 五藏论). Upon further comparison, Fan found that P. 2755V bore many similarities to the *Five Viscera Theory* (Wǔ Zàng Lùn, 五藏论) cited by Chen Ziming in *Great Herbal Formulas for Women* (Fù Rén Liáng Fāng, 妇人良方). Although most scholars at the time believed that the *Five Viscera Theory* (Wǔ Zàng Lùn, 五藏论) cited by Chen was the *Jivaka's Five Viscera Theory* (Qí Pó Wǔ Zàng Lùn, 耆婆五脏论), Fan agreed with this view and consequently identified P. 2755V as the *Jivaka's Five Viscera Theory* (Qí Pó Wǔ Zàng Lùn, 耆婆五脏论).

However, this conclusion was not the final word. After the victory in the War of Resistance against Japan, Fan Xingzhun traveled to Shanghai to visit the library of the Chinese Medical Association and took the opportunity to visit Yuan Tongli's private library. During this visit, he detailed to Yuan his research findings and Yuan's "mistake."

In 1951, Fan Xingzhun published a milestone paper in the *Journal of Medical History* (Yī Shǐ Zá Zhì, 医史杂志), titled *A Study on Expository Medical Texts for Physicians: A Study of the Wu Zang Lun* (医家训蒙书一五脏论的研究). This paper was not only a deep dive into the history of *Five Viscera Theory* (Wǔ Zàng Lùn, 五藏论) but also unveiled a startling fact: the history of texts like the *Five Viscera Theory* (Wǔ Zàng Lùn, 五藏论) is much older than previously thought. Fan's research indicated that the *Five Viscera Theory* (Wǔ Zàng Lùn, 五藏论) found in the Dunhuang artifacts dates back to the Sui and Tang dynasties, revealing its long-standing significance in ancient Chinese medicine.

In his paper, Fan meticulously listed at least 14 different versions of the *Five Viscera Theory* (Wǔ Zàng Lùn, 五藏论) that existed during the Sui and Tang dynasties, as recorded in various historical annals. These versions attest to the significant standing and widespread circulation of the *Five Viscera Theory* (Wǔ Zàng Lùn, 五藏论) in ancient medical practice. These versions include the following:

- *Five Viscera Theory* (Wǔ Zàng Lùn, 五藏论), one volume, in the *Book of Sui* (Suí Shū, 隋书) and *Old Book of Tang* (Jiù Táng Shū, 旧唐书).
- *Five Viscera Theory by Anonymous Author* (Wáng Míng Shì Wǔ Zàng Lùn, 亡名氏五脏论), one volume, in *Old Book of Tang* (Jiù Táng Shū, 旧唐书).
- *Five Viscera Theory Corresponding to Phenomena* (Wǔ Zàng Lùn Yīng Xiàng, 五脏论应象), one volume, written by Wu Jing, in *New Book of Tang* (Xīn Táng Shū, 新唐书).
- *Five Viscera Theory* (Wǔ Zàng Lùn, 五藏论), one volume, written by Pei Lian, in *New Book of Tang* (Xīn Táng Shū, 新唐书).
- *Shennon's Five Viscera Theory* (Shén Nóng Wǔ Zàng Lùn, 神农五脏论), one volume, in *Comprehensive Catalogue of Literature During the Song Dynasty* (Chóng Wén Zǒng Mù, 崇文总目).
- *Yellow Emperor's Five Viscera Theory* (Huáng Dì Wǔ Zàng Lùn, 黄帝五脏论), one volume, in *Comprehensive Catalogue of Literature During the Song Dynasty* (Chóng Wén Zǒng Mù, 崇文总目).
- *Zhang Zhongjing's Five Viscera Theory* (Zhāng Zhòng Jǐng Wǔ Zàng Lùn, 张仲景五脏论), one volume, in *Comprehensive Catalogue of Literature During the Song Dynasty* (Chóng Wén Zǒng Mù, 崇文总目).
- *Jivaka's Five Viscera Theory* (Qí Pó Wǔ Zàng Lùn, 耆婆五脏论), one volume, in *Comprehensive Catalogue of Literature During the Song Dynasty* (Chóng Wén Zǒng Mù, 崇文总目).
- *Five Viscera Theory* (Wǔ Zàng Lùn, 五藏论), one volume, written by Zhang Shangrong, in *Comprehensive Catalogue of Literature During the Song Dynasty* (Chóng Wén Zǒng Mù, 崇文总目).
- *Little Five Viscera Theory* (Xiǎo Wǔ Zàng Lùn, 小五脏论), one volume, writer missing, in *Comprehensive Catalogue of Literature During the Song Dynasty* (Chóng Wén Zǒng Mù, 崇文总目).
- *Lian Fang's Five Viscera Theory* (Lián Fāng Wǔ Zàng Lùn, 连方五脏论), one volume, writer missing, in *Comprehensive Catalogue of Literature During the Song Dynasty* (Chóng Wén Zǒng Mù, 崇文总目).
- *Five Viscera Theory by Various Scholars* (Zhū Jiā Wǔ Zàng Lùn, 诸家五脏论), five volumes, in *Comprehensive Records • Monographs on Arts and Literature* (Tōng Zhì • Yì Wén Lüè, 通志•艺文略).
- *Xuannü's Five Viscera Theory* (Xuán Nǚ Wǔ Zàng Lùn, 玄女五脏论), one volume, in *Monographs on Arts and Literature* (Yì Wén Lüè, 艺文略).
- *Qibo's Five Viscera Theory* (Qí Bó Wǔ Zàng Lùn, 岐伯五脏论), one volume, in *Catalog of the Green Bamboo Hall* (Lǜ Zhú Táng Shū Mù, 绿竹堂书目).

In his paper, Fan further explained that although there were many books historically named *Five Viscera Theory* (Wǔ Zàng Lùn), most of them have vanished without a trace. These texts only began to circulate widely during the Song Dynasty, but many were works falsely attributed to famous historical figures such as Shennong, the Yellow Emperor, Qi Bo, the Xuan Nü, and Zhang Zhongjing. Similarly, many popular medicine properties in poems circulating in the market were also falsely attributed works, a phenomenon not uncommon in ancient literature.

In his work *Expository Medical Texts for Physicians: A Study of the Wu Zang Lun* (医家训蒙书一五脏论的研究), Fan Xingzhun made an important assertion regarding the *Five Viscera Theory* (Wǔ Zàng Lùn, 五藏论) P. 2755V unearthed in Dunhuang. Fan pointed out that Yuan Tongli's earlier identification of this fragment as the *Verses on Medicinal Properties* (Yào Xìng Gē Jué, 药性歌诀) was incorrect. Based on his own research, Fan concluded that this work was actually the *Jivaka's Five Viscera Theory* (Qí Pó Wǔ Zàng Lùn, 耆婆五脏论). He stated:

> After examining the *Five Viscera Theory* (Wǔ Zàng Lùn, 五藏论) fragment found in Dunhuang and comparing it with the little-known *Five Viscera Theory* (Wǔ Zàng Lùn, 五藏论) in the Korean *Categorized Collection of Medical Formulas* (Yī Fāng Lèi Jù, 医方类聚), we have reached a clear conclusion. The *Five Viscera Theory* (Wǔ Zàng Lùn, 五藏论) seen in the Dunhuang collection and the one cited in *Categorized Collection of Medical Formulas* (Yī Fāng Lèi Jù, 医方类聚) are, in fact, the *Jivaka's Five Viscera Theory* (Qí Pó Wǔ Zàng Lùn, 耆婆五脏论). This work is an introduction textbook for physicians. While we cannot assert that those *Five Viscera Theory* (Wǔ Zàng Lùn, 五藏论) written during or after Sui and Tang dynasties are identical in content to the *Jivaka's Five Viscera Theory* (Qí Pó Wǔ Zàng Lùn, 耆婆五脏论), but they were all certainly simple medical books.

Despite Fan Xingzhun being one of the earliest scholars to study the *Five Viscera Theory* (Wǔ Zàng Lùn, 五藏论) manuscripts from Dunhuang, his theory identifying it as the *Jivaka's Five Viscera Theory* (Qí Pó Wǔ Zàng Lùn, 耆婆五脏论) is not beyond question. Similarly, Yuan Tongli's designation of it as the *Verses on Medicinal Properties* (Yào Xìng Gē Jué, 药性歌诀) was proven inaccurate, and likewise, Fan's identification of the *Verses on Medicinal Properties* (Yào Xìng Gē Jué, 药性歌诀) is subject to doubts. Due to limited research conditions, scarcity of materials, and the dispersion of the *Five Viscera Theory* (Wǔ Zàng Lùn, 五藏论) manuscripts from Dunhuang across the world, Fan faced challenges in conducting a comprehensive cross-comparison of these versions. With only the borrowed *Categorized Collection of Medical Formulas* (Yī Fāng Lèi Jù, 医方类聚) and photographs reproduced from Beijing, Fan could hardly have imagined that the incomplete P. 2755V Dunhuang manuscript was the long-lost *Five Viscera Theory* (Wǔ Zàng Lùn, 五藏论) by Zhang Zhongjing, missing for a millennium.

Another distinguished scholar, a leading authority in the field of Chinese medical history and the discoverer of the ancient Artemisia annua formula, Ma Jixing,[9] also held a profound interest in the Dunhuang medical manuscripts. Ma devoted 30 years to studying ancient Chinese medical texts, particularly those from Dunhuang, and authored *Annotations on the Ancient Medical Texts from the Dunhuang Cave Library* (Dūn Huáng Gǔ Yī Jí Kǎo Shì, 敦煌古医籍考释). In this book, Ma used the practice of avoiding taboo words to deduce the transcription date of the Dunhuang manuscript P. 2755V housed in France. He noted that in the text, the character "莫" (mò) was replaced with "莲" (lián) and "治" (zhì) with "疗" (liáo) to avoid the taboo names of Emperors Taizong and Gaozong of the Tang Dynasty. However, the text did not avoid the taboo name of Emperor Muzong of Tang (the character "恒" [héng]), suggesting that its transcription likely dates back to the early Tang period.

Additionally, Ma Jixing compared the content of P. 2755V with other versions of Zhang Zhongjing's *Five Viscera Theory* (Wǔ Zàng Lùn, 五藏论) unearthed in Dunhuang and those included in the Korean medical masterpiece *Categorized Collection of Medical Formulas* (Yī Fāng Lèi Jù, 医方类聚). He found that the content of P. 2755V was strikingly similar to other versions of Zhang Zhongjing's *Five Viscera Theory* (Wǔ Zàng Lùn, 五藏论). Therefore, Ma concluded that P. 2755V was neither the *Verses on Medicinal Properties* (Yào Xìng Gē Jué, 药性歌诀) nor the *Jivaka's Five Viscera Theory* (Qí Pó Wǔ Zàng Lùn, 耆婆五脏论) but rather, another version of Zhang Zhongjing's *Five Viscera Theory* (Wǔ Zàng Lùn, 五藏论).

Regarding the content of Zhang Zhongjing's *Five Viscera Theory* (Wǔ Zàng Lùn, 五藏论) P. 2755V, the first 35 lines of text are essentially consistent with the content of two other Dunhuang manuscript fragments of Zhang Zhongjing's *Five Viscera Theory* (Wǔ Zàng Lùn, 五藏论), P. 2115 and S.5614, representing basic theories in materia medica. However, the subsequent 23 lines of text, while not found in the P. 2115 and S.5614 fragments, do appear in the *Five Viscera Theory* (Wǔ Zàng Lùn, 五藏论) contained in volume 4 of *Categorized Collection of Medical Formulas* (Yī Fāng Lèi Jù, 医方类聚), with a similar arrangement and sequence of the text.

It's noteworthy that some of the content in these latter 23 lines is the same or similar to the earlier 35 lines, suggesting a possible repetition. These 23 lines follow the phrase "pure and impure, (those) hundred herbs (are all from) mountains," which coincidentally is the concluding sentence in each of the manuscripts P. 2115, S.5614, and P. 2378. This could imply that the latter 23 lines were additions made at a later time. Moreover, these lines exhibit differences from the source material of P. 2115, S.5614, and P. 2378 yet show a connection with the content found in *Categorized Collection of Medical Formulas* (Yī Fāng Lèi Jù, 医方类聚).

The following is a literal translation of the full text of Zhang Zhongjing's *Five Viscera Theory* (Wǔ Zàng Lùn, 五藏论) P. 2755V. The translation process strictly adheres to the original text, translating word for word, sentence by sentence, to ensure that every character and every sentence remains faithful to the original manuscript:

☒，相使还须白止。择写、树☒耳目聪明；远枳、人参，巧合开心益智。

[*unrecognizable*], but it must be combined with Bai Zhi (白芷, dahurian Angelica root) to have mutual support effect. Ze Xie (泽泻, alisma tuber) and tree [*unrecognizable*] can benefit hearing and vision; Yuan Zhi (远枳 or 远志, Thinleaf milkwort root) and Ren Shen (人参, ginseng root) magically open the heart to make people smart.

赤痛宜涂鸡子，白癞须附越桃，火烧宜怙水荓，杖打稍加螢实。非尸走疰，速用雄黄；忽尔惊耶，急求龙齿。头风旋闷，须访椈花；脚弱行迟，宜求石斛。欲令见鬼，久服麻花；拟去白虫，柒和鸡子，墙薇却其疥癣，解黄嗜去瘰疮，通草巧疗耳聋，石胆唯除眼寞。

Red ulcer should apply Ji Zi (鸡子, chicken eggs); tuberculoid leprosy needs to use Yue Tao (越桃 or "Zhi Zi" 栀子, gardenia fruit); burns to be treated by applying Shui Ping (水萍 or "Fu Ping" 浮萍, floating duckweed) topically; wounds from caning can use Ying Shi (螢实 or "Qiang Wei Zi" 蔷薇子, multiflora Rose Fruit). Pestilential illness uses Xiong Huang (雄黄, realgar) right away; sudden frightening should ask for Long Chi (龙齿, fossilized animal teeth) immediately. Head wind with dizziness must use Ju Hua (菊花, chrysanthemum flower); weakness of limbs caused difficult walking should seek for Shi Hu (石斛, dendrobium stem). Prolonged consumption of Ma Hua (麻花, cannabis flowers) will make (people) see ghosts; if you want to eliminate white parasite, use Qi (漆, lacquer) and Ji Zi (鸡子, chicken eggs); Qiang Wei (蔷薇, multiflora Rose Fruit) can get rid of fungal infection; Xie Huang (蟹黄, crab yolk) can eliminate eczema; Tong Cao (通草, rice paper plant pith) can magically treat deafness; Shi Dan (石胆, chalcanthite) eliminates cataract.

胶秦结罗纹之状，干柒作蜂窠之形。丹砂会取光明，升麻只求青绿。秦胶须行，礬石须刨，杜仲削去胶皮，桂心取其有味。石英研之似粉，杏人别擣如膏。菟丝酒渗乃凉，朴消火烧方好。防葵唯轻唯上，狼毒唯重唯加。黄零以附肠为精，蕳茹柒头为用。石南采叶，甘椈收花。五茄割取其皮，母丹搥其去骨。鬼箭破血，仍有射鬼之零；神屋除温，非带报口之验。

Qin Jiao (秦胶 or "Qin Jiao" 秦艽, largeleaf gentian root) pertains spiral shape; Gan Qi (干漆, dried lacquer) looks like honeycomb. Dan Sha (丹砂 or "Zhu Sha" 朱砂, cinnabar) should be shiny; Sheng Ma (升麻, largetrifoliolious bugbane Rhizome) seeks only green and verdant. Qin Jiao (秦椒, prickly ash peel) need to be steamed; Fan Shi (礬石, white alum-stone) should be roasted; Du Zhong (杜仲, eucommia bark) must peel off the outer skin; Gui Xin (桂心 or "Rou Gui" 肉桂, cinnamon bark) must have intense fragrance. Shi Ying (石英, Cristobalite) must be powdered; Xing Ren (杏仁, apricot seed) should be grinded until gets creamy. Tu Si (菟丝, Chinese dodder seed) must be soaked with alcohol; Pu Xiao (朴硝, a crude form of sodium sulfate) must be calcinated. Fang Kui (防葵, white flower hog fennel root) the lighter the better; Lang Du (狼毒, Bracteole-lacked Euphorbia root) the heavier the better. Good Huang Qin (黄芩, Baical skullcap root) looks like rotten intestine; only use Lin Ru's (蕳茹, Euphorbia Lanru root) top part. Shi Nan (石南, Chinese photinia Leaf) should pick its leaves; Gan Ju (甘菊, sweet chrysanthemum flower) uses its flower; Wu Jia (五加, Slenderstyle Acanthopanax Bark) only uses the bark; Mu Dan (牡丹, tree peony bark), hammer its stem and take the bone out. Gui Jian (鬼箭 or "Gui Jian Yu" 鬼箭羽, winged branches) must cut to bleed to have the effect of shooting the ghost spirit; Shen Wu (神屋 or "Gui Ban" 龟板, tortoise carapace and plastron) must be warm process to generate [*missing*] (*miraculous*) effect.

呕口汤煎干葛, 新转酒煮木瓜。目赤须点黄连, 口疮宜含黄蘗。脾专应痛, 须访茵芋; 躁痒皮肤, 汤口蒴藋。伤寒发汗, 要用麻黄; 壮热不除, 宜加竹叶。恒山鳖甲, 大有差疟之功; 蛇蜕绿丹, 善除癫痫之用。雄黄除黑干, 木兰能去死皮, 歔草煞齿内之虫, 黎芦烂鼻中宿肉。黄连断痢除疳, 子支悦偷面皮, 桃花润泽痛肉。芎藭、 枳实, 心急即用加之; 紫菀、缓冬, 气嗽要须当用。虻虫、水蛭, 即有破血之功; 白术、槟榔, 有散气消食之效。菖蒲强寄, 鳖甲通神。

Decoct Gan Ge (干葛 or "Ge Geng" 葛根, dried pueraria root) to treat vomiting [*missing*]; use alcohol to decoct Mu Gua (木瓜, Chinese quince fruit) for muscle spasm. Use Huang Lian (黄连, yellow coptis root) to make eye drops for red eyes. Hold Huang Bo (黄蘗 or 黄柏, phellodendron bark) in the mouth for mouth ulcer. Painful arthritis uses Yin Yu (茵芋, Japanese skimmia stem and leaf); severe skin itch uses Shuo Huo (蒴藋, Chinese elder) decoction [*missing*]. Promote sweat during Shang Han, exogenous pathogenic cold-induced diseases, uses Ma Huang (麻黄, ephedra stem). Constant high fever can benefit from Zhu Ye (竹叶, bamboo leaves). Heng Shan (恒山 or "Chang Shan" 常山, dichroa root) and Bie Jia (鳖甲, Chinese soft-shelled turtle shell) have great function to relieve malaria; She Tui (蛇蜕, snake slough) and Lü Dan (绿丹, aluminum pill) relieve seizure attacks. Xiong Huang (雄黄, realgar) is to treat gangrene; Mu Lan (木兰, lily magnolia bark) can remove dead skin; Wang Cao (菵草 or "Mang Cao" 莽草, leaf of poisonous eightangle tree) treats cavity inside the teeth; Li Lu (藜芦, veratrum root and rhizome) can treat chronic nasal infection. Huang Lian (黄连, yellow coptis root) stops dysentery disease and eliminates malnutrition; Zi Zhi (子支 or "Zhi Zi" 栀子, gardenia fruit) benefits facial skin; Tao Hua (桃花, peach blossom) can moisten body skin. Xiong Qiong (芎藭 or "Chuan Xiong" 川芎, Sichuan lovage rhizome) and Zhi Shi (枳实, immature range fruit) treat anxiety; Zi Wan (紫菀, tatarian aster root) and Kuan Dong (款冬, Common coltsfoot flower) are used for asthma and cough. Mang Chong (虻虫, horse fly) and Shui Zhi (水蛭, leech) are to break blood stagnation; Bai Zhu (白术, white atractylodes tuber) and Bing Lang (槟榔, betel nut, or areca seed) relieve bloating and promote digestion. Chang Pu (菖蒲 or "Shi Chang Pu" 石菖蒲, grassleaf sweetflag rhizome) enhances memory; Bie Jia (鳖甲, Chinese soft-shelled turtle shell) promotes spiritual function.

阴疮汤煮蛇床，淋涩须加滑石。仙零脾能去腰痛，然则忘杖而归家。大鼠膏巧疗耳聋，得草麻而加妙。蛇咬宜封人粪，蜂螫荜茇妙除。零羊角通噎驱耶，青羊肝疗疳明目。石脂加颜发色，白及卷面除皮。知母通痢开胸，空青消癥止泪。孔公孽消食肥檡，密陀僧去疥癞，人压石寄假蜂房。水肿唯须杖戟，肠结通须甘遂。患眼宜取蕤人，安胎必籍紫紫葳，伤身要须地髓。脑闷偏加木笔，血闭急□蒲黄。连翘却累□疮痈，地胆破癥瘕息肉。斑苗能除鼠漏，松热抽恶刺风疽。牵□小泻排脓，葶苈代卑池水。桃人绝其鬼气，石南复去诸风。瘿□昆布咸除，痈肿囟砂食却。肠痈必须消石，脱公宜用鳖头，下贱虽曰地浆，天行病饮者皆愈；黄龙汤出其厕内，时气病服者能除。贫□虽号小方，不及君臣，取写有处出处，有零有验，有贵有贱，有高有下，净秽百草山中药。

Vaginal discharge, exterior vaginal itching, and redness, use She Chuang (蛇床, common cnidium fruit) to decoct. Urgent or hesitate urination, add Hua Shi (滑石, talc). Xian Lin Pi (仙灵脾 or "Yin Yang Huo" 淫羊藿, horny goat weed or epimedium) relieves lower back pain so that the patient can walk back home without the crutches. Syrup made from Da Shu (大鼠 or "Bian Fu" 蝙蝠, bat) treats deafness, to add Bi Ma (蓖麻, castor leaf or bean) for better results. Topically cover with Ren Fen (人粪 or "Ren Zhong Huang" 人中黄, human excrement) for snake bite; bee sting can be treated by Bi Ba (荜茇, piper longum). Ling Yang Jiao (零羊角 or 羚羊角, antelope's horn) is for esophageal obstruction and to eliminate evil. Qing Yang Gan (青羊肝, goral liver) treats malnutrition and brightens vision. Shi Zhi (石脂, halloysite) darkens hair; Bai Ji (白及, bletilla tuber) removes dead skin and regenerates new skin. Zhi Mu (知母, common anemarrhena rhizome) treats dysentery and opens chest; Kong Qing (空青, azurite) relieves bloating and stops tearing. Kong Gong Nie (孔公孽, Calcite) helps digest food and gains weight. Mi Tuo Seng (密陀僧, lithargite) treats eczema and skin infection. Feng Fang (蜂房, honeycomb) used to calm down the rebellious Qi caused by taking Ru Shi (乳石, stalactite). Edema can use Da Ji (大戟, Peking spurge root). Intestinal obstruction uses Gan Sui (甘遂, gansui root). Eye disease uses Rui Ren (蕤人, hedge prinsepia nut). Calm down fetus must use Zi Wei (紫葳, Chinese Trumpetcreeper Flower); Di Sui (地髓 or "Gan Di Huang" 干地黄, drying rehmannia root) is for physical exhaustion. Mentally depress use Mu Bi (木笔 or "Xin Yi Hua" 辛夷花, magnolia flower); amenorrhea [*missing*] (uses) Pu Huang (蒲黄, cat-tail pollen) immediately. [*missing*] scrofula and boils (use) Lian Qiao (连翘, weeping forsythia Capsule); Di Dan (地胆, a kind of blister beetles) treats mass, nodules, and polyps. Ban Mao (斑猫, mylabris) can treat chronic skin abscess; Song Re (松热 or "Song Zhi" 松脂, pine resin) is anti-infection. It can promote discharge of pus. Qian Niu (牵牛, morning glory) is a strong diuretic to reduce swelling. It also helps discharge pus; Ting Li (葶苈 or "Ting Li Zi" 葶苈子, tansymustard seed) and Da Zao (大枣, Chinese date) eliminate edema. Tao Ren (桃人 or 桃仁, peach kernel) stops evil energy; Shi Nan (石南, Chinese photinia Leaf) to eliminate all kinds of internal wind. Kun Bu (昆布, kombu) relieves goiter [*missing*]; Nao Sha (硇砂, sal ammoniac) treats abscess and swelling. Xiao Shi (消石 or "Mang Xiao" 芒硝, nitrate from saline alkali land) treats intestinal abscess; Bie Tou (鳖头, soft-shell turtle head) treats rectal prolapse. Regardless of the degrading name of "Di Jiang" (地浆, Earth Slurry), Tian Xing Bing (epidemic diseases caused by natural factors) gets healed by taking Di Jiang (地浆, Earth Slurry). Although Huang Long Tang (黄龙汤, Yellow Dragon Decoction) came from toilet, it can treat infectious disease. Although small [*missing*] (*formula*) was considered lower class, it doesn't even have King and Minister herbs in the formulation (still, you know) where the formula originally come from. And the formula is clinically proven, the medicine could be expensive or cheap, and the herbs could be higher or lower class and clean or dirty. They are all come from the nature.

琥珀拾芥，乃辨其真；磁石引针，方知不伪。石得鸩粪，乃烂如泥；柒遇蟹黄，便化为水。三棱破癖，本出河途；刘寄燸疮，起于田猎。牡蛎助佰仁之力，地黄益门冬之功。白敛反乌头之情，栀子解踯躅之毒。苦参、酸枣，以味为名；白术，黄芪，将色为号。蜈蚣、蜀柒，缘地标名；狗脊、狼牙，因形为记。

Real Hu Po (琥珀, amber) can pick up tiny things; if the Ci Shi (磁石, magnetite) can attract needles, then we know it is not fake. Zhen Fen (鸩粪, the excrement of a legendary poisonous bird) can make stones melt like mud; Xie Huang (蟹黄, crab yolk) can make Qi (漆, paint) melt like water. San Leng (三棱, common burreed tuber) can break the nodule; this comes from He Tu; Liu Ji Nu (刘寄奴, diverse wormwood herb) heals the wound. This function was discovered from field hunting. Mu Li (牡蛎, oyster shell) can help the function of Bo Ren (柏仁, Oriental arborvitae seed kernel); Di Huang (地黄, rehmannia root) can benefit the function of Tian Men Dong (天门冬, Cochinchinese asparagus root). Bai Lian (白蔹, Japanese ampelopsis root) is incompatible with Wu Tou (乌头, Sichuan aconite root); Zhi Zi (栀子, gardenia fruit) is the antidote of Zhi Zhu (踯躅, Chinese azalea flower). Ku Shen (苦参, light-yellow sophora root) and Suan Zao (酸枣, Chinese sour jujube) are named after their tastes; Bai Zhu (白术, white atractylodes tuber) and Huang Qi (黄芪, astragalus root) are named after their colors; Wu Gong (蜈蚣, centipede) and Shu Qi (蜀漆, Sichuan dichroa leaf) are named after their place of origin; Gou Ji (狗脊, cibot rhizome) and Lang Ya (狼牙, the underground winter bud of Agrimonia root) are named after their shapes.

伤寒发汗，要用麻黄；久热不除，宜加竹叶。卒逢鬼注，访觅牛黄；忽尔惊邪，要须龙齿。杜仲、萆薢，能去腰疼；枳实、芎藭，善除心痛；当归、芍药，能除腹内之疴；紫菀、款冬，善除咳嗽之疾；槟榔、白术，能除宿食而不消；芒硝、大黄，泻癥瘕之热病。黄连阿胶断痢，通草钟乳发声。蔷薇可以除疮，水蛭尤能破血。桃槐蕤仁明目，秦皮决明去翳。牛膝去冷膝，鹅脂开耳聋。蜂房消肿，芜荑杀虫。桔梗能除虫毒，乱发止于衄如竹反入鼻出血血。滑石通草，能恙五淋。茵草绝得牙疼，海藻能除瘿气。知母、栝楼止消渴，麦门冬去心除温。甘草补五脏，人参定精神。丹参养魂魄，地黄通血脉。黄芪长肌肉，茯苓开胸膈。署蓣益聪明，泽泻相随客。仙虚心脚若。牛膝相成益，心风忘前后，远能相敌。黄菊愈头风，上气生姜击。

To promote sweat during Shang Han, exogenous pathogenic cold-induced diseases should use Ma Huang (麻黄, ephedra stem). Constant high fever can benefit from Zhu Ye (竹叶, bamboo leaves). If suddenly get unspecified deep abscesses, looking for Niu Huang (牛黄, cow bezoar, or cattle gallstone). Sudden frightening should ask for Long Chi (龙齿, fossilized animal teeth) immediately. Du Zhong (杜仲, eucommia bark) and Bi Xie (萆薢, hypoglauca yam) can treat back pain; Zhi Shi (枳实, immature range fruit) and Xiong Qiong (芎藭 or "Chuan Xiong" 川芎, Sichuan lovage rhizome) are good for heartache. Dang Gui (当归, Chinese angelica root) and Shao Yao (芍药, white peony root) can heal the disease in the abdomen; Zi Wan (紫菀, tatarian aster root) and Kuan Dong (款冬, Common coltsfoot flower) are good to eliminate cough. Bing Lang (槟榔, betel nut) and Bai Zhu (白术, white atractylodes tuber) can treat food stagnation; Mang Xiao (芒硝, Nitrate from saline alkali land) and Da Huang (大黄, rhubarb root) can reduce the heat from abdominal mass. Huang Lian (黄连, yellow coptis root) and E Jiao (阿胶, donkey-hide glue) stop dysentery disease; Tong Cao (通草, rice paper plant pith) and Zhong Ru (钟乳 or "Zhong Ru Shi" 钟乳石, stalactite) help to open up voice. Qiang Wei (蔷薇, multiflora Rose Fruit) can heal ulcer; Shui Zhi (水蛭, leech) can break blood stagnation. Tao Ren (桃仁, peach kernel), Huai Zi (槐子, pagodatree pod), and Rui Ren (蕤仁, hedge prinsepia nut) can brighten the eyes; Qin Pi (秦皮, fraxinus bark) and Jue Ming (决明, cassia seeds) will treat cataract. Niu Xi (牛膝, twotoothed achyranthes root) helps cold knees; E Zhi (鹅脂, goose fat) treats deafness. Feng Fang (蜂房, honeycomb) reduces swelling; Wu Yi (芜荑, large-fruited elm seed) kills parasites. Jie Geng (桔梗, platycodon root) can treat insect poison. Luan Fa Hui (乱发灰, human hair ash) can stop bleeding (like the bleeding caused by bamboo poked into the nose). Hua Shi (滑石, talc) and Tong Cao (通草, rice paper plant pith) can treat Lin syndrome. Wang Cao (茵草, leaf of poisonous eightangle tree) stops toothache; Hai Zao (海藻, seaweed) reduces goiter. Zhi Mu (知母, common anemarrhena rhizome) and Gua Lou (栝楼 or "Tian Hua Fen", 天花粉, trichosanthes root) quench thirst. Mai Men Dong (麦门冬, dwarf lilyturf tuber) clears the heart and eliminates irritability. Gan Cao (甘草, licorice root) nourishes five Zang; Ren Shen (人参, ginseng root) replenishes the vital energy. Dan Shen (丹参, salvia root) calms the Hun and Po; Di Huang (地黄, rehmannia root) unblocks the blood vessels. Huang Qi (黄芪, astragalus root) helps to grow muscles; Fu Ling (茯苓, Indian bread, or poria) opens chest. Shu Yu (署蓣 or "Shan Yao" 山药, dioscrea rhizome) enhances intelligence. Ze Xie (泽泻, alisma tuber) accompanies the traveler, just like a fairy gently treading in the void. Niu Xi (牛膝, twotoothed achyranthes root) can complement each other and enhance efficacy, allowing one to forget past and future worries, and its effects can far surpass those of other competitors. Huang Ju (黄菊, yellow chrysanthemum flower) heals head wind; Shang Jiang (生姜, fresh ginger) attacks rebellious Qi.

只如八味肾气，补六极而差五劳；四色神丹，荡千疴而除万病。槟榔汤下虫除气，玉壶丸破积癖消玄。李子预有杀鬼之（方）名，刘涓子有鬼遗之录。耆婆童子，药性妙述千端。踰附医王，神方万品。是以有命者必差，虢太子死而更苏；无命者难理，晋景公于焉智死。养病如积火于薪中，薪去于火而得全，如病人得活。薪不去火，虚被焚烧；人患不除，徒劳丧命者矣。

Just like Ba Wei Shen Qi (八味肾气, Eight-Ingredient Kidney Qi Pills) nourishes the six exhaustions and cures the five overstrains, Si Se Shen Dan (四色神丹, Four-Color Magic Pills) eliminates thousands of diseases and cures 10,000 illnesses. Bing Lang Tang (槟榔汤, Areca Nut Decoction) can eliminate parasites and relieve bloating; Yu Hu Wan (玉壶丸, Jade Pot Pills) is able to eliminate long-accumulated bad habits or stubborn thoughts. Li Ziyu was known to kill ghosts. Liu Juanzi has a record of expelling ghosts. Jivaka understood medical theory profoundly. He was known as the king of the medicine; he had many magical formulas. Those destined to live will recover from illness. Like the Prince of Guo (Guo is one of the ancient feudal states), he was resurrected even though he was considered dead already. Those destined to die are difficult to save, like the death of Duke Jing of Jin. Treating an illness is like a fire within a pile of firewood; removing the fire keeps the firewood intact, removing the illness allows the person to live. If the firewood is not removed from the fire, it will be burned in vain; if a person's illness is not treated, they will lose their life in vain.

REFERENCES

1. Shanghai Chinese Classics Publishing House and Bibliotheque Nationale de France, *Dunhuang and Other Central Asian Manuscripts in the Bibliotheque Nationale de France: Volume 18 Fonds Pelliot chinois 2729–2824* (Shanghai: Shanghai Chinese Classics Publishing House, 2001), 105–107.
2. [法] 保罗·伯希和，*伯希和西域探险日记[M]* (1906–1908) [M]，耿昇译（北京：中国藏学出版社, 2014), 491.
3. 袁同礼，*国立北平图书馆现藏海外敦煌遗籍照片总目[M]*（北平：国立北平图书馆/图书馆季刊 单行本), 613.
4. 黄永武，*敦煌宝藏[M]，第124册：伯2752–2876号*（台北: 新文丰出版公司, 1981), 7.
5. 范行准，*医家训蒙书-五脏论的研究[A]*. 见：*王咪咪.，范行准医学论文集[M]*（北京：学苑出版社， 2011), 27.
6. 焨铂，"图书馆学家袁同礼的北大时代 [J]. " *档案天地*, No. 5 (2015): 34–37.
7. 刘波，林世田，"国立北平图书馆拍摄及影印出版敦煌遗书史事钩沉[J]." ***敦煌研究***, No. 2 (2010): 119–125.
8. 范行准，*医家生平[A]*. 见：王咪咪.，范行准医学论文集[M]（北京：学苑出版社, 2011), 4.
9. 王晓易，"马继兴：发现青蒿古方的人[N]." *北京晚报* (December 21, 2015).

6 The Thought-Provoking Anonymous *Wu Zang Lun* – P. 2378 Collected in France

"The remnants of P. 2755, P. 2378, and S. 5614 from Dunhuang represent three distinct versions of Zhang Zhongjing's 'Wu Zang Lun.'"

– Luo Fuyi

Among the treasured collections of the National Library of France in Paris lies an ancient scroll known as the *Five Viscera Theory* (Wǔ Zàng Lùn, 五藏论) (catalog number: Pelliot chinois Toven-Hoving 2378, abbreviated as P. 2378).[1] This scroll, measuring 23.6 cm in height, is meticulously hand-copied on both sides with a brush, showcasing the delicate touch of ancient scribes. The front side displays an unknown and incomplete Taoist scripture. The reverse side contains 46 lines of text, constituting the concluding part of a medical text, written in a fluid running script with neat, unaltered handwriting. Despite the incompleteness or fading of the earlier part of the medical text, the last page is inscribed in deep-black ink with the words "Wu Zang Lun, one volume," without the author's name. Who was the author of this document? Who hand-copied this ancient book? These mysteries have sparked deep thought and speculation among countless scholars. For years, enthusiasts of Dunhuang studies have relentlessly pursued these historical enigmas, aiming to unravel these puzzles.

When discussing the P. 2378 manuscript, it's essential to mention an outstanding scholar from Japan, Genji Kuroda (December 4, 1886–January 13, 1957).[2] He was the founder and head of one of the earliest institutions dedicated to the study of traditional Chinese medicine in the modern world – the East Asian Medical Research Institute. Kuroda's exploration into the history of East Asian medicine was nothing short of an obsession. His expertise was widely recognized in the fields of Chinese, Japanese, and Korean medicine. The number of medical documents he collected and researched is immeasurable, reflecting his deep commitment and profound influence in the realm of medical historical studies.

As a professor of physiology, Genji Kuroda, while serving as the director of the East Asian Medical Research Institute, devoted immense passion to the study of Chinese medicine. Records indicate that the Institute alone housed an impressive collection of 3,774 Chinese medical texts. Kuroda's approach to ancient medical literature was distinct compared to his contemporaries. He firmly believed that to truly

DOI: 10.1201/9781032698205-6

grasp the value of Chinese medicine, one must start from its deep roots, delving into its heritage and developmental journey. In collaboration with Tameto Okanishi, Kuroda co-authored *Compilation of Dunhuang Stone Chamber Medical Formulas from the National Library of France* (巴黎国立图书馆藏敦煌石室医方书类纂), a significant work included in their *Comprehensive Catalog of Medical Books from the Song Dynasty* (宋代医书目一览). This publication was released in 1933 as a mimeographed edition.[3] And it was this publication that catalyzed Chinese scholar Luo Fuyi to write *Compilation of Ancient Medical Formula Fragments from the Western Frontier* (Xī Chuí Gǔ Fāng Jì Shū Cán Juàn Huì Biān, 西陲古方技书残卷汇编). Kuroda's compilation served as a vital resource, aiding Luo in his scholarly endeavors and, in the process, shedding light on the true identity and value of this previously unnamed and invaluable manuscript.

According to the preface of Luo Fuyi's *Compilation of Ancient Medical Formula Fragments from the Western Frontier* (Xī Chuí Gǔ Fāng Jì Shū Cán Juàn Huì Biān, 西陲古方技书残卷汇编),[4] in 1948, while Luo was in Shenyang, he obtained a copy of *Compilation of Dunhuang Stone Chamber Medical Formulas from the National Library of France* (巴黎国立图书馆藏敦煌石室医方书类纂) hand-copied by Genji Kuroda through his connection with the Japanese scholar Mutsu Takeuchi. This manuscript, compiled by Kuroda during his time in Europe, included 21 Dunhuang medical documents. Luo believed that it might have recorded some lost texts, so he borrowed it from Takeuchi and planned to transcribe them. However, less than a month later, Luo had to leave the Northeast Museum and return to Beijing, with Kuroda's hand-copied original manuscript still with him.

Upon returning to Beijing, Luo Fuyi discovered that the National Peiping Library houses numerous photocopies of Dunhuang manuscripts scattered overseas. He meticulously compared these precious document photographs with Genji Kuroda's handwritten manuscript, uncovering some content that Kuroda had not recorded. With special permission from the Beijing Library, Luo borrowed these documents and asked the help of his brother-in-law, Shang Jingxun, for the transcription work.

To ensure accuracy, they strictly adhered to the original layout of the manuscripts. When encountering possible errors in the original text, Luo chose not to make corrections, staying true to the original transcription. For the reduced document photographs, they enlarged and transcribed them while still retaining the original line format. Where the original manuscripts included annotations in red ink, they mirrored this in the transcriptions. They also marked the end of paragraphs with Luo's own transcription notes and added previous scholars' revision comments at the end of each paragraph. For sections not previously annotated, they provided supplementary explanations based on Luo's understanding. They meticulously recorded the original cataloging by Paul Pelliot and Aurel Stein and the dimensions of the manuscript papers, providing references for readers.

In the collection of the National Library of France in Paris, there were eight items whose photographs were not included in the National Peiping Library's collection. Luo had to rely solely on Kuroda's manuscript for these records. Undertaking this complex task with commitment, Shang Jingxun diligently worked for six months and successfully completed the demanding transcription process.

Luo Fuyi ingeniously organized these precious manuscripts into five volumes, categorizing them into four major types: 1) medical formulas from the Han and Jin dynasties, 2) medical classics from the Tang Dynasty, 3) materia medica from the Tang Dynasty, and 4) medical formulas from the Tang Dynasty. This magnificent compilation was aptly titled *Compilation of Ancient Medical Formula Fragments from the Western Frontier* (Xī Chuí Gǔ Fāng Jì Shū Cán Juàn Huì Biān, 西陲古方技书残卷汇编), encompassing 40 different medical documents. Remarkably, the content curated by Luo Fuyi in this collection was more than double that of Genji Kuroda's handwritten manuscript.

Although the documents included in the compilation were only fragments and broken pieces, the medical wisdom they contained represented some of the oldest in traditional Chinese medicine still preserved today. Through these fragmented texts, we gain insight into the long history of Chinese medicine and the unique styles of medical books before the Tang Dynasty. Notably, Luo Fuyi humbly admitted in his book to having limited knowledge of traditional Chinese medicine. He harbored a sincere hope that medical experts would delve deeply into these texts, much like Liu Xiang did when revising the *Abstracts* (Bié Lù, 别录) during the Han dynasty. Luo's work focused on gathering as many medical manuscript fragments from the Han and Tang periods as possible, providing future scholars and experts with invaluable research material.

Luo Fuyi's *Compilation of Ancient Medical Formula Fragments from the Western Frontier* (Xī Chuí Gǔ Fāng Jì Shū Cán Juàn Huì Biān, 西陲古方技书残卷汇编) stands as the first specialized work on Dunhuang medical literature, holding immense historical value. Yet what's even more captivating is that during the compilation of this work, Luo made an extremely important discovery through his in-depth study of the connections between various manuscripts.

Firstly, Luo noticed that the manuscript P. 2378, housed in the National Library of France, was titled *Five Viscera Theory* (Wǔ Zàng Lùn, 五藏论) but lacked an author's name. Even more surprisingly, the content of this medical text matched precisely with another medical text in P. 2755, also part of the French collection. Previously, Yuan Tongli had named P. 2755 as *Verses on Medicinal Properties* (Yào Xìng Gē Jué, 药性歌诀), but no title or author's name was found on the fragment itself. This meant that P. 2755 in the French collection was not the *Verses on Medicinal Properties* (Yào Xìng Gē Jué, 药性歌诀) as Yuan had thought, but in fact, like P. 2378, it was an anonymous version of *Five Viscera Theory* (Wǔ Zàng Lùn, 五藏论). This discovery undoubtedly held profound academic significance, reshaping the understanding of these ancient medical texts.

Meanwhile, another Dunhuang fragment caught Luo Fuyi's attention: the British Collection S. 5614, Zhang Zhongjing's *Five Viscera Theory* (Wǔ Zàng Lùn, 五藏论). As previously mentioned, Xiang Da faced challenges at the British Library, where the Dunhuang Chinese documents were not cataloged, and there was no service to browse by number. Instead, the library's staff would personally retrieve the documents for readers, making the borrowing process cumbersome and limiting the amount of material that could be viewed at one time. Fortunately, among the limited Dunhuang manuscript photocopies obtained, there was one numbered S. 5614,

Zhang Zhongjing's *Five Viscera Theory* (Wǔ Zàng Lùn, 五藏论). Intriguingly, its content encompassed that of both P. 2755 and P. 2378 from the French collection.

Through the British Library's S.5614, Luo Fuyi successfully unveiled the true identity of the mysterious French P. 2378. As a result, both P. 2755 and P. 2378 from the French collection were correctly identified. Luo Fuyi made a decisive determination for these three Dunhuang fragments: P. 2755 and P. 2378 from France, along with S.5614 from Britain, were all confirmed as different versions of Zhang Zhongjing's *Five Viscera Theory* (Wǔ Zàng Lùn, 五藏论). This significant research finding was published in 1953 in the *Journal of Chinese Medical History* (Zhōng Huá Yī Shǐ Zá Zhì, 中华医史杂志). Additionally, Luo distinguished Zhang Zhongjing's *Five Viscera Theory* (Wǔ Zàng Lùn, 五藏论) from other texts such as *Mingtang's Five Viscera Theory* (Míng Táng Wǔ Zàng Lùn, 明堂五脏论) (P. 3655 from the French collection) and the German collection's version of *Jivaka's Five Viscera Theory* (Qí Pó Wǔ Zàng Lùn, 耆婆五脏论), further clarifying and categorizing these ancient medical documents.

In the *Compilation of Ancient Medical Formula Fragments from the Western Frontier* (Xī Chuí Gǔ Fāng Jì Shū Cán Juàn Huì Biān, 西陲古方技书残卷汇编), among the 40 types of medical texts included, five versions are named *Five Viscera Theory* (Wǔ Zàng Lùn, 五藏论). This collection encompasses three versions of Zhang Zhongjing's *Five Viscera Theory* (Wǔ Zàng Lùn, 五藏论), as well as *Mingtang's Five Viscera Theory* (Míng Táng Wǔ Zàng Lùn, 明堂五脏论) and the *Jivaka's Five Viscera Theory* (Qí Pó Wǔ Zàng Lùn, 耆婆五脏论). Fan Xingzhun, in his 1951 publication *Expository Medical Texts for Physicians: A Study of the Wu Zang Lun* (医家训蒙书一五脏论的研究), also mentioned that historically, many books were titled *Five Viscera Theory* (Wǔ Zàng Lùn, 五藏论). It's essential to revisit the historical records of medical books categorized under *Five Viscera Theory* (Wǔ Zàng Lùn, 五藏论), which include works by Zhang Zhongjing as well as texts by other authors. Let's take a closer look and enumerate them.

In the verification and preservation of ancient texts, the *Records of Arts and Literature* (Yì Wén Zhì, 艺文志) and *Records of Classics and Books* (Jīng Jí Zhì, 经籍志) sections of the official Chinese histories have played a crucial role by investigating the records from various dynasties' *Records of Arts and Literature* (Yì Wén Zhì, 艺文志) regarding the following: ① the existence of works personally authored by Zhang Zhongjing, ② works titled *Five Viscera Theory* (Wǔ Zàng Lùn, 五藏论) that are not attributed to Zhang Zhongjing, ③ *Five Viscera Theory* (Wǔ Zàng Lùn, 五藏论) attributed to "Zhang Zhongjing," and ④ other works attributed to "Zhang Zhongjing."[5–11] It could be seen that records of Zhang Zhongjing as a person began from the Sui Dynasty, along with accounts of *Five Viscera Theory* (Wǔ Zàng Lùn, 五藏论) not attributed to Zhang Zhongjing. It was not until the Song Dynasty that *Five Viscera Theory* (Wǔ Zàng Lùn, 五藏论) bearing Zhang Zhongjing's name started appearing in the official Chinese histories. This implies that historically, there indeed was a work titled *Five Viscera Theory* (Wǔ Zàng Lùn, 五藏论) authored by Zhang Zhongjing.

The *Comprehensive Catalogue of Literature During the Song Dynasty* (Chóng Wén Zǒng Mù, 崇文总目) is the first document to record Zhang Zhongjing's *Five Viscera Theory* (Wǔ Zàng Lùn, 五藏论). Notably, this catalog also includes another major work of Zhang Zhongjing, titled *Classic of the Golden Casket and the Jade Box* (Jīn Guì Yù Hán, 金匮玉函). It is well-known that Zhang Zhongjing's foremost work is *Treatise on Cold Damage Disorders* (Shāng Hán Lùn, 伤寒论), and his second most renowned work is *Essential Prescriptions from the Golden Cabinet* (Jīn Guì Yào Lüè, 金匮要略), which is derived from *Classic of the Golden Casket and the Jade Box* (Jīn Guì Yù Hán, 金匮玉函).

The *Comprehensive Catalogue of Literature During the Song Dynasty* (Chóng Wén Zǒng Mù, 崇文总目) is meticulously organized, providing explanations for each book and including prefaces and introductions for each category. During the Shaoxing period of Emperor Gaozong of Song, the secretariat published a simplified version that omitted the prefaces, introductions, and explanations, listing only the book titles, volume numbers, and authors. Books missing from the imperial collection were marked with the character "阙" (quē, missing) beneath their titles. The examination of the *Comprehensive Catalogue of Literature During the Song Dynasty* (Chóng Wén Zǒng Mù, 崇文总目) reveals that almost all versions of *Five Viscera Theory* (Wǔ Zàng Lùn, 五藏论) in the simplified edition were marked as "missing," except for Zhang Zhongjing's *Five Viscera Theory* (Wǔ Zàng Lùn, 五藏论), which retained its original description. This confirms that the imperial library of the time indeed possessed Zhang Zhongjing's *Five Viscera Theory* (Wǔ Zàng Lùn, 五藏论). Both the detailed and simplified versions of the catalog coexisted during the Song and Yuan dynasties, but the detailed version gradually disappeared after the Ming and Qing dynasties. Fortunately, a copy of the simplified version from the Ming dynasty is preserved in the Tianyi Pavilion, becoming the earliest surviving catalog from an official library.[12] Regrettably, the Tianyi Pavilion's copy has become a precious relic, making it difficult for ordinary people to access.

Looking into the *Summary of Arts and Literature in the Comprehensive Chronicles of the Song Dynasty* (Sòng Dài Tōng Zhì Yì Wén Lüè, 宋代通志艺文略) and *Records of Arts and Literature in the History of the Song Dynasty* (Sòng Shǐ Yì Wén Zhì, 宋史艺文志), we find clear records about the authors and categorization of *Five Viscera Theory* (Wǔ Zàng Lùn, 五藏论). The *Summary of Arts and Literature in the Comprehensive Chronicles of the Song Dynasty* (Sòng Dài Tōng Zhì Yì Wén Lüè, 宋代通志艺文略) lists Zhang Zhongjing's *Five Viscera Theory* (Wǔ Zàng Lùn, 五藏论) as a separate entry, whereas the *Records of Arts and Literature in the History of the Song Dynasty* (Sòng Shǐ Yì Wén Zhì, 宋史艺文志) places it under the name "Zhang Zhongjing," distinguishing it from other works titled *Five Viscera Theory* (Wǔ Zàng Lùn, 五藏论). The fact that Zhang Zhongjing's *Five Viscera Theory* (Wǔ Zàng Lùn, 五藏论) appears either as an independent entry or under his name in both the *Summary of Arts and Literature in the Comprehensive Chronicles of the Song Dynasty* (Sòng Dài Tōng Zhì Yì Wén Lüè, 宋代通志艺文略) and *Records of Arts and Literature in the History of the Song Dynasty* (Sòng Shǐ Yì Wén Zhì, 宋史艺文志) confirms its acknowledged existence in these historical sources from the Song dynasty.

Meanwhile, there is an interesting shift. Prior to the Sui Dynasty, both texts with the name *Five Viscera Theory* (Wǔ Zàng Lùn, 五藏论) and works by Zhang Zhongjing were exceedingly rare. However, by the Song Dynasty, various versions of *Five Viscera Theory* (Wǔ Zàng Lùn, 五藏论) proliferated, and the number of works attributed to Zhang Zhongjing increased to eight. This change might be linked to the advancements in papermaking and printing technologies, which significantly accelerated the spread and reach of knowledge. Intriguingly, in the historical records of the Yuan and Ming dynasties,[13, 14] apart from works related to *Treatise on Cold Damage Disorders* (Shāng Hán Lùn, 伤寒论) and *Essential Prescriptions from the Golden Cabinet* (Jīn Guì Yào Lüè, 金匮要略), other works by Zhang Zhongjing had largely disappeared. Concurrently, various editions of *Five Viscera Theory* (Wǔ Zàng Lùn, 五藏论) also gradually faded into obscurity. However, during this period, Korea used the advanced woodblock printing technology of the Song era to produce Zhang Zhongjing's *Five Viscera Theory* (Wǔ Zàng Lùn, 五藏论). This book will delve into the Korean version of Zhang Zhongjing's *Five Viscera Theory* (Wǔ Zàng Lùn, 五藏论) in later chapters.

Time swiftly moved into the Qing Dynasty, a period when textual research became the dominant scholarly trend, particularly flourishing in the field of Kaozheng (evidential research). During this era, eight scholars, including the renowned Yao Zhenzong, supplemented the research on the *Records of Arts and Literature in the Later Han Dynasty* (Hòu Hàn Yì Wén Zhì, 后汉艺文志) with their scholarly contributions. However, of these works, only five versions have survived to the present, with Yao Zhenzong's version being particularly celebrated. It is due to these scholars' effort that the earliest historical record of Zhang Zhongjing's *Five Viscera Theory* (Wǔ Zàng Lùn, 五藏论) has been traced back from the original Song Dynasty to the Later Han period.[15–20]

Both Gu Sanhuai's *Supplement to the Later Han Book of Arts and Literature* (Bǔ Hòu Hàn Shū Yì Wén Zhì, 补后汉书艺文志) and Yao Zhenzong's *Later Han Book of Arts and Literature* (Hòu Hàn Shū Yì Wén Zhì, 后汉书艺文志) record Zhang Zhongjing's *Five Viscera Theory* (Wǔ Zàng Lùn, 五藏论) and *Classic of the Golden Casket and the Jade Box* (Jīn Guì Yù Hán, 金匮玉函), without mentioning other medical books of the "Wu Zang Lun" category. This could suggest that Zhang Zhongjing's *Five Viscera Theory* (Wǔ Zàng Lùn, 五藏论) set a precedent for later medical practitioners to write their own versions of *Wu Zang Lun*–type texts.

In summary, Zhang Zhongjing's *Five Viscera Theory* (Wǔ Zàng Lùn, 五藏论) is an independent version, unrelated to other texts with the same title. Like Zhang Zhongjing's *Classic of the Golden Casket and the Jade Box* (Jīn Guì Yù Hán, 金匮玉函), it emerged in the Later Han period following the publication of *Treatise on Cold Damage Disorders* (Shāng Hán Lùn, 伤寒论). This raises the question: So from what time period does Zhang Zhongjing's *Five Viscera Theory* (Wǔ Zàng Lùn, 五藏论), discovered in the Dunhuang Hidden Library, originate? Ma Jixing believes that since the fragment avoids taboo words related to Emperors Taizong and Gaozong of the Tang Dynasty (for instance, changing "治" (zhì), to "疗" (liáo)) but does not avoid the taboo word "恒" (héng) associated with Emperor Muzong of Tang and Emperor Zhenzong of the Northern Song, it suggests that both the S.5614 in the British collection and the P. 2755 in the French collection are likely early Tang Dynasty copies.

The following is a literal translation of the full text of Zhang Zhongjing's *Five Viscera Theory* (Wǔ Zàng Lùn, 五藏论) P. 2378. The translation process strictly adheres to the original text, translating it word by word, sentence by sentence:

⊠草巧⊠，⊠，□胶有结⊠，⊠宲之形。丹沙会⊠，⊠青绿。秦胶须行，矾石⊠。⊠去酸皮，桂心取其有味。石英⊠，杏仁别捣如膏。吐丝酒渎乃□，□消火烧方好。黄葵唯轻唯上，狼□唯重唯加。黄芩以附肠胃为精，藺⊠为用。石南菜叶，甘槲收花。五加削取其皮，母丹搥其去骨。鬼箭破血，仍有射鬼之令；神屋除温，非带报神之验。

[*unrecognizable*](*Tong*) Cao (通草, rice paper plant pith) can magically [*unrecognizable*] (*treat deafness*); [*unrecognizable*]. [*missing*] (*Qin*) Jiao (秦胶 or "Qin Jiao," 秦艽, largeleaf gentian root) pertains spiral shape [*unrecognizable*]; [*unrecognizable*] looks like honeycomb. Dan Sha (丹砂 or "Zhu Sha" 朱砂, cinnabar) should be [*unrecognizable*]; [unrecognizable] blue and green. Qin Jiao (秦椒, prickly ash peel) need to be steamed; Fan Shi (矾石, white alum-stone) [*unrecognizable*]; [*unrecognizable*] peel off the outer skin; Gui Xin (桂心 or 肉桂, cinnamon bark) must have intense fragrance. Shi Ying (石英, Cristobalite) [*unrecognizable*]; Xing Ren (杏仁, apricot seed) should be grinded until get creamy. Tu Si (菟丝, Chinese dodder seed) must be soaked with alcohol [*missing*]; [*missing*] (*Pu*) Xiao (朴硝, a crude form of sodium sulfate) has to be calcinated. Fang Kui (防葵, white flower hog fennel root) the lighter the better; Lang [*missing*] (Du) (狼毒, Bracteole-lacked Euphorbia root) the heavier the better. Good Huang Qin (黄芩, Baical skullcap root) looks like rotten intestine; only use Lin [*unrecognizable*] (*Ru's*) (藺茹, Euphorbia Lanru root) top part. Shi Nan (石南, Chinese photinia Leaf), should pick its leaves; Gan Ju (甘菊, sweet chrysanthemum flower) uses its flower. Wu Jia (五加, Slenderstyle Acanthopanax Bark) only uses the bark; Mu Dan (牡丹, tree peony bark), hammer its stem and take the bone out. Gui Jian (鬼箭 or "Gui Jian Yu" 鬼箭羽, winged branches) must cut to bleed to have the effect of shooting the ghost spirit. Shen Wu (神屋 or 龟板, tortoise carapace and plastron) could eliminate warm process to generate magical effect.

呕吐汤煎干葛，筋转酒煮木瓜。目赤须点黄连，口疮宜含黄蘗。脾搽应痛，须放茵花；臊痒皮肤，汤煎蒴藋。伤寒发汗，要用麻黄；肚热不除，宜加竹叶，恒山鳖甲，大有差疟之功；蛇脱缘丹，善除癫痫之用。雄黄能除黑汗，木兰能除死皮，欺草煞齿内之虫，藜芦除鼻中宿肉。黄莲断痢除甘，子之悦愈面皮，桃花润泽肤体。芎藭、枳实，心急即用加之，紫苑、凝冬，弃嗽要须当用。盲虫、水质，即有破血之功；白术，槟榔，有散气消食之效。菖蒲强记，鳖甲通神。

Decoct Gan Ge (干葛 or "Ge Geng" 葛根, dried pueraria root) to treat vomiting; use alcohol to decoct Mu Gua (木瓜, Chinese quince fruit) for muscle spasm. Use Huang Lian (黄连, yellow coptis root) to make eye drops for red eyes. Hold Huang Bo (黄蘗 or 黄柏, phellodendron bark) in the mouth for mouth ulcer. Painful arthritis uses Yin Yu (茵芋, Japanese skimmia stem and leaf); severe skin itch uses Shuo Huo (蒴藋, Chinese elder) decoction. Promote sweat during Shang Han, exogenous pathogenic cold-induced diseases, uses Ma Huang (麻黄, ephedra stem). Constant high fever can benefit from Zhu Ye (竹叶, bamboo leaves). Heng Shan (恒山 or "Chang Shan" 常山, dichroa root) and Bie Jia (鳖甲, Chinese soft-shelled turtle shell) have great function to relieve malaria. She Tui (蛇蜕, snake slough) and Lü Dan (绿丹, aluminum pill) relieve seizure attacks. Xiong Huang (雄黄, realgar) is to treat gangrene; Mu Lan (木兰, lily magnolia bark) can remove dead skin; Wang Cao (莔草 or "Mang Cao," 莽草, leaf of poisonous eightangle tree) treats cavity inside the teeth; Li Lu (藜芦, veratrum root and rhizome) can treat chronic nasal infection. Huang Lian (黄莲, yellow coptis root) stops dysentery disease and eliminates malnutrition; Zi Zhi (子之 or "Zhi Zi," 栀子, gardenia fruit) benefits facial skin; Tao Hua (桃花, peach blossom) can moisten body skin. Xiong Qiong (芎藭 or "Chuan Xiong," 川芎, Sichuan lovage rhizome) and Zhi Shi (枳实, immature range fruit) treat anxiety; Zi Wan (紫菀, tatarian aster root) and Kuan Dong (款冬, Common coltsfoot flower) are used for asthma and cough. Mang Chong (盲虫 or 虻虫, horse fly) and Shui Zhi (水质 or 水蛭, leech) are to break blood stagnation; Bai Zhu (白术, white atractylodes tuber) and Bing Lang (槟榔, betel nut, or areca seed) relieve bloating and promote digestion. Chang Pu (菖蒲 or "Shi Chang Pu," 石菖蒲, grassleaf sweetflag rhizome) enhances memory; Bie Jia (鳖甲, Chinese soft-shelled turtle shell) promotes spiritual function.

䯝疮汤煎蛇麻，淋涩须加滑石。仙苓脾草能去腰疼，然则忘杖归家。太鼠煎膏，巧疗耳聋，得草麻而加妙。蛇咬宜封人粪，螯蛇荜菝妙除。羚羊角通噎驱耶，青羊肝疗肝明目。石脂加颜发色，白芨卷面除皮。志母通痢开胸，空清消徵止泪。孔公蘖消食肥泽，蜜陀僧去疥癞人。癖石奇假蜂房，水肿唯须杖戟，肠结通唯须甘遂。患眼宜取蕤人，安胎必籍紫葳，伤身要须地髓。脑心闷偏加述笔，血闭息觅蒲黄。疗脚累疮痈，地胆破徵假息肉。斑猫能除鼠漏，松热抽恶刺风疽。牵牛小写排脓，葶苈大枣除水。桃仁绝其鬼气，石南肠去诸风。瘿气昆布妙除，痈肿硇砂石却，肠痈必须消石，脱公宜取鳖头。下贱虽曰地浆，天行病者皆愈；黄龙汤出其厕内之虫，时起病服者能除。贫者须号小方，不及君臣，取写有处出处，有灵有验，有贵有贱，有高有下，净秽而草山中药。

Vaginal discharge, exterior vaginal itching, and redness, use She Ma (蛇麻 or "She Chuang," 蛇床, common cnidium fruit) to decoct. Urgent or hesitate urination, add Hua Shi (滑石, talc). Xian Lin Pi (仙灵脾 or "Yin Yang Huo" 淫羊藿, horny goat weedor epimedium) relieves lower back pain so that the patient can walk back home without the crutches. Syrup made from Tai Shu (太鼠 or "Bian Fu" 蝙蝠, bat) treats deafness, to add Bi Ma (蓖麻, castor leaf or bean) for better results. Topically cover with Ren Fen (人粪 or "Ren Zhong Huang" 人中黄, human feces) for snake bite; bee sting can be treated by Bi Ba (荜茇, piper longum). Ling Yang Jiao (羚羊角, antelope's horn) is for esophageal obstruction and to eliminate evil. Qing Yang Gan (青羊肝, goral liver) treats malnutrition and brightens vision. Shi Zhi (石脂, halloysite) darkens hair; Bai Ji (白芨, bletilla tuber) removes dead skin and regenerates new skin. Zhi Mu (志母, common anemarrhena rhizome) treats dysentery and opens chest; Kong Qing (空青, azurite) relieves bloating and stops tearing. Kong Gong Nie (孔公孽, Calcite) helps digest food and gains weight. Mi Tuo Seng (密陀僧, litharge) treats eczema and skin infection. Feng Fang (蜂房, honeycomb) used to calm down the rebellious Qi caused by taking Ru Shi (乳石, stalactite). Edema can use Da Ji (大戟, Peking spurge root). Intestinal obstruction uses Gan Sui (甘遂, gansui root). Eye disease uses Rui Ren (蕤人, hedge prinsepia nut). Calm down fetus must use Zi Wei (紫葳, Chinese Trumpetcreeper Flower); Di Sui (地髓 or "Gan Di Huang" 干地黄, drying rehmannia root) is for physical exhaustion. Mentally depress use Mu Bi (木笔 or "Xin Yi Hua" 辛夷花, magnolia flower); amenorrhea uses Pu Huang (蒲黄, cat-tail pollen) immediately. Scrofula and boils use Lian Qiao (连翘, weeping forsythia Capsule); Di Dan (地胆, a kind of blister beetles) treats mass, nodules, and polyps. Ban Mao (斑猫, mylabris) can treat chronic skin abscess; Song Re (松热 or "Song Zhi" 松脂, pine resin) is anti-infection. It can promote discharge of pus. Qian Niu (牵牛, morning glory) is a strong diuretic to reduce swelling. It also helps discharge pus; Ting Li (葶苈 or "Ting Li Zi" 葶苈子, tansymustard seed) and Da Zao (大枣, Chinese date) eliminate edema. Tao Ren (桃人 or 桃仁, peach kernel) stops evil energy; Shi Nan (石南, Chinese photinia Leaf) to eliminate all kinds of internal wind.

Kun Bu (昆布, kombu) relieves goiter; Nao Sha (硇砂, sal ammoniac) treats abscess and swelling. Xiao Shi (消石 or "Mang Xiao" 芒硝, nitrate from saline alkali land) treats intestinal abscess; Bie Tou (鳖头, soft-shell turtle head) treats rectal prolapse. Regardless of the degrading name of "Di Jiang" (地浆, Earth Slurry), Tian Xing Bing, epidemic diseases caused by natural factors, gets healed by taking Di Jiang (地浆, Earth Slurry). Although Huang Long Tang (黄龙汤, Yellow Dragon Decoction) came from the worms in the toilet, it can treat infectious disease. Although small formula was considered lower class, it doesn't even have King and Minister herbs in the formulation (still, you know) where the formula originally come from. And the formula is clinically proven, the medicine could be expensive or cheap, and the herbs could be higher or lower class and clean or dirty. They are all come from the nature.

《五脏论》一卷。

One volume of "Wu Zang Lun."

REFERENCES

1. Shanghai Chinese Classics Publishing House and Bibliotheque Nationale de France, *Dunhuang and Other Central Asian Manuscripts in the Bibliotheque Nationale de France: Volume 13 Fonds Pelliot chinois 2363–2432* (Shanghai: Shanghai Chinese Classics Publishing House, 2000), 82–84.
2. 李勤璞, "黑田源次：传记资料与著作目录[J]." 辽宁省博物馆馆刊 (2015): 308–323.
3. 郭秀梅, "冈西为人漫漫医学路笔耕50年纪念冈西为人博士诞生110周年[J]." *中华医史杂志*, Vol. 39, No. 6 (2009): 375–382.
4. 罗福颐, "西陲古方技书残卷汇编[J]." *中华医史杂志*, Vol. 4, No. 1 (1953): 27–30.
5. 班固，*汉书[M]* (北京：中华书局, 1962), 1775.
6. 长生无忌，*隋书经籍志[M]* (上海：商务印书馆, 1936), 92.
7. 宋昫，*旧唐书经籍志[M]* (上海: 商务印书馆, 1936), 82.
8. 欧阳修，*唐书经籍志[M]* (上海: 商务印书馆, 1936), 65
9. 王尧臣，*崇文总目（附补遗）[M]* (上海: 商务印书馆, 1937), 195.
10. 郑樵，*通志[M]* (北京：中华书局, 1987), 810.
11. 元脱脱，*宋史艺文志[M]* (上海: 商务印书馆, 1936), 116.
12. 张固也、唐黎明，"《崇文总目辑释》"补释撰人"考[J]." *文献季刊*, Vol. 7, No. 3 (2011): 58–65.
13. 田汉云. *元史艺文志[A]*. 见：陈文和. *嘉定钱大昕先生全集 [M]* (南京：江苏古籍出版社, 1997), 49.
14. 张廷玉，*明史艺文志[M]* (上海：商务印书馆, 1936), 54.
15. 姚振宗, *三国艺文志[M]*. 见：*张钧衡, 适园丛书第十二集[M]* (上海: 民国乌程张氏刊本, 1916), 76.
16. 钱大昭，*补续汉书艺文志[A]*. 见：*二十五史补编　第二册[M]* (上海: 开明书店, 1937年), 2095.
17. 侯康，*补后汉书艺文志[A]*. 见：*二十五史补编 第二册[M]* (上海: 开明书店, 1937), 2105.
18. 顾三怀，*补后汉书艺文志[A]*. 见：*二十五史补编 第二册[M]* (上海: 开明书店，1937), 2131.
19. 姚振宗，*后汉书艺文志[A]*. 见：*二十五史补编 第二册[M]* (上海: 开明书店, 1937), 2305.
20. 曾朴，*补后汉书艺文志并考[A]*. 见：*二十五史补编　第二册[M]* (上海: 开明书店, 1937), 2447.

7 Under the Name of Zhang Zhongjing – S. 5614 Collected in England

"The 'Categorized Collection of Medical Formulas' cites an anonymous author's 'Wu Zang Lun,' resembling closely Dunhuang manuscripts. I conclude they are the same medical text."

– Mi Morong

The "One Volume of *Wu Zang Lun*" (briefly referred to as S.5614),[1] housed in the British Library in London, UK, is a precious historical document. This ancient scroll has 15 pages, measuring 35 cm in height and 24 cm in width. Each page is densely inscribed with 13 to 14 lines of text, meticulously copied with an ink brush, and each page is framed with single borders and lined. From the seventh to the fourteenth fold, a total of 195 lines of text, there is a continuous record of four medical texts: Zhang Zhongjing *Five Viscera Theory* (Wǔ Zàng Lùn, 五藏论), *Simplified Examples of Pulse Diagnosis* (Píng Mài Lüè Lì, 平脉略例) (version A), *Method of Judging the Yin and Yang Conditions of the Five Zang Pulses* (Wǔzàng Mài Hòu Yīn Yáng Xiāng Shèng Fǎ, 五脏脉候阴阳相乘法) (version A), and *Divination of the Origins of the Five Zangs through Sounds and Colors* (Zhàn Wǔ Zàng Shēng Sè Yuán Hòu, 占五脏声色源候). All these texts are written in line-style calligraphy with a brush, done in one go without any corrections, and the handwriting is clear and neat, seemingly all from the same hand. Zhang Zhongjing's *Five Viscera Theory* (Wǔ Zàng Lùn, 五藏论) comprises 83 lines. At the beginning of the scroll, it boldly states, "*Wu Zang Lun*, One Volume, written by Zhang Zhongjing," clearly indicating it as Zhang Zhongjing's work. Unfortunately, the bottom left and right corners of the first page of *Five Viscera Theory* (Wǔ Zàng Lùn, 五藏论) are torn, giving the page a butterfly-like appearance and a slightly incomplete look.

The previous text mentioned that Luo Fuyi, in his work *Compilation of Ancient Medical Formula Fragments from the Western Frontier* (Xī Chuí Gǔ Fāng Jì Shū Cán Juàn Huì Biān, 西陲古方技书残卷汇编), identified three different versions of Zhang Zhongjing's *Five Viscera Theory* (Wǔ Zàng Lùn, 五藏论) in the Dunhuang manuscripts preserved in the UK (S. 5614) and France (P. 2755 and P. 2378).[2] At that time, since many of the Dunhuang fragments were scattered abroad, it was difficult for Chinese scholars to witness the true appearance of these fragments firsthand.

DOI: 10.1201/9781032698205-7

Research on the S. 5614 fragment was thus based on secondary studies using Luo Fuyi's compilation. Fortunately, another Chinese scholar, Wang Qingshu, had the opportunity to study abroad in London, UK, where she was able to peruse over 12,000 Dunhuang manuscripts housed in both the UK and France. She also categorized the manuscripts in the British Library and took micro-photographs of important documents related to literature, calendars, divination, medicine, and more. Among these photos were 18 volumes, totaling over 80 pages of medical documents, including the S. 5614 fragment of Zhang Zhongjing's *Five Viscera Theory* (Wǔ Zàng Lùn, 五藏论) and *Simplified Examples of Pulse Diagnosis* (Píng Mài Lüè Lì, 平脉略例), totaling eight pieces. In 1958, Wang Qingshu published the micro-photographs of S. 5614 Zhang Zhongjing's *Five Viscera Theory* (Wǔ Zàng Lùn, 五藏论) in the Chinese medical journal *Medical History and Health Organizations* (Yī Xué Shǐ Yǔ Bǎo Jiàn Zǔ Zhī, 医学史与保健组织) (now known as *Chinese Journal of Medical History*).[3, 4] This was the first publication of the photo of S. 5614 manuscript in China, providing valuable original materials for future research.

Japanese scholars have also put great effort into the study of Dunhuang medicine. Interestingly, the development of Dunhuang studies in Japan is strikingly similar to that in China. Japanese research on Dunhuang also began in 1909, when the Asahi Shimbun published an article by Naitō Torajirō about *The Relics Unearthed in the Dunhuang Stone Room* (敦煌石室发见物), which became a foundational work in the field of Japanese Dunhuang studies. Before World War II, Japanese scholars primarily focused on collecting, organizing, and publishing literature related to Dunhuang. However, during the post–World War II period, Dunhuang studies in Japan entered a slump with no significant works published and only occasional scattered articles appearing in newspapers and magazines. It wasn't until the mid-1950s, with the rediscovery of documents from the Ōtani Kōzui expedition to the Western Regions, and the acquisition of microfilms of Dunhuang manuscripts held in London and Beijing, that Japanese Dunhuang studies experienced a new surge in prosperity. In this field, Mi Morong and Miyazaki Saburo stood out as particularly distinguished, considered to be the leading figures in Japanese Dunhuang studies.

In June 1964, Japanese scholar Mi Morong published the groundbreaking *Catalogue of Comprehensive Commentaries of Medical Literatures Unearthed in the Western Regions* (西域出土医药关系文献综合解说目录) in the renowned *The Toyo Gakuho* (东洋学报).[5] In this work, he ingeniously classified all known medical literature from the western regions of China into eight major categories: I. medical texts (including A. formulation, B. Wu Zang [five Zang-organs], C. pulse diagnosis, D. moxibustion), II. materia medica, III. Buddhist medical formulation, IV. Taoist medical formulation, V. documents related to medicine, VI. medical literatures carved in wood slips, VII. medical information in ancient ethnic languages, and VIII. miscellaneous and supplementary. In the catalog, Mi Morong not only detailed the volume number, physical characteristics, main content, and approximate dates of each document but also added his own research insights, greatly facilitating the work of subsequent scholars. Similar to Luo Fuyi's view, Mi Morong also believed that the S.5614 housed in UK, the P. 2755, and P. 2378 housed in France were all versions of Zhang Zhongjing's *Five Viscera Theory* (Wǔ Zàng Lùn, 五藏论).

Another Japanese scholar who achieved remarkable success in the field of Dunhuang studies is Miyazaki Saburo. In 1959, he published a groundbreaking paper titled *About Zhang Zhongjing's Five Viscera Theory* (关于张仲景五藏论) in the *Journal of Kampo Medicine* (汉方临床).[6] In this paper, Miyazaki Saburo translated and analyzed the original text of Zhang Zhongjing's *Five Viscera Theory* (Wǔ Zàng Lùn, 五藏论). Although he was not entirely satisfied with his work, feeling that the study and interpretation of the original text were not detailed enough, he was undoubtedly the first scholar to comprehensively introduce, verify, correct, translate, and annotate Zhang Zhongjing's *Five Viscera Theory* (Wǔ Zàng Lùn, 五藏论). His work represented a valuable contribution to the global academic community.

In 1964, Miyazaki Saburo published a profoundly influential paper in the 35th volume of the *The Toyo Gakuho* (东洋学报), titled *A Collation, Translation, and Annotation of the Dunhuang Manuscript of Zhang Zhongjing's Wu Zang Lun* (敦煌本"张仲景五藏论"校译注).[7] In this paper, he used the S.5614 Dunhuang fragment of Zhang Zhongjing's *Five Viscera Theory* (Wǔ Zàng Lùn, 五藏论) as the basis for a detailed collation and translation of the entire document. He meticulously compared and studied the three Dunhuang manuscripts S.5614, P. 2755, and P. 2378 and also juxtaposed the content of *Five Viscera Theory* (Wǔ Zàng Lùn, 五藏论) from the Korean *Categorized Collection of Medical Formulas* (Yī Fāng Lèi Jù, 医方类聚) sentence by sentence with the original text, aiming to restore the original appearance of this long-lost historical document as much as possible through these multifaceted comparisons. Miyazaki Saburo's attempt was crucial; he even linked the *Five Viscera Theory* (Wǔ Zàng Lùn, 五藏论) from *Categorized Collection of Medical Formulas* (Yī Fāng Lèi Jù, 医方类聚) with Zhang Zhongjing's *Five Viscera Theory* (Wǔ Zàng Lùn, 五藏论) from Dunhuang and speculated that both might be the same medical text, namely, the historically lost *Five Viscera Theory* (Wǔ Zàng Lùn, 五藏论) of Zhang Zhongjing. The correctness of this view will be further discussed in later chapters of the book.

Is the Zhang Zhongjing's *Five Viscera Theory* (Wǔ Zàng Lùn, 五藏论) unearthed in Dunhuang truly written by Zhang Zhongjing himself? The texts "Wrote by Zhang Zhongjing" clearly printed on this ancient document seems to leave no room for doubt. However, true academic exploration never stops at appearances. The question arises: Was this *Five Viscera Theory* (Wǔ Zàng Lùn, 五藏论) personally penned by Zhang Zhongjing, or was it written by later individuals under the auspices of his revered name? Miyazaki Saburo, in his study of the Dunhuang manuscripts, pointed out that the term used for the herb "Xin Yi" is a key clue in determining the author's identity. In *Five Viscera Theory* (Wǔ Zàng Lùn, 五藏论), the herb "Xin Yi" is referred to as "Mu Bi," a name with distinct regional characteristics, typically used by northerners. It is well known that Zhang Zhongjing was from Henan. During the Eastern Han Dynasty, Henan was in the northern part of the country, implying Zhang Zhongjing could be considered a "northerner." While this does not directly prove that *Five Viscera Theory* (Wǔ Zàng Lùn, 五藏论) was written by Zhang Zhongjing himself, this unique regional linguistic feature indeed increases the likelihood that Zhang Zhongjing personally authored *Five Viscera Theory* (Wǔ Zàng Lùn, 五藏论).

Speaking of which, the name Zhang Zhongjing has been mentioned countless times. Many are familiar with Zhang Zhongjing's medical writings; it can be said that without Zhang Zhongjing, traditional Chinese medicine would have a completely different face. Given his significance, let's talk about Zhang Zhongjing himself. Zhang Zhongjing, whose given name was Ji, and styled as Zhongjing, was a famous medical scholar of the Eastern Han Dynasty.[8] He was born around the first year of the Heping era of Emperor Huan (around 150 AD) and passed away in the 24th year of the Jian'an era of Emperor Xian (219 AD), hailing from Nieyang in Nanyang County, Henan Province. From an early age, Zhang Zhongjing showed a strong interest in learning and profound thinking. At the age of 10, he was already praised by his fellow townsman He Yong, who commented, "With your thoughtful nature and understated style, you are destined to become an outstanding physician," as quoted in *The Biography of He Yong* (Hé Yóng Bié Zhuàn, 何颙别传).

Zhang Zhongjing's passion for medicine was unparalleled. He was diligent in his studies and read extensively. Influenced and inspired by the ancient famous physician Bian Que, Zhang also sought instruction from Zhang Bozu, a renowned local doctor. His intelligence and relentless effort soon led him to surpass his teacher. Even after becoming well-known, he maintained his enthusiasm for learning and would travel long distances to seek guidance from any skilled physician he heard of. This tireless spirit of exploration ultimately made Zhang Zhongjing not only an outstanding physician but also revered as a "saint" in the field of medicine by later generations.

Although the *Book of the Later Han* (Hòu Hàn Shū, 后汉书) and the *Records of the Three Kingdoms* (Sān Guó Zhì, 三国志) do not contain a biography of Zhang Zhongjing, stories about him are widely circulated among the people. It is said that Zhang Zhongjing was not keen on a career in the officialdom and was reluctant to enter public service. However, under his father's urging, he became the county magistrate (xiao lian) during the reign of Emperor Ling (around 168–188 AD), thus beginning his official career. Despite rumors that he was appointed as the prefect of Changsha during the Jian'an period (196–219 AD),[9] there is no concrete historical evidence for this claim.

A well-known story describes how Zhang Zhongjing combined his medical skills with his official duties. At that time, officials usually did not interact with the common people, let alone treat their illnesses. To address this issue, Zhang adopted a unique approach: on the first and 15th days of each lunar month, he would open his office, suspend official duties, and allow sick people to come in. He would sit upright in the hall, carefully diagnosing and treating each person. This practice caused a great sensation locally, earning widespread praise and admiration from the people. It became a custom, and on every first and 15th day of the lunar month, many people seeking medical advice would gather in front of his office. Consequently, medical activities conducted in an office came to be known as "Zuo Tang" (sitting in the hall), leading to the tradition of calling some pharmacies "Tang," such as Tong Ren Tang, Chang Chun Tang, and Hu Qing Yu Tang. The physicians in these pharmacies thus came to be known as "Zuo Tang doctors" (doctors sitting in the hall). Zhang Zhongjing was revered as Zhang Changsha, and his herbal formulas were referred to as Changsha prescriptions, possibly deriving from his supposed position as prefect.

In 1981, an ancient tombstone was discovered at the Nanyang Medical Sage Temple, which was later designated as a national second-level cultural relic. The back of the stone base is engraved with the words "The Fifth Year of Xianhe," corresponding to the year 330 AD. The central inscription of the stone reads, "Tomb of Zhang Zhongjing, the Medical Sage and Prefect of Changsha of the Han Dynasty."

In the late Eastern Han Dynasty, the state fell into chaos and war, bringing immense suffering to the people's lives. It was during this era that Zhang Zhongjing witnessed the Yellow Turban Rebellion and the fierce struggles among the regional warlords. Continuous warfare led to endless displacement and misery, compounded by rampant epidemics that claimed countless lives, even to the point where "nine out of ten households were empty." Wang Can, one of the "Seven Scholars of Jian'an," depicted the suffering of the people in his poem *Seven Laments* (Qī Āi Shī, 七哀诗), writing:

> When I step outside, I see nothing but white bones scattered across the fields. Along the roadsides, there are starving women abandoning their children in the bushes. Even when they hear their children's cries, the mothers, wiping away their tears, do not turn back. I can only spur my horse and leave, unable to bear these sorrowful sighs.

Cao Zhi, in his *On the Epidemic Qi* (Shuō Yì Qì, 说疫气), described, "Every family experiences the pain of death, every household is immersed in sorrow. Some families have all perished from illness, some lineages have been completely wiped out."

Zhang Zhongjing's hometown was not spared from the turmoil and suffering of that tumultuous era. Originally a prosperous and thriving family, the Zhang family had over 200 members during the Jian'an period. However, within less than a decade, two-thirds of the family tragically perished, with 70% dying from typhoid fever. As a physician, Zhang Zhongjing felt deep grief and self-reproach for this tragic and irreversible loss, as he expressed in the preface of his *Treatise on Cold Damage Disorders* (Shāng Hán Lùn, 伤寒论): "I am mourning for all the deaths in the past and heartbroken over those who have died because I couldn't save them." This inspired him to diligently study medicine. He devoted himself day and night to studying medical classics, learning various formulations, referencing texts like the *Basic Questions* (Sù Wèn, 素问), *Divine Pivot* (Líng Shū, 灵枢), *Yellow Emperor's Canon of 81 Difficult Issues* (Huáng Dì Bā Shí Yī Nàn Jīng, 黄帝八十一难经), *Records of Fetal and Neonatal Medicine* (Tāi Lú Yào Lù, 胎胪药录), and *Differentiation of the Even Pulse* (Píng Mài Biàn Zhèng, 平脉辨证), among others.

Eventually, he completed the renowned medical work *Treatise on Cold Damage and Miscellaneous Disorders* (Shāng Hán Zá Bìng Lùn, 伤寒杂病论), comprising 16 volumes. According to the preface of the *A-B Canon of Acupuncture and Moxibustion* (Zhēn Jiǔ Jiǎ Yǐ Jīng, 针灸甲乙经), in *Treatise on Cold Damage and Miscellaneous Disorders* (Shāng Hán Zá Bìng Lùn, 伤寒杂病论), Zhang Zhongjing not only used prescriptions from *Canon of Decoctions* (Tāng Yè Jīng Fǎ, 汤液经法) but also integrated theories from the *Inner Canon of the Yellow Emperor* (Huáng Dì Nèi Jīng, 黄帝内经). In *Treatise on Cold Damage and Miscellaneous Disorders* (Shāng Hán Zá Bìng Lùn, 伤寒杂病论), diseases are classified into two major categories: externally contracted cold damage and internally caused miscellaneous diseases.

After the completion of *Treatise on Cold Damage and Miscellaneous Disorders* (Shāng Hán Zá Bìng Lùn, 伤寒杂病论), parts of the original text were lost due to the frequent wars during the Three Kingdoms period. The *Treatise on Cold Damage Disorders* (Shāng Hán Lùn, 伤寒论) that has been passed down to later generations was actually compiled by Wang Shuhe, a medical scholar of the Western Jin Dynasty. Wang Shuhe accidentally saw this incomplete medical masterpiece, which, despite only having scattered chapters remaining, still demonstrated supreme wisdom. Utilizing his position as the Imperial Physician, Wang Shuhe dedicated himself to collecting all copies of *Treatise on Cold Damage and Miscellaneous Disorders* (Shāng Hán Zá Bìng Lùn, 伤寒杂病论). He eventually gathered the complete part concerning cold damage and organized it, naming it *Treatise on Cold Damage Disorders* (Shāng Hán Lùn, 伤寒论). However, the sections of the original work on "miscellaneous diseases" remained lost. *Treatise on Cold Damage Disorders* (Shāng Hán Lùn, 伤寒论) consists of 22 chapters, describing 397 treatment methods and containing 113 formulas, totaling over 50,000 characters. The contribution of Wang Shuhe to *Treatise on Cold Damage Disorders* (Shāng Hán Lùn, 伤寒论) was such that, in the words of Xu Dachun, a famous physician of the Qing Dynasty, "Without Shuhe, this book would not exist."

Wang Shuhe also left us the earliest written record about Zhang Zhongjing in the preface of the *Pulse Classic* (Mài Jīng, 脉经):

> The treatments we provide are about the life and death of a patient. Miraculous like Yi He and Bian Que still need careful deliberation before making diagnosis; Saints like Zhongjing not only takes pulses but also co-references the pulse diagnosis with patient's chief complaint and constitution. Whenever there was doubt, Zhongjing looked into classics and conducted further investigation in order to make his treatment work.

This passage reflects Zhang Zhongjing's rigorous attitude in medical practice and academic research.

Subsequently, *Treatise on Cold Damage Disorders* (Shāng Hán Lùn, 伤寒论) gradually became widely circulated among the public and highly esteemed in the medical community. Tao Hongjing, a famous medical scholar during the Southern and Northern dynasties, commented: "Of all, only Zhang Zhongjing's work is the ancestor of all formulas." Therefore, *Treatise on Cold Damage Disorders* (Shāng Hán Lùn, 伤寒论) is also revered as to be fundamental to the development of Chinese medicine formulation throughout history. The book systematically elaborates the theory of "differential diagnosis," making an extremely important contribution to the development of the etiology and formulation studies in traditional Chinese medicine.

As time flowed by, in the blink of an eye, it was the Song Dynasty, about 800 years after the death of Zhang Zhongjing. During the reign of Emperor Renzong of Song, a Hanlin Academy scholar named Wang Zhu discovered a damaged ancient book in the library of the Hanlin Academy. This book was divided into three volumes: the first volume discussed cold damage (Shang Han), the second volume elaborated on miscellaneous diseases, and the third volume recorded prescriptions and treatments for gynecological diseases. This book was named *Essentials and Formula Discussions of the Golden Cabinet and Jade Case* (Jīn Guì Yù Hán Yào Lüè Fāng Lùn, 金匮玉函要略方

论). Interestingly, part of its content was similar to *Treatise on Cold Damage Disorders* (Shāng Hán Lùn, 伤寒论), while another part discussed miscellaneous diseases.

Later, physicians such as Lin Yi and Sun Qi, under the imperial commission, revised *Treatise on Cold Damage Disorders* (Shāng Hán Lùn, 伤寒论). They compared it with *Essentials and Formula Discussions of the Golden Cabinet and Jade Case* (Jīn Guì Yù Hán Yào Lüè Fāng Lùn, 金匮玉函要略方论) and eventually confirmed that both works were authored by Zhang Zhongjing. Consequently, they renamed the part concerning miscellaneous diseases as *Essential Prescriptions from the Golden Cabinet* (Jīn Guì Yào Lüè, 金匮要略) and published it. *Essential Prescriptions from the Golden Cabinet* (Jīn Guì Yào Lüè, 金匮要略) consists of 25 chapters, containing 262 prescriptions.

Therefore, in the Song Dynasty, both *Treatise on Cold Damage Disorders* (Shāng Hán Lùn, 伤寒论) and *Essential Prescriptions from the Golden Cabinet* (Jīn Guì Yào Lüè, 金匮要略) underwent significant revision processes. The versions we see today are those revised during the Song Dynasty. The two works together contain 269 formulas, involving 214 types of medicinal ingredients. These formulas almost encompass all the common diseases seen in clinical practice. Along with the *Yellow Emperor's Classic of Internal Medicine* (Huáng Dì Nèi Jīng, 黄帝内经) and the *Shennong's Classic of Materia Medica* (Shén Nóng Běn Cǎo Jīng, 神农本草经), they are revered as the "Four Great Classics" of traditional Chinese medicine, two of which were solely authored by Zhang Zhongjing.

Attentive readers may have noticed that in addition to *Treatise on Cold Damage and Miscellaneous Disorders* (Shāng Hán Zá Bìng Lùn, 伤寒杂病论), Zhang Zhongjing authored many other works, such as *Zhang Zhongjing's formula for gynecological disorders* (Zhāng Zhòng Jǐng Liáo Fù Rén Fāng, 张仲景疗妇人方) in two volumes, *Zhang Zhongjing's Formula* (Zhāng Zhòng Jǐng Fāng, 张仲景方) in 15 volumes, Zhang Zhongjing's *Five Viscera Theory* (Wǔ Zàng Lùn, 五藏论) in one volume, *Zhang Zhongjing's Treatise on treating the yellow* (Zhāng Zhòng Jǐng Liáo Huáng Jīng, 张仲景疗黄经), *Zhang Zhongjing's Theory of Mouth and Tooth* (Zhāng Zhòng Jǐng Kǒu Chǐ Lùn, 张仲景口齿论), and *Zhang Zhongjing's Discussion about Diseases and Essential Formula* (Zhāng Zhòng Jǐng Píng Bìng Yào Fāng, 张仲景评病要方), in one volume, among others.[10] However, due to years of wars, the original books mentioned earlier, except for *Five Viscera Theory* (Wǔ Zàng Lùn, 五藏论), were all lost.

Although papermaking technology was invented during the Han Dynasty, the widespread use of paper was still in its early stages. Therefore, the main writing material at that time was still bamboo slips, which were inexpensive and easily available. Given that the area where Zhang Zhongjing lived was abundant in bamboo forests, it is reasonable to speculate that his works, including *Five Viscera Theory* (Wǔ Zàng Lùn, 五藏论), were originally inscribed on bamboo slips.

However, these volumes of bamboo slips could hardly withstand the turmoil of wars and chaos. Many works, including *Treatise on Cold Damage and Miscellaneous Disorders* (Shāng Hán Zá Bìng Lùn, 伤寒杂病论), began to scatter and disperse, and it was inevitable that some would become fragmented or lost. In that era, books were primarily disseminated through manual copying. Due to repeated transcription by many people over time, omissions and errors in copying were common occurrences. Thus, it is reasonable that various versions of these texts emerged in later generations.

In the process of organizing and studying Zhang Zhongjing's works by later generations of physicians, the emergence of various versions was due to differences in the understanding and emphasis on the pathology of cold damage diseases, as well as differing styles of book compilation. Taking *Treatise on Cold Damage Disorders* (Shāng Hán Lùn, 伤寒论) as an example. Some well-known surviving editions are Chen Wuji's *Annotated Treatise on Cold Damage Disorders* (Shāng Hán Lùn Zhù Shì, 伤寒论注释), the Song Dynasty edition copied by Zhao Kaimei, the Kang Ping edition, and the Gui Lin edition.

Having introduced Zhang Zhongjing, let's return to Dunhuang. About 100 types of medical manuscripts were unearthed in Dunhuang, among which eight are works of Zhang Zhongjing. Based on our current knowledge, the transcription of these Dunhuang medical manuscripts dates back no later than the end of the Five Dynasties. This allows us to clarify several long-debated issues. Ma Jixing, in his book *Annotations on the Ancient Medical Texts from the Dunhuang Cave Library* (Dūn Huáng Gǔ Yī Jí Kǎo Shì, 敦煌古医籍考释),[11] put forward several key arguments, which will be discussed in the following sections.

1. The remnants of Zhang Zhongjing's works unearthed in Dunhuang not only confirm the integrity of his writings but also provide significant evidence for the authenticity of their dates of composition.

The earliest existing version of *Treatise on Cold Damage Disorders* (Shāng Hán Lùn, 伤寒论) is from the Song Dynasty. Regarding the creation dates of the chapters "Bian Mai Fa" (Pulse Diagnose Method) and "Shang Han Li" (Clinical Cases of Shang Han external disorders) in this book, there have been varied opinions. For example, Qing Dynasty scholars Yu Chang, Qian Huang, Wei Litong, Shen Jinbie, and others believed that "Bian Mai Fa" was an original work of Zhang Zhongjing, while Japanese scholar Kimura Nagahisa believed that "Shang Han Li" was authored by Zhang Zhongjing. Ming Dynasty scholars like Huang Zhongli, Fang Youzhi, and Ke Qin thought that both chapters were compiled by Wang Shuhe; Qing Dynasty scholar Cao He believed that "Shang Han Li" was adapted by common doctors during the Tang and Song dynasties; Fang Youzhi thought that "Shang Han Li" was compiled by Cheng Wuji of the Jin Dynasty; while Japanese scholar Kawagoe Seishoku believed that both chapters were adaptations by Gao Jichong of the Five Dynasties. However, the medical manuscripts unearthed in Dunhuang include parts of "Bian Mai Fa" and "Shang Han Li" written during the Sui and Tang dynasties, proving that these two articles were written at least before the Five Dynasties and Song Dynasty. Although we cannot definitively determine whether these two chapters were authored by Zhang Zhongjing or Wang Shuhe, we can at least rule out the claims that they were written by "ordinary doctors of the Tang and Song periods" as believed by Cao He or by Cheng Wuji and Gao Jichong. This provides important evidence for determining the latest possible date of these articles' composition.

2. The works of Zhang Zhongjing unearthed in Dunhuang also provide conclusive evidence for the dates of composition of other non–Zhang Zhongjing works.

The creation date of *Master Lei's Discourse on Medicinal Processing* (Léi Gōng Pào Zhì Lùn, 雷公炮炙论) has long been a point of contention among scholars. According to Zhao Xiqi's record in the *Postscript of Reading at the County Magistrate's Residence* (Jùn Zhāi Dú Shū Hòu Zhì, 郡斋读书后志) during the Southern Song Dynasty, the book was written by Lei Xiao and revised by Hu Qia. Considering Hu Qia was a figure from the Liu Song period, scholars like Li Shizhen generally believe that *Master Lei's Discourse on Medicinal Processing* (Léi Gōng Pào Zhì Lùn, 雷公炮炙论) was authored by Lei Xiao during the Liu Song period. However, there are different views on the date of composition of this work. For instance, the entry on "Hua Shi" (talc) in *Illustrated Pharmacopoeia* (Běn Cǎo Tú Jīng, 本草图经) mentions: "Although Lei Xiao was a person of the Sui Dynasty, some herb names mentioned in his book are from the Tang Dynasty and later, possibly added by later people." Additionally, there are views that the book was written during the Zhao Song period or the late Tang Dynasty, and some scholars even believe it was composed in the 10th century.

Considering that the transcription date of the Zhang Zhongjing's *Five Viscera Theory* (Wǔ Zàng Lùn, 五藏论) fragment (marked as P. 2115) found in Dunhuang can be traced back to the early Tang Dynasty, this document clearly contains the original text stating, "Lei Gong's exquisite canon, fully describing the appropriateness of medicinal processing." This discovery effectively refutes the previous notion that *Master Lei's Discourse on Medicinal Processing* (Léi Gōng Pào Zhì Lùn, 雷公炮炙论) was composed after the Tang Dynasty. Therefore, we can infer that the composition of *Master Lei's Discourse on Medicinal Processing* (Léi Gōng Pào Zhì Lùn, 雷公炮炙论) must have been earlier than the Tang Dynasty.

Let us recall the famous academic principle of "dual evidence method" proposed by Wang Guowei, which involves combining recently unearthed materials with existing paper documents for comparison and analysis, in order to unravel the layered mysteries of history. With the ongoing deepening and expansion of archaeological work, a large amount of medical literature has been discovered that is either awaiting organization or still to be excavated. These new findings hold the promise of answering those historical questions that remain unresolved.

Many significant events in history have often occurred due to fortuitous coincidences. For instance, about 2,000 years ago during the Jin Dynasty, Wang Shuhe accidentally discovered fragments of *Treatise on Cold Damage and Miscellaneous Disorders* (Shāng Hán Zá Bìng Lùn, 伤寒杂病论). This prompted him to start an exhaustive collection of various copies of this book, eventually gathering the complete section on cold damage. After organizing it, he named it *Treatise on Cold Damage Disorders* (Shāng Hán Lùn, 伤寒论) by Zhang Zhongjing.

About a thousand years ago, during the Song Dynasty, a Hanlin Academy scholar named Wang Zhu unexpectedly discovered a fragment of an ancient book titled *Essentials and Formula Discussions of the Golden Cabinet and Jade Case* (Jīn

Guì Yù Hán Yào Lüè Fāng Lùn, 金匮玉函要略方论) in the library of the Hanlin Academy. This discovery facilitated the publication of Zhang Zhongjing's *Essential Prescriptions from the Golden Cabinet* (Jīn Guì Yào Lüè, 金匮要略), leaving this invaluable medical work as a legacy for future generations.

Around a hundred years ago, in the early 20th century, a Taoist named Wang Yuanlu accidentally discovered the Dunhuang Scripture Caves, bringing several hand-copied manuscripts of Zhang Zhongjing's *Five Viscera Theory* (Wǔ Zàng Lùn, 五藏论) back into the light. The wheel of history thus turns full circle. Whether there exists a version of *Five Viscera Theory* (Wǔ Zàng Lùn, 五藏论) authored by Zhang Zhongjing himself has always been a mystery for scholars. Although there are records of Zhang Zhongjing's *Five Viscera Theory* (Wǔ Zàng Lùn, 五藏论) in official records, it remains unclear how much of the content we see today was personally written by Zhang Zhongjing and how much was later added or modified by others based on their understanding. Despite this, Zhang Zhongjing's *Five Viscera Theory* (Wǔ Zàng Lùn, 五藏论), as one of the earliest introduction books of Chinese medicine, has had an immeasurable impact and significance for subsequent generations.

Based on the examination of the transcription dates, Luo Fuyi proposed: "Judging from the style of the characters and decorations, these manuscripts seem to have originated from the Five Dynasties or the early Song Dynasty." However, it is noteworthy that in these manuscripts, there are instances of avoiding taboo words related to Emperor Taizong and Emperor Gaozong of the Tang Dynasty. For example, the character "葉" (yè) is changed to "X," and "治" (zhì) is altered to "疗" (liáo). However, there is no avoidance of the taboo characters "旦" (dàn) associated with Emperor Ruizong of Tang and "恒" (héng) related to Emperor Muzong of Tang and Emperor Zhenzong of the Northern Song Dynasty. Therefore, it is more likely that these are manuscripts from the early Tang Dynasty.

The S.5614 version of *Five Viscera Theory* (Wǔ Zàng Lùn, 五藏论) housed in the British Library is a relatively complete manuscript. Its content is similar to the P. 2115 version, indicating that both might have originated from the same source or were copied from each other. However, there are a considerable number of missing characters in the S.5614 version (over 300 characters). Fortunately, these missing contents can be found in another two versions of *Five Viscera Theory* (Wǔ Zàng Lùn, 五藏论), the *Categorized Collection of Medical Formulas* (Yī Fāng Lèi Jù, 医方类聚) version and the *Five Viscera Theory* (Wǔ Zàng Lùn, 五藏论) manuscripts found in the Zhejiang region in China.

Following is a direct, word-for-word translation of the British Library's S.5614 version of *Five Viscera Theory* (Wǔ Zàng Lùn, 五藏论). The translation process will strictly adhere to the original text, translating each word and sentence, ensuring that every word and sentence remains faithful to the original text:

《五脏论》一卷 张仲景撰

Wu Zang Lun, One Volume, authored by Zhang Zhongjing

普名之部，出本于医王，皇帝☒，□有一千余卷，耆婆童子，妙闲□□，☒，何能备矣。
Medicine is contributed from the works of (later) various kings of medicine. Yellow Emperor [*unrecognizable*] (*made "The Canon of Acupuncture"*) [*missing*] consists of one thousand volumes, Jivaka has a miracle skill to adept [*missing*]

(*the medicinal function of herbs.*) [*unrecognizable*] (*Moreover, how could one from ordinarily family*) have mastered that!

天有五星，地有五岳，运有五行，人有□□。⊠军，脾为大夫，心为帝王，肝为丞相，⊠。□与胆合，脾与为通，小肠连心，膀胱□□。□□则目赤，心热则口干，肾虚则耳聋，肺风⊠。□□肝候，舌是心观，耳作肾思，鼻为肺应。⊠，⊠肤，肝主于磊，肾主于骨。骨假磊立，肉假皮存，面肿关脾，皮因骨长。故知骨患由肾，磊患则出肝，肉患则伤心，皮患则由肺。

The heaven has five stars, the earth has five mountains, the movement has five phases, and the human body has [*missing*] (*five zang*). [*unrecognizable*] [*So that the lung (liver) is like*] a general, the spleen is like an officer, the heart is like an emperor, the liver (lung) is like a prime minister, [*unrecognizable*] (*the kidney is like a woman with moral integrity*). [*missing*] (*The liver*) works with the gallbladder; the spleen connects with the stomach together. The small intestine links to the heart; and the urinary bladder [*missing*] (*works together with the kidney*). [*Missing*] (*Therefore, liver excess*) causes red eyes; heart heat causes dry mouth; kidney deficiency causes deafness; lung wind [*unrecognizable*] (*causes nose stiffness; spleen disorder causes lip scorched*). [*missing*] (*The eyes are*) the gate of the liver; the tongue is the window of the heart; the ears are the thinker for the kidney; and the nose is the reactor of the lung. [*unrecognizable*] (*The heart rules the blood vessels*); [*unrecognizable*] (*the spleen rules muscle; the lung rules*) the skin; the liver rules the tendons; the kidney rules the bones. Bones depend on tendon to stand straight, muscle depends on skin to exist, face swelling related to spleen, skin depends on bone to grow. Therefore, the bone disorders are resulted from the kidney; the tendon disorders are resulted from the liver; the muscle disorders will damage the heart; the skin disorders are resulted from the lung.

只是十二经脉，上下巡还，八脉寄经，内外流转。三燋六府，四海七身，膔膈咽喉，唇舌牙齿，臂肘指爪，膝胫脚踝，背胁项股，归鼻主，须眉鬓发，俱有患处，并有所因，莫不内积虚劳，外员风习者也。察其颜色，即便寒温；听之音声，便之□□。

There are 12 meridians circulate upward and downward, and eight extraordinary meridians flow in the human body internally and externally. There are also triple burners and six Fu-organs; four seas and seven spirits; the space between the flesh, diaphragm, pharynx, and throat; lips, tongue, and teeth; arm, elbows, fingers, and nails; knees, lower leg, feet, and ankles; back, hypochondriac area, and neck; (head, chin, forehead,) nose; sideburns, eyebrow, mustache, and hair, all the aforementioned places could suffer from illness, and the illness must have their causes, which are either internal deficiency and impairment or external caught wind. By looking at the facial color, you will be able to tell if it is cold syndrome or warm syndrome. By listening to the voice, you will know [*missing*] (*the person has excess or deficiency*).

⊠心病，多火者肾耶，啼哭者患肝，声吟者□□。⊠冷，波青者是风，颜黑者是温，面黄者□□。⊠妄，脾虚则戏饥，肾冷则腰疼，肺⊠。□□者患冷，声沉者患风，声轻者患虚，⊠。□毛则知骨，见爪则知磊，看目则知肝，⊠。⊠齿黑，血伤则皮燋，磊绝则爪干，声⊠，⊠血。余是患者，植表其原，寻原⊠，⊠脏腑，如此委细，乃是良医。⊠，应病与药，无病不除。世无□□，⊠。

[*unrecognizable*] (*Talking a lot could means*) heart sickness; yawn too much means there is kidney evil; whimper and cry are due to the illness of liver, moan and groan [*missing*] (*are because of the illness of spleen*). [*unrecognizable*] (*Pale *skin indicates*) cold in the body; blue skin tone indicates wind invasion; dark facial color indicates warmth in the body; sallow face [*missing*] (*indicates the heat in the body*). [*unrecognizable*] (*The heart wind causes*) preposterous; the spleen deficiency causes hunger; the kidney cold causes the lumbar pain, the lung [*unrecognizable*] [*(liver) excess causes anger*]. [*missing*] (*A soft voice indicates*) suffering from cold, a deep voice indicates suffering from wind, a weak voice indicates suffering from deficiency, [*unrecognizable*] (*and a rough voice indicates suffering from heat*). [*missing*] (*Looking*) at hair can know about the bone (lung), looking at nail can know about tendons, looking at eyes can know about the liver, [*unrecognizable*] (*looking at the teeth can know about bone*). [*unrecognizable*] (*The bone injury causes*) the teeth to turn dark color; the blood injury causes the skin looks burned; the tendon damage causes the nail to be dried. The hoarse voice [*unrecognizable*] (*indicates insufficient qi*), [*unrecognizable*] (*the shouting voice produces swift*) blood flow. Therefore, the patient has external manifestation and internal causes. To find the causes [*unrecognizable*] (*to treat the illness*), [*unrecognizable*] (*to see outside to investigate the inside*) (zang fu organ); if do so, you are a good doctor. [*unrecognizable*] [*(A good doctor) also needs to come up with medical formula carefully.*] You must prescribe the medicine according to the illness. (If do so), no [*missing*] (*disease can't be cured!*). [*unrecognizable*] (*But there is no good doctor now. Half of the patients died due to improper treatments.*)

⧅，□□为贵，头圆法天，足方法地。天有□□，⧅。天有六律，人有六腑。天有七星，人有□□。⧅。□□十二时，人有十二经。天有二十四气，人有二十四□。⧅，⧅六十骨节。天有昼夜，人有睡眠。天有雷□，⧅。⧅，人有眼目。地有草木，人有血脉，地有九□，⧅。⧅石，人有骨齿。地有草木，人有毛发。四大五□，⧅，⧅调，百病俱起。

[*unrecognizable*] (*Between heaven and the earth*), [*missing*] (*the human being*) is the most valued. The head is round shaped that imitates the heaven; the feet are square shaped that imitates the earth. (On the analogy concept), the heaven has [missing] (*four seasons*), [*missing*] (*correspondingly, human has four limbs*); [*unrecognizable*] (*the heaven has five elements, so does human has five zang organs*); the heaven has six rhyms, so does human has six fu organs; the heaven has seven stars, so does human has [*missing*] (*seven orifices*); [*unrecognizable*] (*the heaven has eight kinds of winds, so does human has eight (big) joints*); [*missing*] (*The heaven has*) 12 two-hour periods, so does human has 12 meridians; the heaven has 24 divisions of the solar year, so does human has 24 [*missing*] (*acupuncture shu points*). [*unrecognizable*] (*The heaven has 360 days*), [*unrecognizable*] (*so does human has*) 360 joints; the heaven has day and night, so does human knows when to sleep, the heaven has thunder [*missing*] (*and lightning*), [*unrecognizable*] (*so does human has anger*). [*unrecognizable*] (*The heaven has sun and moon*), so does human has eyes; The earth has spring water, so does human has blood vessels. The earth has nine [*missing*] (*states*), [*unrecognizable*] (*so does human has nine orifices*). [*unrecognizable*] (*The earth has mountains and*) rocks, so does human has bones and teeth. The earth has grass and trees, so does human has hair. The human body is created by four greats and five [*missing*] (*ordinalities*). [*unrecognizable*] (*If one does not*) balance, it will cause hundreds of illnesses.

经曰：神农本草，辩⊠；□□注经，说酸咸而陈冷热。雷公妙典，咸述刨⊠。⊠方，委说根茎之用。周公药对，虚谈犯触□□。⊠，直说五风之妙。扁鹊能回丧车、起死人，⊠；画地割骨除根，患者悉得抽愈。刘涓子秘述，学在鬼边。徐百一之丹方，偏疗小儿之效。淮南葛氏之法，秘要不传；集验之方，人间行用。药疗也，疗人万病，肥白俱解，子孙昌盛，众从爱敬，皆由药性。

Medical classic canon indicated: "Shen Nong Ben Cao" (*Shennong's Classic of Materia Medica*) differentiated [*unrecognizable*] (*the earth to manifest as King and Minister*). [*missing*] (*In "Variorum of the Classic of Materia Medica," Tao Hongjing*) explained sour and salty, discussed cold and hot nature (of the herbs). Lei Gong's marvelous classic talked in detail about herbal processing. [*unrecognizable*] (*Zhang ZhongJing's*) formulas tirelessly discussed the use of stems and roots. "Zhou Gong's pair herbs" concisely talked about the contraindications. [*unrecognizable*] ("*Song Xia Zheng Fang*") directly discusses the wonder of the five winds. Bian Que can call back the funeral canopy, and rescue the people back to life from death, [*unrecognizable*] (*all rely on magical formulas.*) Hua Tuo scratched the bones to eliminate the root of poison. That's why patients can get fully recovered. Liu Juanzi's secret talk was from his learning by the side of the ghost. Xu Baiyi's medical pill formulas, specialized for children's illness. Scholar Ge who came from south of Huai River, kept his formulas secret. Formulas from "The Collection of Clinical Effective Formulas" (Ji Yan, 集验) were used widely. The effect of the herbs and formulas can treat many human illnesses. People recover from taking the medicine. The descendants can be prosperous. They can respect and love each other all because of the effect of the medicine.

只如八味肾气，补六极而差五劳；四色神丹，荡千阿而除万病。有命者必差，虢太子死苏生；无命者难为，秦景公于焉致死。人之养病，如火积薪中，去火如薪得全，去病人皆得活。薪不去火，虚被焚烧；有病不医，徒劳丧命。贵人之所贵，贱人之所贱，昔季康子会药，夫子拜而受之。上故贤圣，由敬其药。是以上中□□，⊠同；甘苦酸咸，随其本性。若能君臣行用，玄疾能□；⊠，□他身命。

For example, Ba Wei Shen Qi (八味肾气丸, Eight-Ingredient Kidney Qi Pills) tonifies six types of extreme deficiencies to recover from five exhaustions. Si Se Shen Dan (四色神丹, Four-Color Magic Pills) cleans up thousands of illnesses to eliminate tens of thousands of diseases. Those destined to live will recover from illness. That's why Prince Guo was revived from death. Those destined to die are difficult to save. That's the reason why Qin Jing Gong died. Treating an illness is like a fire within a pile of firewood; removing the fire keeps the firewood intact, removing the illness allows the person to live. If the firewood is not removed from the fire, it will be burned in vain; if a person's illness is not treated, they will lose their life in vain. One should treat valuable things as being precious and treat valueless things as being worthless. In ancient times, Ji Kangzi gave medicines to Confucius. Confucius bowed and received the medicine with respect. Since ancient times, the saints and intelligence all respected medicine. The plants were divided into upper, middle, [*missing*] (*and lower classes*). [*unrecognizable*] (*Each class treats different conditions*); sweet, bitter, sour, and salty, follows the plant's nature. If one could also use the principle of King and Minister in a formula, even some very difficult diseases could [*missing*] (*be cured*). [*unrecognizable*] (*If prescribed wrong medicine,*) people's life [*missing*] (*could be impaired*).

故本草云：零瑞之草，然则长先；钟乳⊠，⊠。□角有抵触之义，故能趁疰驱耶。牛黄怀⊠，⊠魄。蓝田玉屑，镇压精神；中台射香，差除□□。⊠，□□冷而去腰疼；上蔡防风，愈头风而肠痛。⊠，⊠去头疼；太山伏苓，发阴阳而延年益寿。⊠，⊠之名；大黄宣引众公，乃得将军之号。⊠，⊠藉生姜；当归有致痛之能，相使还⊠。⊠，⊠目聪明；远志、人参，巧含开心益智。

Thus, in "Materia Medica," it said: Ling Rui Zhi Cao (灵瑞之草 or "Ling Zhi" 灵芝, lucid ganoderma) could make people live forever. Taking Zhong Ru (钟乳, stalactite) [*unrecognizable*] (*could make people happier*). Xi Jiao (犀角, rhinoceros horn) has the power to fight against illness, so it can eliminate chronic infectious disease and disperse evil. Niu Huang (牛黄, cattle gallstone) has [*unrecognizable*] [*the function like Chen Xiang (沉香, Chinese eaglewood) to calm the Hun (ethereal soul) and*] the Po (corporeal soul). Yu Xie (玉屑, Jade Chips) from Lan Tian can tranquilize the mind. She Xiang (麝香, musk) from Zhong Tai can drive out [*missing*] (*evil*). [*unrecognizable*] [*Niu Xi (牛膝, twotoothed achyranthes root), from He Nei*], [*missing*] (*treats*) cold knee and relieves lower back pain. Fang Feng (防风, siler root, or divaricate saposhnikovia root) from Shang Cai heals the head wind, also relieves the hypochondriac pain. [*unrecognizable*] [*Long Gu (龙骨, dragon bone fossil, or fossilized animal bone) from Jin Di can stop greediness so to*] relieve headache. Fu Ling (茯苓, Indian bread, or poria) from Tai Shan Mountain balances Yin and Yang to achieve longevity. [*unrecognizable*] [*Gan Cao (甘草, licorice root) has the function of harmonizing*]; thus, it has been called [*unrecognizable*] (*the "Guo Lao"*), a respected elder in the kingdom. Da Huang (大黄, rhubarb root) has the function of opening and inducing the elimination. That's why it was called the "Marshall General." [*unrecognizable*] [*Ban Xia (半夏, pinellia tuber) dissolves phlegm*], raw ginger can [*unrecognizable*] (*counteract its toxicity*). Dang Gui (当归, Chinese angelica root) can stop pain, but it must be combined [*unrecognizable*] [*with Bai Zhi (白芷, Dahurian angelica root)*]. [*unrecognizable*] [*Ze Xie (泽泻, alisma tuber) and Zhu Yu (茱萸 or "Shan Zhu Yu" 山茱萸, cornus fruit) can benefit hearing and vision.*] [*unrecognizable*] [*Yuan Zhi (远志, Thinleaf milkwort root) and Ren Shen (人参, ginseng root) magically open the heart to* make people smart.

赤⊠，⊠。火烧宜怗水苹，杖打稍加营实。非⊠，⊠；⊠耶，急求龙齿。头风起闷，须访菊花；脚⊠，⊠。□□见鬼，久服麻花，拟去白虫，柒和鸡子。墙薇⊠，⊠去柒疮。通草巧疗耳龙，石胆唯除眼莫。

Red [*unrecognizable*] [*ulcer should apply Ji Zi (鸡子, chicken eggs)*]; [*unrecognizable*] [*tuberculoid leprosy needs to use Yue Tao (越桃 or "Zhi Zi" 栀子, gardenia fruit)*]; burns to be treated by applying Shui Ping (水萍 or "Fu Ping" 浮萍, floating duckweed) topically; wounds from caning can use Ying Shi (营实 or "Qiang Wei Zi" 蔷薇子, multiflora Rose Fruit). [*unrecognizable*] [*Pestilential illness uses Xiong Huang (雄黄, realgar) immediately. Sudden frightening*] should ask for Long Chi (龙齿, fossilized animal teeth) immediately. Head wind with dizziness must use Ju Hua (菊花, chrysanthemum flower). [*unrecognizable*] (*Weakness of limbs caused difficult*) walking [*unrecognizable*] [*will be benefit from Shi Hu (石斛, dendrobium stem)*]. If see ghost, consume Ma Hua (麻花, cannabis bud) long-term. If you want to eliminate white parasite, use Qi (漆, lacquer) and Ji Zi (鸡子, chicken eggs). Qiang Wei (蔷薇, multiflora Rose Fruit) [*unrecognizable*] (*can get rid of fungal infection*); [*unrecognizable*] [*Xie Huang (蟹黄, crab yolk) can*] eliminate eczema. Tong Cao (通草, rice paper plant pith) can magically treat deafness; Shi Dan (石胆, chalcanthite) eliminates cataract.

⊠，干柒作蜂窠之刑。丹砂会取光明，升麻只求□□。⊠包。杜仲削去腠皮，桂心取其有味。石英研之□□，⊠。菟丝酒滲乃良凉，朴消火烧方好。防葵为轻□□，⊠唯加。黄芩以附肠为精，藺茹柒头为用。石南□□，□菊收花。五加割取其皮，母丹槌其去骨。鬼箭破血，仍有射鬼之零。神屋除温，非带报神之验。

[*unrecognizable*] [*Qin Jiao (秦艽, largeleaf gentian root) pertains spiral shape*]; Gan Qi (干漆, dried lacquer) looks like honeycomb. Dan Sha (丹砂 or 朱砂, cinnabar) should be shiny; Sheng Ma (升麻, largetrifoliolious bugbane Rhizome) should be [*missing*] (*blue and green*). [*unrecognizable*] [*Qin Jiao (秦椒, prickly ash peel) needs to be steamed; Fan Shi (矾石 or 明矾, a sulfate of alum-stone, or white alum-stone) should be roasted;*] Du Zhong (杜仲, eucommia bark) must peel off the outer skin; Gui Xin (桂心 or 肉桂, cinnamon bark) must have intense fragrance. Shi Ying (石英, Cristobalite) must be powdered; [*unrecognizable*] [*Xing Ren (杏仁, apricot seed) should be grinded until gets creamy*]. Tu Si (菟丝, Chinese dodder seed) must be soaked with alcohol; Pu Xiao (朴硝, a crude form of sodium sulfate) must be calcinated. Fang Kui (防葵, white flower hog fennel root) the lighter [*missing*] (*the better*); [*unrecognizable*] [*Lang Du (狼毒, Bracteole-lacked Euphorbia root) the heavier*] the better. Good Huang Qin (黄芩, Baical skullcap root) looks like rotten intestine; only use Lin Ru's (藺茹, Euphorbia Lanru root) top part. Shi Nan (石南, Chinese photinia Leaf) [*missing*] (*should pick its leaves*); Gan Ju (甘菊, sweet chrysanthemum flower) uses its flower. Wu Jia (五加, Slenderstyle Acanthopanax Bark) only uses the bark; Mu Dan (牡丹, tree peony bark), hammer its stem and take the bone out. Gui Jian (鬼箭 or "Gui Jian Yu" 鬼箭羽, winged branches) can break up the blood stasis thus to kill ghost toxins. Shen Wu (神屋 or "Gui Ban" 龟板, tortoise carapace and plastron) clears the heat and has magical effect.

呕吐汤煎干葛，磊转酒煮木瓜。目赤须点黄连，口疮宜含黄蘗。腂转应痛，须访茵芋；甚痒皮痛，汤煎蒴□。伤寒发汗，要用麻黄；壮热不除，宜加竹葉。恒山鳖甲，大有差疟之功；蛇脱绿丹，善除癫痫之用。雄黄除黑干，木兰能去死皮。莽草煞齿内之虫，藜芦除烂鼻中宿肉。黄连断痢除疳。子支悦愈面皮，桃花润泽肤体。芎藭、枳实，心急即用加之；紫菀、凝冬，气嗽要须當用。虻虫、水犄，即有破血之□。白述、槟榔，有散气消食之效。昌莆强寄，鳖甲通神。

Decoct Gan Ge (干葛 or "Ge Geng" 葛根, dried pueraria root) to treat vomiting; use alcohol to decoct Mu Gua (木瓜, Chinese quince fruit) for muscle spasm. Use Huang Lian (黄连, yellow coptis root) to make eye drops for red eyes. Hold Huang Bo (黄蘗 or "Huang Bo" 黄柏, phellodendron bark) in the mouth for mouth ulcer. Painful arthritis uses Yin Yu (茵芋, Japanese skimmia stem and leaf); [*missing*] (*severe skin itch uses*) Shuo Huo (蒴藋, Chinese elder) decoction. Promote sweat during Shang Han, exogenous pathogenic cold-induced diseases, use Ma Huang (麻黄, ephedra stem). Constant high fever can benefit from Zhu Ye (竹叶, bamboo leaves). Heng Shan (恒山 or "Chang Shan" 常山, dichroa root) and Bie Jia (鳖甲, Chinese soft-shelled turtle shell) have great function to relieve malaria. She Tui (蛇蜕, snake slough) and Lü Dan (绿丹, should be 铝丹, aluminum pill) relieve seizure attacks.

(雄黄, Realgar) is to treat gangrene; Mu Lan (木兰 or "Hou Po" 厚朴, lily magnolia bark) can remove dead skin; Mang Cao (莽草, leaf of poisonous eightangle tree) treats cavity inside the teeth; Li Lu (藜芦, veratrum root and rhizome) can dissolve polyps in the nose. Huang Lian (黄连, yellow coptis root) stops dysentery disease and eliminates malnutrition; Zi Zhi (子支 or Zi Zhi 栀子, gardenia fruit) benefits facial skin; Tao Hua (桃花, peach blossom) can moisten body skin. Xiong Qiong (芎藭 or "Chuan Xiong" 川芎, Sichuan lovage rhizome) and Zhi Shi (枳实, immature range fruit) treat anxiety; Zi Wan (紫菀, Tatarian aster root) and Kuan Dong (款冬, Common coltsfoot flower) are used for asthma and cough. Mang Chong (虻虫, horse fly) and Shui Zhi (水蛭, leech) are to break blood stagnation; Bai Zhu (白术, white Atractylodes tuber) and Bing Lang (槟榔, areca nut) relieve bloating and promote digestion. Chang Pu (菖蒲 or "Shi Chang Pu" 石菖蒲, grassleaf sweetflag rhizome) enhances memory; Bie Jia (鳖甲, Chinese soft-shelled turtle shell) promotes spiritual function.

阴疮汤□蛇床，淋涩须加滑石。仙零脾草能去腰疼，然则忘杖归家。犬鼠煎膏巧疗耳聋，得蓖麻而加妙。蛇咬宜封人粪，蜂螫荜茇妙除。零羊角通噎驱耶，青羊肝疗疳明目。石脂加颜发色，白及卷面除皮。知母通痢开胸，空青消徵止泪。孔公孽消食肥择，密陀僧去疥癞人。压石寄假蜂房，水肿惟须仗□。肠结通惟须甘遂，患眼宜取蕤仁。安胎必藉紫威，伤身要须地髓。恼心闷偏加木笔，血闭急觅蒲黄。□翘脚累□疮痈，地胆破徵瘕息宍。斑猫能除鼠漏，松脂抽恶刺风疽。牵牛写水排脓，葶苈伐枣池水。桃人绝其鬼气，石南伤去诸风。瘿气菎布妙除。仕瘴必须硝石，脱公宜取鳖头。下贱虽曰地浆，天行病飲者皆愈；黄龙汤出其厕内，时气病者能除。贫者虽号小方，不及君臣，取写有处，出处有灵有验，有贵有贱，有高有下，净秽亢草山中药。

Vaginal discharge, exterior vaginal itching, and redness, use She Chuang (蛇床, common cnidium fruit) to decoct. Urgent or hesitate urination, add Hua Shi (滑石, talc). Xian Lin Pi (仙灵脾 or "Yin Yang Huo" 淫羊藿, horny goat weed, or epimedium) relieves lower back pain so that the patient can walk back home without the crutches. Syrup made from Tian Shu (天鼠 or "Bian Fu" 蝙蝠, sky rat, or bat) treats deafness, to add Bi Ma (蓖麻, castor leaf or bean) for better results. Topically cover with Ren Fen (人粪 or "Ren Zhong Huang" 人中黄, human excrement) for snake bite; bee sting can be treated by Bi Ba (荜茇, long pepper, or piper longum). Ling Yang Jiao (零羊角 or 羚羊角, antelope's horn) is for esophageal obstruction and to eliminate evil. Qing Yang Gan (青羊肝, goral liver) treats malnutrition (anemia) and brightens vision. Shi Zhi (石脂, halloysite) darkens hair; Bai Ji (白芨, bletilla tuber) removes dead skin and regenerates new skin. Zhi Mu (知母, common anemarrhena rhizome) treats dysentery and opens chest; Kong Qing (空青, azurite) relieves bloating and stops tearing. Kong Gong Nie (孔公孽, Calcite) helps digest food and gains weight. Mi Tuo Seng (密陀僧, lithargite) treats eczema and skin infection. Feng Fang (蜂房, honeycomb) used to calm down the rebellious Qi caused by taking Ru Shi (乳石, stalactite). Edema can use [*missing*] [*Da Ji (大戟, Peking spurge root)*]. Intestinal obstruction uses Gan Sui (甘遂, gansui root). Eye disease uses Rui Ren (蕤仁, hedge prinsepia nut). Calm down fetus must use Zi Wei (紫威or 紫薇, Chinese Trumpetcreeper Flower); Di Sui (地髓 or Gan Di Huang 干地黄, drying rehmannia root) is for physical exhaustion. Mentally depress use Mu Bi (木笔 or "Xin Yi Hua" 辛夷花, magnolia flower); amenorrhea uses Pu Huang (蒲黄, cat-tail pollen) immediately. Scrofula and boils use (连翘, weeping forsythia Capsule); Di Dan (地胆, a kind of blister beetles) treats mass, nodules, and polyps. Ban Mao (斑猫, mylabris, or blister) can treat chronic skin abscess; Song Zhi (松脂, pine resin) is anti-infection. It can promote discharge of pus. Qian Niu (牵牛, morning glory) is a strong diuretic to reduce swelling. It also helps discharge pus; Ting Li (葶苈 or "Ting Li Zi" 葶苈子, tansymustard seed) and Da Zao (大枣, Chinese date) eliminate edema. Tao Ren (桃人 or 桃仁, peach kernel) stops evil energy; Shi Nan (石南, Chinese photinia Leaf) to eliminate all kinds of internal wind. Kun Bu (昆布, kombu, or sea tangle) relieves goiter; Xiao Shi (硝石or "Mang Xiao" 芒硝, nitrate from saline alkali land) treats intestinal abscess; Bie Tou (鳖头, soft-shell turtle head) treats rectal prolapse. Regardless of the degrading name of "Di Jiang (地浆, Earth Slurry)," Tian Xing Bing, epidemic diseases caused by natural factors, gets healed by taking Di Jiang (地浆, Earth Slurry). Although Huang Long Tang (黄龙汤, Yellow Dragon Decoction) came from toilet, it can treat infectious disease. Although small formula was considered lower class, it doesn't even have King and Minister herbs in the formulation (still, you know) where the formula originally come from. And the formula is clinically proven, the medicine could be expensive or cheap, and the herbs could be higher or lower class and clean or dirty. They are all come from the nature.

《五脏论》一卷

"Wu Zang Lun," one volume.

REFERENCES

1. The British Library and The Dunhuang-Turfan Academic Society of China, Dunhuang Manuscripts Editorial Committee and The Institute of History, Chinese Academy of Social Sciences and The School of Oriental and African Studies, University of London, *Dunhuang Manuscripts in British Collections* (Chinese texts other than Buddhist scriptures): Volume 8 (S.5551-S.5644) (Chengdu: Sichuan People's Publishing House, 1992), 151–154.
2. 罗福颐,"西陲古方技书残卷汇编[J]." *中华医史杂志*, Vol. 4, No. 1 (1953): 27–30.
3. 王慶菽,"英國倫敦不列顛博物館藏敦煌卷子中的古代醫方(一) [J]." *医学史与保健组织*, No. 1 (1958): 64–71.
4. 王慶菽,"英國倫敦不列顛博物館藏敦煌卷子中的古代醫方(二) [J]." 医学史与保健组织, No. 4 (1958): 315–316.
5. 三木栄,"西域出土医薬関係文献総合解説目録[J]." *東洋學報*, Vol. 47, No. 6 (1964): 140–164.
6. 宫下三郎,"張仲景五蔵論について[J]." *漢方の臨床*, Vol. 6, No. 4 (1959): 187–192.
7. 宫下三郎,"敦煌本張仲景《五藏論》校譯注[J]." *東方學報(京都)*, Vol. 35, No. 3 (1964): 289–330.
8. 姜春华,"伟大医学家张仲景[J]." *自然杂志*, Vol. 6, No. 5 (1983): 375–378.
9. 廖国玉,"张仲景官居长沙太守的三项根据[J]." *中医杂志*, No. 4 (1982): 71–72.
10. 姜春华,"张仲景著作略考[J]." 上海中医药杂志, No. 7 (1962): 12.
11. 马继兴, *敦煌古医籍考释[M]* (南昌: 江西科学技术出版社, 1988), 28.

8 Survived through the Wars – The *Categorized Collection of Medical Formulas* Edition

"In the 12th year during the reign of Goryeo Munjong, newly carved . . . and 'Zhang Zhongjing Wu Zang Lun' were all received by the Imperial Archives."

– Chŭngbo munhŏn pigo kwŏn

This version of *Five Viscera Theory* (Wǔ Zàng Lùn, 五藏论) is a medical text included in volume 4, "Wu Zang" (Five Viscera) section of the Korean medical compendium *Categorized Collection of Medical Formulas* (Yī Fāng Lèi Jù, 医方类聚). The author is not mentioned in the book.

The version cited in this chapter is the Jiuzhou edition,[1] published in August 2002, exactly 520 years following the initial printing of *Categorized Collection of Medical Formulas* (Yī Fāng Lèi Jù, 医方类聚). This was a collaborative publication by the China Association for Culture Studies and Beijing Jiuzhou Press. During the printing process, they referred to the version stored in Japan's Imperial Household Agency and used the Kitamurana Ohira's "Bunkyū gannen" edition as the blueprint, creating a facsimile edition identical in size to the original.

In the previous chapter, we mentioned Japanese scholar Miyazaki Saburo as the first to undertake an in-depth study of Zhang Zhongjing's *Five Viscera Theory* (Wǔ Zàng Lùn, 五藏论) among the Dunhuang manuscripts. He meticulously examined and compared three precious Dunhuang manuscripts: S.5614, P. 2755, and P. 2378. Additionally, he included, sentence by sentence, the content of *Five Viscera Theory* (Wǔ Zàng Lùn, 五藏论) found in the Korean *Categorized Collection of Medical Formulas* (Yī Fāng Lèi Jù, 医方类聚) into his research paper. It was during this research that Miyazaki Saburo discovered striking similarities between the Dunhuang manuscript of Zhang Zhongjing's *Five Viscera Theory* (Wǔ Zàng Lùn, 五藏论) and the version in *Categorized Collection of Medical Formulas* (Yī Fāng Lèi Jù, 医方类聚).[2] This led him to speculate that these two texts might have originated from the same medical book. This poses an intriguing question: Why does Zhang Zhongjing's *Five Viscera Theory* (Wǔ Zàng Lùn, 五藏论) from China appear in the Korean *Categorized Collection of Medical Formulas* (Yī Fāng Lèi Jù, 医方类聚)?

Medical exchanges between China and Korea have deep historical roots.[3] According to ancient records, Korea, around the 1st century AD, was split into the

DOI: 10.1201/9781032698205-8

kingdoms of Goguryeo, Silla, and Baekje. In Baekje, notably, there was a dedicated "Medicine Department" for handling herbs, where the medicinal materials were strikingly similar to those in China. The rich tapestry of Chinese medical literature, including works like *Supplementary Records of Famous Physicians* (Míng Yī Bié Lù, 名医别录) by Tao Hongjing from the Liang Dynasty, even delve into fascinating comparisons between Korean ginseng varieties from Baekje and Goryeo and their Chinese counterpart from Shangdang.

During the Southern and Northern dynasties period, Emperor Wu of Liang responded to Baekje's request by sending doctors to Korea to conduct medical activities. This move not only signified a strengthening of ties but also marked the introduction and spread of acupuncture techniques in Korea. Fast forward to the Tang Dynasty, an epoch of Chinese history renowned for its flourishing economy, political harmony, and swift advancements in medical and health sectors. This golden age became a magnet for merchants, monks, and scholars from across the globe, drawn by the dynasty's stability and cultural richness.

During this period, several medical classics, such as *Basic Questions* (Sù Wèn, 素问), *Treatise on Cold Damage Disorders* (Shāng Hán Lùn, 伤寒论), *A-B Canon of Acupuncture and Moxibustion* (Zhēn Jiǔ Jiǎ Yǐ Jīng, 针灸甲乙经), *Shennong's Classic of Materia Medica* (Shén Nóng Běn Cǎo Jīng, 神农本草经), *General Treatise on Causes and Manifestations of All Diseases* (Zhū Bìng Yuán Hòu Lùn, 诸病源候论), *Essential Formulas for Emergencies [Worth] a Thousand Pieces of Gold* (Qiān Jīn Yào Fāng, 千金要方), and *Arcane Essentials from the Imperial Library* (Wài Tái Mì Yào, 外台秘要), were introduced into Silla. As a vassal state of the Tang Dynasty, Silla's medical system was modeled after the Tang's, including the establishment of medical educational institutions and the position of medical doctor (physician). Texts such as *Basic Questions* (Sù Wèn, 素问), the *Canon of Difficult Issues* (Nàn Jīng, 难经), *A-B Canon of Acupuncture and Moxibustion* (Zhēn Jiǔ Jiǎ Yǐ Jīng, 针灸甲乙经), and *Shennong's Classic of Materia Medica* (Shén Nóng Běn Cǎo Jīng, 神农本草经) were used as teaching materials to train professional doctors.

With the establishment and unification of the Korean Peninsula under the Goryeo Dynasty in 918, an end came to the eras of Silla and Baekje, ushering in a new phase in the relationship between Korea and China. After Zhao Kuangyin founded the Song Dynasty in 960, Goryeo began paying tribute to the Song Dynasty. In 963, Goryeo officially adopted the Song Dynasty's era name, thereby becoming a vassal state of the Song Dynasty.

During the reign of Emperor Zhenzong of the Song Dynasty, specifically in the ninth year of Dazhong Xiangfu (1016) and the fifth year of Tianxi (1021), the Song Dynasty gifted the medical classic *Taiping Holy Prescriptions for Universal Relief* (Tài Píng Shèng Huì Fāng, 太平圣惠方) to Goryeo on two separate occasions. Following this, other significant medical texts like the *Illustrated Pharmacopoeia* (Běn Cǎo Tú Jīng, 本草图经) and *Prescriptions of the Bureau of Taiping People's Welfare Pharmacy* (Tàipíng Huì Mín Hé Jì Jú Fāng, 太平惠民和剂局方) also made their way to Goryeo. Goryeo not only treasured these medical books from China but also reprinted and published them, facilitating a wider spread and development of traditional Chinese medicine in the region. Through such exchanges, Traditional

Chinese Medicine deeply ingrained itself in Goryeo, becoming an integral part of the local healthcare system.

However, this period of prosperity was short-lived. During the same era as the Song Dynasty, formidable forces, the Liao Dynasty and the Jin Dynasty, successively emerged along the northern borders of mainland China. In the history of China, the Northern Song Dynasty had the smallest territory of any centralized empire in the Central Plains, bordered to the north by today's Haihe River, Bazhou in Hebei, and Yanmen Pass in Shanxi, sharing borders with the Liao. This meant that the Liao, located to the north of the Song, effectively blocked overland routes between the Song Dynasty and Goryeo, leaving the Song to rely solely on maritime routes for communication with Goryeo. The Liao Dynasty was later conquered by the Jin Dynasty. Consequently, Goryeo found itself neighbored by Liao and then Jin on land. Pressured by the military might of Liao and Jin, Goryeo was compelled to pay tribute and acknowledge vassalage to these states. Under the obstruction and interference of Liao or Jin, the relationship between the Song and Goryeo fluctuated, experiencing periods of both harmony and disconnection, with tribute missions at times even ceasing entirely.

In the early 11th century, Goryeo entered a longer period of peace, during which its relations with the Song, Liao, and Jin were often cautiously neutral. Both the Goryeo and Song dynasties subjectively hoped to maintain security between their nations through economic and cultural exchanges. However, given the political complexities, interactions between the Song and Goryeo relied more on private, people-to-people exchanges.

In the 33rd year of Goryeo's King Munjong's reign (1079), Munjong, who was suffering from an ailment caused by wind (possibly a reference to a neurological or respiratory condition), sent a formal request through Goryeo's Ministry of Rites to the Dazaifu in Japan. In this request, Munjong earnestly asked the Dazaifu to select a renowned physician from Japan who was skilled in treating such illnesses. He hoped that this doctor could be dispatched to Goryeo in the early spring of the following year to treat his condition.

King Munjong's quest for medical help from Japan might have been sparked by an enchanting tale from King Seongjong's time, a story that later found its way into the "Genkō Shakusho." It revolves around a queen, famous for her stunning beauty and dearly loved by the king. Despite her youth, she was troubled by her prematurely greying hair, and no remedy seemed to work. Then one night, she dreamt of the powerful Kannon at Japan's Katsuo-ji Temple. Moved by the dream, she prayed earnestly towards Japan. That night, she dreamt again, this time of a luminous mountain in Japan, and woke up to find her hair had magically turned black again. Overjoyed, King Seongjong expressed his gratitude by sending lavish gifts like golden drums and bells to Katsuo-ji Temple, a gesture that became a part of this enduring legend.

The year following King Munjong's request for medical assistance from Japan, the merchant Wang Zezhen brought his plea to Japan, presenting it through the Dazaifu to the Japanese imperial court. After several deliberations, the Japanese court officials not only declined the medical assistance request from the Goryeo king but also issued an official response that sternly criticized the improprieties in the request submitted by Goryeo. This incident, historically known as "The Incident of King Munjong of Goryeo's Request for a Physician," showcased the complex and nuanced diplomatic relations between the two countries at the time.

Interestingly, a year prior to reaching out to Japan, King Munjong had made a similar request for medical assistance to China.[4] In stark contrast to Japan's cool response, Emperor Shenzong of the Song Dynasty expressed deep concern for King Munjong's health. The following year, he sent a medical team of 88 members to Goryeo to provide treatment. Additionally, the Song Dynasty gifted over a hundred varieties of precious medicinal herbs to Goryeo. This gesture marked the formal resumption of diplomatic relations between the Song Dynasty and Goryeo, which had been disrupted for decades due to pressure from the Liao Dynasty. Consequently, diplomatic exchanges between the two countries became more frequent. The Song Dynasty also sent medical officials to Goryeo several times to impart medical knowledge and techniques.

Until 1122, when Goryeo once again requested medical assistance from the Song Dynasty, the Song government responded by dispatching two medical officials. They returned after two years, and following this, the "Han Medicine" system in Goryeo, primarily based on traditional Chinese medicine, began to flourish. Numerous medical institutions were established across Goryeo, such as the Office of Benefitting People (Hyeminguk, 혜민국), Bureau of Saving People (Hwalinseo, 활인서), the Palace Dispensary (Naeuiwon, 내의원), and the Palace Medical Office (Jeonuigam, 전의감). These were founded in imitation of the Song Dynasty's medical system. Therefore, it can be said that King Munjong's request to the Song Dynasty for physicians and medicinal materials has become a symbolic event marking the restoration of diplomatic relations between the Song and Goryeo kingdoms.

Apart from sending physicians to Goryeo to provide treatment and impart medical knowledge, the exchange of texts also played a crucial role. Before the Song Dynasty, due to the lack of printing technology, book production was extremely limited, and distribution was restricted. At that time, the exchange of books between China and the Korean Peninsula was mainly conducted through religious organizations or official channels. However, with the advent and popularization of printing technology during the Song era, the complexity and cost of book production significantly decreased. Books gradually became an important commodity in trade, transforming what was primarily official cultural exchange into a commercial activity. This shift opened up new avenues for the dissemination of knowledge and ideas between the two regions.

Goryeo always held Chinese medical texts in high regard. During their tributary missions to China, Goryeo's envoys frequently requested books as gifts. The emperors of the Song Dynasty not only bestowed many significant texts upon Goryeo but also included a variety of other books, such as works on philosophy, history, geomancy, geography, and calendars. Moreover, they allowed Goryeo's envoys to copy these books, which was a significant gesture of intellectual exchange. Additionally, the Song Dynasty opened up its book markets, permitting Goryeo's envoys to purchase the books they needed. This open access to literature played a vital role in enhancing the knowledge and cultural connections between the two kingdoms.

With the continuous influx of Chinese medical texts, Goryeo gradually embraced and inherited numerous classics of traditional Chinese medicine. These included seminal works like *Basic Questions* (Sù Wèn, 素问), *A-B Canon of Acupuncture and Moxibustion* (Zhēn Jiǔ Jiǎ Yǐ Jīng, 针灸甲乙经), *Shennong's Classic of Materia Medica with Collected Commentaries* (Shén Nóng Běn Cǎo Jīng Jí Zhù, 神农本草经集注), *General Treatise on Causes and Manifestations of All Diseases* (Zhū Bìng Yuán Hòu Lùn, 诸病源候论), *Essential Formulas for Emergencies [Worth] a Thousand Pieces of Gold* (Qiān Jīn Yào Fāng, 千金要方), and *Arcane Essentials from the Imperial Library* (Wài Tái Mì Yào, 外台秘要). Goryeo's medical education system, modeled after the Tang Dynasty, utilized texts such as *Shennong's Classic of Materia Medica* (Shén Nóng Běn Cǎo Jīng, 神农本草经), *A-B Canon of Acupuncture and Moxibustion* (Zhēn Jiǔ Jiǎ Yǐ Jīng, 针灸甲乙经), *Basic Questions* (Sù Wèn, 素问), *Classic of Acupuncture* (Zhēn Jīng, 针经), *Pulse Classic* (Mài Jīng, 脉经), *Yellow Emperor's Classic of Mingtang* (Huáng Dì Míng Táng Jīng, 黄帝明堂经), and *Yellow Emperor's Canon of 81 Difficult Issues* (Huáng Dì Bā Shí Yī Nàn Jīng, 黄帝八十一难经) as core teaching materials. This approach significantly enriched and advanced Goryeo's medical knowledge and practices.

On the other hand, when officials or professionals from the Song Dynasty visited Goryeo, they brought back some precious books to China, including medical works that had been lost in China itself. For instance, the *The Yellow Emperor's Classic of Acupuncture* (Huáng Dì Zhēn Jīng, 黄帝针经), gifted by Goryeo to the Northern Song Dynasty, was a book that had become untraceable in China at that time. In fact, *The Yellow Emperor's Classic of Acupuncture* (Huáng Dì Zhēn Jīng, 黄帝针经) is what is widely known today as *Yellow Emperor's Classic of Internal Medicine • Divine Pivot* (Huáng Dì Nèi Jīng • Líng Shū, 黄帝内经•灵枢).

While political relations between the Song Dynasty and Goryeo sometimes saw ups and downs, the two empires consistently nurtured a warm and close cultural bond. A notable highlight in this cultural exchange is detailed in the *History of Goryeo* (Gāo Lì Shǐ, 高丽史): In 1058, during King Munjong's twelfth year and the third year of Emperor Renzong's Jiayou era in the Northern Song Dynasty, Goryeo received exquisitely carved new editions of seven medical classics. These treasures included *Yellow Emperor's Canon of 81 Difficult Issues* (Huáng Dì Bā Shí Yī Nàn Jīng, 黄帝八十一难经), *Chuan Yu Ji* (川玉集), *Treatise on Cold Damage Disorders* (Shāng Hán Lùn, 伤寒论), *Summarization of the Essentials of Materia Medica* (Běn Cǎo Kuò Yào, 本草括要), *Chao's Etiology of Children's Diseases* (Xiǎo'ér Cháo Shì Bìng Yuán, 小儿巢氏病源), *Eighteen Discussions of the Medications, Symptoms, and Causes of Pediatric Diseases* (Xiǎo'ér Yào Zhèng Bìng Yuán Yī Shí Bā Lùn, 小儿药证病源一十八论), and Zhang Zhongqing's *Five Viscera Theory* (Zhāng Zhòng Qīng Wǔ Zàng Lùn, 张仲卿五脏论). Crafted on 99 woodblocks from the Song era, these texts were revered as invaluable cultural assets and were carefully preserved in the Imperial Archives of Goryeo.[5]

Another work titled *Supplemented Documents for Reference* (Chŭngbo munhŏn pigo kwŏn, 增补文献备考) meticulously categorizes and organizes all cultural and institutional artifacts from the ancient period of Goryeo to the end of the Korean Empire. This book also documents the batch of medical classics presented to

Goryeo in the twelfth year of King Munjong's reign, including a mention of Zhang Zhongjing's *Five Viscera Theory* (Zhāng Zhòng Jǐng Wǔ Zàng Lùn, 张仲景五脏论).[6] This record indicates that the Goryeo royal family indeed owned Zhang Zhongjing's *Five Viscera Theory* (Wǔ Zàng Lùn, 五藏论). Although the historical texts do not detail the specific contents of these medical books, lending a layer of mystery to this version of *Five Viscera Theory* (Wǔ Zàng Lùn, 五藏论), it is reasonable to infer, given the status of these medical carvings as prized gifts to the Goryeo royal family, that they were unlikely to be forgeries.

At that time, Song Dynasty was facing crises along its northern borders, while Goryeo endeavored to strike a balance between the Liao Dynasty and the Song Dynasty, thus maintaining a neutral stance with both. In fact, a month before the Goryeo received those 99 woodblock carvings of medical texts, including Zhang Zhongjing's *Five Viscera Theory* (Zhāng Zhòng Jǐng Wǔ Zàng Lùn, 张仲景五脏论), the Jurchens from the Liao Dynasty (Khitan) also gifted precious thoroughbred horses and treasured swords to Goryeo as symbols of diplomatic goodwill.

At the same time, a merchant from the Huang family in Quanzhou, part of the Song Dynasty, brought gifts to Goryeo. The *Baoqing Siming Records* (Bǎo Qìng Sì Míng Zhì, 宝庆四明志) of the Song era detail this interaction. Huang Shen, a merchant from Anhai in Quanzhou, Fujian, changed his name to Huang Zhen, also known as Huang Jin, because his birth name shared the temple name of Emperor Xiaozong of the Song. Since the Southern Tang period (937–975 AD), Quanzhou had been an important center for managing overseas trade, particularly maintaining robust maritime trade links with Goryeo. Huang Shen's father, Huang Guanglüe, had once traveled to Goryeo as an envoy from the Southern Tang but sadly died there, leaving his family to continue the trade legacy. Throughout the Song Dynasty, the Huang family remained actively engaged in maritime commerce with Goryeo.

Song Dynasty merchants played a crucial role in rekindling diplomatic ties between the Song and Goryeo kingdoms, making a notable impact on the evolution of their relationship. Emperors of the Song specifically chose these merchants as envoys to Goryeo. King Munjong of Goryeo enthusiastically welcomed these special merchant emissaries, offering them a grand reception. Together, they deliberated on re-establishing diplomatic links between the two countries. Merchants like Huang Shen, as mentioned earlier, were instrumental in fostering this diplomatic thaw, carrying imperial messages that helped bridge the Northern Song and Goryeo kingdoms. Hence, gifts like Zhang Zhongjing's *Five Viscera Theory* (Wǔ Zàng Lùn, 五藏论), presented by the Song to the Goryeo royalty, were not just symbols of cultural exchange but also tangible markers of the renewed friendship between the two countries.

On the other hand, officials or professionals from the Song Dynasty, upon visiting Goryeo, brought back to China some valuable books as well, including medical works that had already been lost in mainland China. One example is the *The Yellow Emperor's Classic of Acupuncture* (Huáng Dì Zhēn Jīng, 黄帝针经) that Goryeo presented to the Northern Song. This book was untraceable in Song Dynasty China at the time. In November of the eighth year of the Dae'an reign of Goryeo's King Yejong (1092, the seventh year of Emperor Zhezong's Yuanfeng reign in China), Goryeo sent envoys to China, offering the *The Yellow Emperor's Classic of Acupuncture* (Huáng Dì Zhēn Jīng, 黄帝针经) among other books, with a request to exchange for the *Comprehensive Mirror to Aid in Government* (Zī Zhì Tōng Jiàn, 资治通鉴) and the *Primary [divination] tortoise of the records office* (Cè Fǔ Yuán Guī, 册府元龟). This proposal for a book exchange met with firm opposition from the renowned Su Dongpo, who petitioned against it five times. However, Emperor Zhezong of the Northern Song did not heed his advice. Emperor Zhezong even issued a decree to have the *The Yellow Emperor's Classic of Acupuncture* (Huáng Dì Zhēn Jīng, 黄帝针经) that Goryeo presented published and distributed throughout China, thus reintroducing the *The Yellow Emperor's Classic of Acupuncture* (Huáng Dì Zhēn Jīng, 黄帝针经) back to China,[7] which is widely known today as *Yellow Emperor's Classic of Internal Medicine • Divine Pivot* (Huáng Dì Nèi Jīng • Líng Shū, 黄帝内经•灵枢).

Woodblock printing, a pioneering technique that emerged during the Tang Dynasty in China, often employed high-quality hardwoods like rosewood for their fine grain and durability. The method starts with slicing the wood into individual blocks. The intended text is first written on thin paper, which is then affixed face-down to the block. Artisans meticulously carve the text in relief, ensuring each character protrudes from the block's surface, ready for printing. These meticulously carved blocks, once finished, are used to produce books. Known as "irreplaceable editions," these blocks are unique; if damaged or lost, they cannot be replaced, rendering many books as rare, once-in-a-lifetime editions. This rarity is why ancient collectors especially treasured books from the Song Dynasty.

As woodblock and movable clay type printing technologies made their way into Goryeo, the kingdom's book printing industry flourished significantly. There was a growing appetite for Chinese classics, notably Confucian and Buddhist scriptures, to the point where Goryeo was acclaimed for having the most refined Confucian scholarship among all overseas regions. The influx of books from China soon fell short of meeting Goryeo's burgeoning demand. This led to Goryeo's own initiative of reprinting Chinese texts, employing woodblock or movable type printing methods. These freshly printed editions were either safeguarded in the imperial archives, distributed to government agencies, or presented as gifts to officials and the elite. Through such endeavors, Goryeo not only augmented its cultural treasury but also played a pivotal role in the preservation and propagation of ancient Chinese cultural heritage.

The spread of Chinese literature in Goryeo reached remarkable heights by the Song Dynasty, amassing an extraordinary collection that included texts long lost within China itself. In his work *Gui Er Ji* (贵耳集), Zhang Duanyi recounts a mission during the Xuanhe period to Goryeo, where an envoy discovered that Goryeo's collection of books from China spanned from the pre-Qin era through the dynasties of Jin, Tang, Sui, and Liang, comprising a vast array of works from thousands of authors and spanning thousands of volumes, all preserved from the ravages of war. This unparalleled collection was so extensive and comprehensive that it was possibly unmatched even within China. Consequently, the Song Dynasty turned to Goryeo in search of books that had disappeared from China, a testament to Goryeo's significant role in safeguarding and perpetuating Chinese cultural heritage. Among Goryeo's contributions, the *Categorized Collection of Medical Formulas* (Yī Fāng Lèi Jù,

医方类聚) stands out as a luminous jewel in its medical literature, reflecting the depth and richness of its cultural preservation efforts.

The *Categorized Collection of Medical Formulas* (Yī Fāng Lèi Jù, 医方类聚), an extensive medical compilation, was conceived under the directive of Sejong, the fourth ruler of the Goryeo Dynasty, involving a collaboration between civil servants and medical experts. Initiated in the 25th year of Sejong's reign (1443),[8] this ambitious project unfolded over three years, culminating in its finalization and printing in 1477, during the eighth year of King Seongjong's reign. This inaugural edition was limited to a mere 30 copies, encapsulating 153 medical texts from Korea and China – 152 from China and just one Korean work. These texts spanned a historical breadth of about 2,000 years, from the pre-Qin era through to the early Ming Dynasty. Comprising 266 volumes across 264 books and containing over 9.5 million characters with more than 5,000 formulas, its enormity rivals that of the Ming Dynasty's *Universal Relief Prescription* (Pǔ Jì Fāng, 普济方), known for its comprehensive collection of medical prescriptions. Today, unfortunately, only a single complete set remains, housed not in Korea but within the rare collections of the Shoryobu (Archives and Mausolea Department Building) in Japan, marking it as an extraordinarily precious artifact.

Why would a Korean national treasure find its home in Japan? To answer this, we must look back to the turbulent period between 1592 and 1598, when Toyotomi Hideyoshi, a Japanese military leader, launched two invasions into Korea, events historically remembered as the Imjin War. It was during these invasions that daimyō Kato Kiyomasa of Japan seized the *Categorized Collection of Medical Formulas* (Yī Fāng Lèi Jù, 医方类聚) as war booty and transported it back to Japan. After arriving in Japan, this invaluable medical manuscript underwent a series of handovers. Initially, it was housed with Sendai's physician Kyūkei Kudō, then circulated through institutions such as the Edo Medical School, the University Eastern School's Library, the Asakusa Bookstore, and the Ueno Imperial Museum before ultimately being safeguarded by the Shoryobu (Archives and Mausolea Department Building).

During its time at the Edo Medical School, the *Categorized Collection of Medical Formulas* (Yī Fāng Lèi Jù, 医方类聚) was meticulously replicated under the supervision of the renowned traditional Chinese medicine practitioner Kitamurana Ohira. This effort culminated in the famous 1861 edition of the *Categorized Collection of Medical Formulas* (Yī Fāng Lèi Jù, 医方类聚). This version was later gifted back to Korea by a Japanese envoy and then, in 1965, Lee Jong-kyu, the president of Dongyang Medical College (now Kyung Hee University's College of Medicine) in South Korea, organized a monumental effort involving thousands of people to sort and ultimately publish this work. After more than half a year of dedicated work, this collection, weathered by over 500 years of history, was once again published in its homeland, Korea, where it received widespread application and recognition.

In China, significant achievements have been made in the study and reproduction of the *Categorized Collection of Medical Formulas* (Yī Fāng Lèi Jù, 医方类聚). In 1981, a team of scholars led by Sheng Zengxiu from the Zhejiang Institute of traditional Chinese medicine meticulously proofread the 1861 edition of the *Categorized Collection of Medical Formulas* (Yī Fāng Lèi Jù, 医方类聚), which was published by the People's Medical Publishing House. Following this, in 2002, the Chinese Cultural Society collaborated with Beijing Jiuzhou Publishing House to publish a facsimile of the *Categorized Collection of Medical Formulas* (Yī Fāng Lèi Jù, 医方类聚) that matched the original in size. The version referenced in this chapter is precisely this edition.

By 2006, the Zhejiang Academy of traditional Chinese medicine undertook a meticulous re-examination of the 1981 proofread edition, resulting in a revised version published and distributed by the People's Medical Publishing House. This new edition also included an additional volume of indexes, designed to facilitate easier reference and research for readers.[9]

The *Categorized Collection of Medical Formulas* (Yī Fāng Lèi Jù, 医方类聚) encompasses a wide range of texts, including renowned medical works like *Basic Questions* (Sù Wèn, 素问), *Divine Pivot* (Líng Shū, 灵枢), *Canon of Difficult Issues* (Nàn Jīng, 难经), *Treatise on Cold Damage Disorders* (Shāng Hán Lùn, 伤寒论), *Essential Prescriptions from the Golden Cabinet* (Jīn Guì Yào Lüè, 金匮要略), *Pulse Classic* (Mài Jīng, 脉经), *General Treatise on Causes and Manifestations of All Diseases* (Zhū Bìng Yuán Hòu Lùn, 诸病源候论), *Essential Formulas for Emergencies [Worth] a Thousand Pieces of Gold* (Qiān Jīn Yào Fāng, 千金要方), *Taiping Holy Prescriptions for Universal Relief* (Tài Píng Shèng Huì Fāng, 太平圣惠方), *Confucians' Duties to Parents* (Rú Mén Shì Qīn, 儒门事亲), and *Clear Synopsis on Recipes* (Xuān Míng Lùn Fāng, 宣明论方) among others. It adopts a classification system primarily based on the type of disease while also considering the location and cause of the illness. The entire collection is divided into 95 categories, covering diseases across various clinical disciplines such as internal medicine, surgery, gynecology, pediatrics, otorhinolaryngology, emergency medicine, and dermatology, making it a comprehensive and in-depth medical encyclopedia.

The *Categorized Collection of Medical Formulas* (Yī Fāng Lèi Jù, 医方类聚) adheres to a stringent academic standard when citing references: whenever it quotes from a book, it always clearly states the title first, followed by an exact transcription of the original text, with no alterations or omissions. Among the 152 Chinese medical texts referenced in the compilation, 35 original works have been lost in China, and the status of another two is still uncertain. It is precisely because of this faithful preservation of the original texts that the *Categorized Collection of Medical Formulas* (Yī Fāng Lèi Jù, 医方类聚) provides invaluable material for the reconstruction and study of those lost works. Thanks to its citations, these medical texts are preserved to varying degrees, ensuring their continued relevance and accessibility.

According to cataloging works such as *Chinese Medicine Bibliography Researched* (Zhōng Guó Yī Jí Kǎo, 中国医籍考) and *Examination of Medical Literature Prior to the Song Dynasty* (Sòng Yǐ Qián Yī Jí Kǎo, 宋以前医籍考), Japanese scholars including Motokata Taki have conducted research on the *Categorized Collection of Medical Formulas* (Yī Fāng Lèi Jù, 医方类聚), resulting in the reconstruction of 13 lost medical texts. These works include *Chuan Yu Ji* (川玉集), *Wei Sheng Shi Quan Fang* (卫生十全方), *Xiao Er Yao Zheng* (小儿药证), *Qian Jin Yue Ling* (千金月令), *Five Viscera Theory* (Wǔ Zàng Lùn, 五藏论), *Shen Qiao Wan Quan Fang* (神巧万全方), *Jing Yan Mi Fang* (经验秘方), *Jing Yan Liang Fang* (经验良方), *Yan Xia Sheng Xiao Fang* (烟霞圣效方), *Bao Tong Mi Yao* (保童秘要), *Shi Tu Duan Xiao Fang*

(施图端效方), *Tong Zhen Zi Shang Han Kuo Yao* (通真子伤寒括要), and *Jian Yao Ji Zhong Fang* (简要济众方).[10]

We note that the *Categorized Collection of Medical Formulas* (Yī Fāng Lèi Jù, 医方类聚) sequences the entries according to the era in which each medical text was compiled. This approach furnishes us with a distinct historical documentary reference framework. The compilation begins with the *Basic Questions* (Sù Wèn, 素问), with the tenth entry being the *Treatise on Cold Damage Disorders* (Shāng Hán Lùn, 伤寒论), the eleventh is the *Commentary on the "Treatise on Cold Damage Disorders"* (Shāng Hán Lùn Zhù Jiě, 伤寒论注解), the twelfth is the *Five Viscera Theory* (Wǔ Zàng Lùn, 五藏论), the thirteenth is *Essential Prescriptions from the Golden Cabinet* (Jīn Guì Yào Lüè, 金匮要略), the fourteenth is *Wang Shuhe's Pulse Classic* (Wáng Shū Hé Mài Jué, 王叔和脉诀), and the fifteenth is *Wang's Pulse Classic* (Wáng Shì Mài Jīng, 王氏脉经). This order, while not directly proving that the *Five Viscera Theory* (Wǔ Zàng Lùn, 五藏论) was written by Zhang Zhongjing, indeed strongly hints at the possibility.

From both a historical and academic perspective, this method of arrangement likely reflects the compilers' deep understanding of these texts and their views on the interrelationships among them. The placement of the *Five Viscera Theory* (Wǔ Zàng Lùn, 五藏论) indicates that the compilers believed this work to be closely related to Zhang Zhongjing's medical philosophy and likely considered it to be a product of the same era as his other works.

This arrangement also provides us with deeper insights into understanding Zhang Zhongjing's medical philosophy. The placement of the *Five Viscera Theory* (Wǔ Zàng Lùn, 五藏论) hints at its significance within Zhang Zhongjing's medical system and suggests that our study of his work should not be confined to the *Treatise on Cold Damage Disorders* (Shāng Hán Lùn, 伤寒论) and *Essential Prescriptions from the Golden Cabinet* (Jīn Guì Yào Lüè, 金匮要略) alone. Instead, it should encompass a thorough exploration of the *Five Viscera Theory* (Wǔ Zàng Lùn, 五藏论) to achieve a more comprehensive understanding of his medical theories and practices.

In the *Categorized Collection of Medical Formulas* (Yī Fāng Lèi Jù, 医方类聚), the arrangement of medical texts seems to take into account not only the compilation era but also the authors. Within this framework, the placement of the *Five Viscera Theory* (Wǔ Zàng Lùn, 五藏论) is particularly worth mentioning. While the *Categorized Collection of Medical Formulas* (Yī Fāng Lèi Jù, 医方类聚) does not specify the authors of the works it compiles, its organization – placing it adjacent to other known works by Zhang Zhongjing and close to those by Wang Shuhe – may reveal the compilers' belief in a tight connection between the *Five Viscera Theory* (Wǔ Zàng Lùn, 五藏论) and Zhang Zhongjing's medical philosophy. It suggests that the work might originate from the same era, possibly emerging from the same school of thought or intellectual tradition; it might even share the same authorship period. This offers researchers a unique perspective: the *Five Viscera Theory* (Wǔ Zàng Lùn, 五藏论) is not merely an independent medical document but an integral part of Zhang Zhongjing's medical system. Alongside works like the *Treatise on Cold Damage Disorders* (Shāng Hán Lùn, 伤寒论) and *Essential Prescriptions from the*

Golden Cabinet (Jīn Guì Yào Lüè, 金匮要略), it contributes to a broader and more in-depth theoretical framework of medicine.

In the study of ancient medical literature, discovering such connections is crucial. It aids us in gaining a more comprehensive understanding of the evolution of ancient medical thought, as well as the interplay and connections between different medical works. By delving into the *Five Viscera Theory* (Wǔ Zàng Lùn, 五藏论) and its relationship with Zhang Zhongjing's other writings, we can attain a deeper insight into the medical knowledge and practices of that era, offering valuable historical references for modern medicine.

The *Five Viscera Theory* (Wǔ Zàng Lùn, 五藏论) included in the *Categorized Collection of Medical Formulas* (Yī Fāng Lèi Jù, 医方类聚) is found under the fourth volume, titled "'Wu Zang' (five viscera) section." Its content starts immediately after the last line of the "Song of the Five Qi Insufficiencies," which reads, "This is spleen deficiency. The prognosis will be good if treated as soon as possible. The healer." Remarkably, this section bears a striking resemblance to the version of Zhang Zhongjing's *Five Viscera Theory* (Wǔ Zàng Lùn, 五藏论) discovered in the Dunhuang manuscripts. This significant discovery was first unveiled by Chinese scholar Fan Xingzhun in 1951, who noticed the extraordinary similarity between the *Five Viscera Theory* (Wǔ Zàng Lùn, 五藏论) in the Dunhuang manuscript P. 2755 and the version contained within the *Categorized Collection of Medical Formulas* (Yī Fāng Lèi Jù, 医方类聚).

In 1988, Chinese scholar Ma Jixing referred to the version of Zhang Zhongjing's *Five Viscera Theory* (Wǔ Zàng Lùn, 五藏论) found in the *Categorized Collection of Medical Formulas* (Yī Fāng Lèi Jù, 医方类聚) as the "Yi Fang Lei Ju version," using it to collate and organize the version of Zhang Zhongjing's *Five Viscera Theory* (Wǔ Zàng Lùn, 五藏论) discovered among the Dunhuang medical manuscripts.

Here is a direct translation of the full text of Zhang Zhongjing's *Five Viscera Theory* (Wǔ Zàng Lùn, 五藏论) from the *Categorized Collection of Medical Formulas* (Yī Fāng Lèi Jù, 医方类聚) edition. The translation process strictly adheres to the original text, translating word for word and sentence by sentence:

医方类聚卷之四
"Categorized Collection of Medical Formulas" Volume Four
五藏門
"Wu Zang" (five viscera) section
五藏論
Wu Zang Lun

夫天地之精氣，化萬物之形。父之精氣為魂，魂則黑；母之精氣為魄，魄則白也。以分晝夜。一月懷其胎，如酪。二月成其果，而果李相似。三月有形象。四月男女分。五月筋骨成。六月髮鬢俱生。七月遊其魂而能動右手，是男於母左，是女於母右。八月遊其魄能動左手。九月二轉身。十月滿足，母子分解祷。其中亦有延月者，有相富貴；而有月不足者，下賤而貧窮。子生經六十日，瞳子成，能喜笑。二百一十日，掌骨成而能匍匐。三百日，髀骨成而能獨立。三百六十日為一歲，膝骨成而能行動。若不能依此者，男女不安，必有疾病。又兒女三十二日為一變，六十四日為再變。父母三年之中，迴乾就濕，嚥苦吐甘，始得離父母之懷抱，割損母之形像，毀傷母之筋骨，以成其身。夫內有五藏，外應五行，頭圓像天，足方像地，因緣而生。

The essence of heaven and earth has transformed the shape of everything. The Jing Qi from father is called Hun, and the Hun is black; the Jing Qi from mother is called Po, and the Po is white. Like day and night, (Jing Qi can be divided into yin and yang). The first month of pregnancy, (the embryo) is like cheese. The second month of pregnancy, (embryo) begins to take shape, and it looks like a plum. Into the third month, (the fetus) began to form humanoid. The fourth month, the gender of the baby can be revealed. Into the fifth month, tendons, ligaments, and bones of the fetus begin to form. Hair grows in the sixth month. Into the seventh month, Hun awakes, the fetus can move the right hand; boy situated in the left side of mother's womb, while girl lies on the right side of mother's womb. During the eighth month, Po awakes, and the fetus can move the left hand. The 9-month-old fetus starts to be very active, turning the body many times. After ten months of pregnancy, the fetus is separated from the mother. If the child is born beyond the gestation period, there are signs of wealth; if it is a premature baby, there are signs of poverty. 60 days after the child is born, the child's pupils form. He/she can see, can feel joy, and can laugh. 210 days after the birth (about seven months), metacarpal bones are formed, and the baby can crawl. After 300 days, the femur is formed, and the baby can stand alone. 360 days after the birth marked 1 year old, the child's knee bone is formed, and he/she can walk. If the baby does not develop according to this progress, no matter if it's a boy or girl, it must have illnesses. An infant has the initial growth spurt around 32 days after birth, then another one around 64 days. In the first three years after the child is born, the parents (take care of the baby in every possible way). They let the child live in a dry place while they are bearing the pain from living in a damp place; the parents eat simple foods themselves but feed the baby with nutritious foods. To help the child to grow so that he/she can walk independently, the mother's appearance deteriorated; her muscles and bones were damaged. In human body, there are five internal organs, which corresponds to the five elements on earth. The head is round, which symbolizes the sky. The foot is rectangular, which symbolizes the ground. (The existence of all things) is produced by the union of destiny.

因依足根，以拄著踝骨，以拄脛骨。因依脛骨，以拄膝骨，拄腿骨。因依腿骨，以拄髀骨、胯骨、腰脊骨、膂骨、項骨、頭骨、髑髏骨、肩骨、臂骨、肘骨、腕骨、掌骨、指骨。

The heel is the base point to support the ankle bone, and the ankle bone supports the tibia. The tibia is the base point to support the knee bone, and the knee bone supports the leg bone. The leg bone is the base point to support the femur, hip joint, lumbar spine, thoracic spine, cervical spine, skull, scapula, humerus, ulna and radius, wrist bones, metacarpal bones, and finger bones.

已上指骨，都共有三百六十五骨節，以應天三百六十五度。身上有五百筋脉，復有八萬毛孔，復有八萬戶此户字合是尸虫，虫戶八萬種，譬如窟中無所不成，名字各異。

Including the phalanges, the human body has 365 joints, corresponding to 365 days in a year. The human body has 500 veins, plus 80,000 pores, and 80,000 insects. And the insects have 80,000 species. It seems that all kinds of insects can grow in the "cave" and all have different names.

五藏者：心 肝 脾 肺 腎上是陰陽也。

The five Zang-organs refers to the heart, liver, spleen, lung, and kidney. (Kidney has kidney Yin and kidney Yang.)

六府者: 大腸 小腸 膽 胃 膀胱是三焦也。

The six Fu-organs refers to the large intestine, small intestine, gallbladder, stomach, and bladder (the bladder has the function of triple burner).

肝合於膽，膽者中精之腑。
心合於小腸，腸受盛之腑。
脾合於胃，胃者水穀之腑。
肺合於大腸，大腸者傳導之腑。
腎合於膀胱，膀胱者津液之腑。

The liver and gallbladder are connected, and the gallbladder is the Fu-organ that stores pure essence (bile). The heart is connected to the small intestine; the small intestines is the Fu-organ to digest and absorb nutrients. The spleen is connected to the stomach; the stomach is the Fu-organ to receive food and water. The lung is connected to the large intestine; the large intestine is the Fu-organ to transport the waste. The kidney is connected to the bladder; the bladder is the Fu-organ to excrete water.

三焦者，中腑水道出於膀胱，膀胱者為三焦之腑。血氣之津液皆出於血，血海有餘，自然無疾；血海不足，身少顏色，面無精光。氣海有餘，胷面具赤；氣海不足，少氣力，不多言。水穀之海有餘，則消食腸滿；水穀之海不足，則多飢，不消食。髓海有餘，輕便多力；髓海不足，則肝轉耳鳴。

The triple burner is in charge of the internal water metabolism, and the fluids end up in the bladder, so the bladder is the Fu-organ of the triple burner. The fluid of blood and Qi both come from blood. If the sea of blood is full, there will be no sickness. If the sea of blood is insufficient, the body will have little color, and the face will be pale and dull. If there is too much in the sea of Qi, the excess Qi accumulates in the upper part of the body, resulting in a red face and chest. If the sea of Qi is deficient, the person may have no strength and be unwilling to speak. If the sea of grain is sufficient, one will be able to digest food while also can feel full. If the sea of grain is weak, one will often be hungry but unable to digest food. If the sea of marrow is sufficient, the body feels light and energetic; if the sea of marrow is deficient, one will feel dizzy, and tinnitus may occur.

肝屬東方甲乙木，外應於眼。
心屬南方丙丁火，外應於舌。
肺屬西方庚辛金，外應於鼻。
腎屬北方壬癸水，外應於耳。
脾屬中央戊巳土，外應於唇。

Liver corresponds to the direction of east, the first and second of heavenly stem, and the five elements of wood, and connected to the eyes on the outside. Heart corresponds to the direction of south, the third and fourth of heavenly stem, and the five elements of fire, and connected to the tongue on the outside. Lung corresponds to the direction of west, the seventh and eighth of heavenly stem, and the five elements of gold, and connected to the nose on the outside. Kidney corresponds to the direction of north, the ninth and tenth of heavenly stem, and the five elements of water, and connected to the ears on the outside. Spleen corresponds to the direction of middle, the fifth and sixth of heavenly stem, and the five elements of earth, and connected to the lips on the outside.

六神配五藏

Six Shen and five Zang-organs relations

胆為滕蛇。心為帝王监領四方。肺為將軍應四方。肝為尚书有流淚。腎為列女命主之門。脾為大夫王在四時。

The gallbladder is like a flying snake. The heart is the emperor, who supervises and controls all four directions. The lung is the general, who manages far and near. The liver is the minister, who weep sometimes. The kidney is like an upright woman with moral integrity, and it is the entrance to life. The spleen is a senior official, who is in charge of the end of four seasons.

夫五藏象天，六腑象地，上下相對，以合陰陽之氣，外有耳、鼻、舌、口、眼，內有五藏六腑。

The five Zang-organs corresponds to the heaven, and the six Fu-organs corresponds to the earth. The heaven and the earth are facing each other, and the Yin and Yang energy integrates. There are ears, nose, tongue, mouth, and eyes on the outside of human body, while inside, there are five Zang-organs and six Fu-organs.

心病則口焦，肝病則目暗，脾病嘔逆不下食，肝病則鼻塞不通，腎病則耳聾。心主於血，肺主於涕，肝生於淚，腎生於津液，脾生於涎。心是神，肺是魄，肝是魂，腎是志，脾是意。色脉為心，毛髮為肺，爪甲為肝，脂肉為腎，化食為脾。心逆則憂，肺逆則滿，肝逆則怒，腎逆則蹇，脾逆則嘔。心順面赤，肺順面白，肝順目明，腎順耳目精明，脾順則變化飲食。久坐濕地，強力入水，傷腎；愁憂必慮，傷心；形寒飲冷，傷肺；恚怒逆不可食，傷肝；飲食勞倦，傷脾。

Heart disease manifests as dry mouth; liver disease manifests as diminished vision; spleen disease manifests as vomiting, hiccups, and inability to take food; liver (might mean "lung") disease manifests as nasal congestion; and kidney disease manifests as deafness. Heart dominates blood, lung dominates nasal mucus, liver dominates tears, kidney dominates fluid, and spleen dominates saliva. Heart houses Shen (mind), lung houses Po (the corporeal soul), liver houses Hun (the ethereal soul), kidney houses Zhi (the will-power), and spleen houses Yi (the intellect). The health of heart reflects through complexion and blood vessels. The health of lung is reflected through hairs. The health of liver reflects through nails. The health of kidney reflects through adipose tissues and muscles. And the health of spleen reflects through the ability of digesting food. Imbalance in the heart will cause depression, imbalance in the lung will cause chest tightness, imbalance in the liver will cause irritability, imbalance in the kidney will cause blockage of urination, and imbalance in the spleen will cause vomiting. Heart being healthy makes the skin rosy, lung being healthy makes the skin pale, liver being healthy makes the eyes clear, kidney being healthy makes the ears and eyes sharp, and spleen being healthy makes the body digest and absorb food. Sitting in a humid place for a long time, or entering the water after overwork, will hurt the kidney; depressed and worried about everything will hurt heart; the body catching cold or eating cold food will hurt the lung; being angry to an extend that one does not want to eat, this will hurt liver; and intemperate diet, or overwork, can hurt the spleen.

夫五勞、七傷、六極、五藏敗、九候、十絕及婦人產後餘疾，悉緣內積風冷所致。

Five strains, seven impairments, six exhaustions, five Zang-organs damages, nine dangerous symptoms, ten critical conditions, and diseases caused by childbirth are all caused by the accumulation of wind and coldness in the body.

五劳者

The five kinds of strains are as follows:

一、忽喜怒，大便苦難，口內生瘡，此為心勞；二、短氣面腫，鼻不聞香，咳嗽餘痰，兩脇脹痛，喘息不定，此為肺勞；三、面目乾黑，口中復苦，精神不定，不能獨臥，目視不明，如隔羅幕，頻頻下淚，此為肝勞；四、口苦，舌卷強直，不得嘔逆，醋心氣脹，脣焦，此為脾勞；五、小便黃赤，兼有餘瀝，腰痛耳鳴，夜間多夢，此為腎勞。

1. Sudden mood change, constipation, and sore in the mouth, these are the manifestations of heart strain; 2. shortness of breath, puffy face, loss of smell, cough out phlegm, intercostal tightness and pain, and breathlessness, these are the manifestations of lung strain; 3. dark complexion, dry eyes, bitter taste in mouth, restlessness, can't sleep alone, eyes can't see clearly like there is curtain in front, and tears often, these are the manifestations of liver strain; 4. bitter taste in mouth, tongue stiffness, often vomiting, heartburn, flatulence, and dry lips, these are the manifestations of spleen strain; and 5. yellow or dark urine, dribbling urination, back pain, tinnitus, insomnia and dreaminess, these are the manifestations of kidney strain.

七伤者

The seven types of impairments are as follows:

一陰汗；二精寒；三精清；四精少；五囊下濕癢；六小便數；七夜夢陰。

1. sweaty in male's genital area; 2. cold semen; 3. thin seminal plasma; 4. sparse semen; 5. wet and itchy scrotum; 6. frequent urination; and 7. nocturnal emission.

六極者 筋、骨、血、肉、精、氣。

The six exhaustions are (the overstrain of) tendons, bones, blood, muscles, essence, and Qi.

筋極則數轉筋，十指爪甲皆痛；骨極則牙齒痛，手足疼，不能久立；血極則令人面元顏色，頭髮墮悲；肉極則令人身上往往如鼠走，體上乾黑；精極則令人氣少無力，漸漸內虛，身上無潤澤，翕翕羸瘦，眼元精光，立不能定，身中若癢，搔之生瘡；氣極則令人胷脇逆滿，邪氣沖胷，恒欲大怒，氣少不能言。此為六極。

The tendon exhaustion will cause frequent cramps, and the fingers and nails will be painful; the bone exhaustion will cause toothache; the hands and feet are also painful so that one cannot stand for long; the blood exhaustion will cause pale complexion and the thinning of hair; the muscle exhaustion will make one feels foreign objects crawling on the body, and the body is dry and dark; the essence exhaustion will cause fatigue, then gradually feels weak inside, and the skin is not shiny; the body emaciated like an old person, dull eyes, unstable posture or tremor, itching, and sores may develop after scratching; the Qi exhaustion will cause chest fullness, rebellious Qi in the chest, easily burst in anger to an extend that one cannot even speak. These are the six exhaustions.

九候者

The nine dangerous symptoms are as follows:

一手足青；二手足久腫；三脉枯齒禁；四語聲散，鼻虛張聲勢；五脣寒冷宣露；六脣腫齒焦；七手順衣縫；八汗出不流；九舌捲卵縮。

1. The hands and feet are blue; 2. chronic edema on the hands and feet; 3. the blood vessels dry up and the teeth are clenched; 4. the voice is scattered and the nose flaps; 5. the lips are cold, and the gums are atrophied; 6. the lips are swollen, and the teeth are black; 7. the hands unconsciously smooth out the corner of clothes; 8. the sweat stays on the skin, does not drip; and 9. the tongue curls and the scrotum retracts.

五敗者

The five (Zang-organ) damages are as follows:

手足腫，無交文，心敗；唇反黑無文，肺敗；面黑有瘡，肝敗；陰腫囊縮，腎敗；臍腫滿，脾敗。

Edema on hands and feet. The edema is so severe that there is no wrinkle on skin, this is heart damage; darkened lips with no luster, this is lung damage; darkened complexion with sores outbreak, this is liver damage; swollen or contracted scrotum, this is kidney damage; full and swollen belly button, this is spleen damage.

十絕者

The ten critical conditions are as follows:

氣短，目視亭亭無精光，心絕；口鼻虛張聲勢，氣復短，肺絕；面青，眼視人不具數出淚，肝絕；面黑，眼睛黃，素汁流，腎絕；泄涎唾不覺，時時忘語，脾絕；手上爪甲青黑，惡罵不休，筋絕；背脊酸疼，腰中復重，骨絕；面無精光，頭髮自落，血絕；舌捲卵縮如紅丹，嚥唾不得，足踝小腫，肉絕；髮直如竿，汗出不止，腸絕。

Shortness of breath, straight and dull look in the eyes, this is heart failure; mouth and nose are feebly open with shortness of breath, this is lung failure; a bluish color to the skin, eyes are not focused and watery, this is liver failure; face is dark, eyes are yellow, spontaneous sweat, this is kidney failure; unconsciously drooling and often forget words, this is spleen failure; the nails on the hands are blue and black, constantly cursing, this is tendon failure; the back is sore, there is heavy sensation around the waist, this is bone failure; dull complexion with eyes lacking in luster, hair loss, this is blood failure; the tongue is curled, the scrotum is retracted like a red pellet, having trouble of swallowing saliva, and the ankle is swollen, this is muscle failure; hair is stiff like a bamboo pole, sweat continuously, this is intestine failure.

五氣不足歌五言

Song of the Five Qi Insufficiencies (five characters to a line)

心氣若不足，衄血眼中黃。悲愁及喜怒，煩悶即荒忙。夢寤不自覺，心熱須水漿。喉嚨中滿痛，舌強口誇張。冷汗出不止，忘語忽驚忙。此為損心氣，不療轉加傷。

If heart Qi is deficient, will have nose bleeding and eyes will turn yellow. Sometimes sad, sometimes worried, sometimes happy, and sometimes angry. One moment being bothered, and in a flurry the next. Dreamful sleep but does not remember the dreams, dysphoria with thirst. Pain in the throat, stiff tongue, mouth wide open. Continuous cold sweat, forgetful and has sudden panic. This is the deficiency of the heart and will be more serious if left untreated.

肺氣若不足，肚脹不能安。嘔逆及上氣，悲思數多端。形寒似飲冷，肺損唾痰涎。皮毛不覺起，恚怒數千般。肩脊背強痛，夢裹鬼相牽。鼻中不覺氣，尋常骨膈乾。此為肺不足，不療病成難。

If lung Qi is deficient, there will be fullness in the stomach so that it is hard to feel comfortable. Nauseous, vomiting, and belching, often feels sad and worried. Body feels chilly like drinking cold water. Because the lung is damaged, which leads to excessive amount of sputum and saliva. The hair on the skin erected unconsciously and often gets angry. The shoulders, spine, and back are stiff and painful. There are ghosts in the dream. Nasal obstruction and dryness. This is the deficiency of the lung. If it is not treated, the disease will be more difficult to treat.

肝氣若不足，遠視目失力。兩脇氣脹滿，上下連胷臆。四肢熱復冷，肚痛不能食。眼前見火生，冷淚頻頻拭。不療恐失明，此為肝不足。

If liver Qi is deficient, it is difficult to see from a distance. The hypochondriac area feels full, and the chest is also affected by the tightness of the surrounding areas. The limbs are one moment hot and cold right after. Pain in the abdomen is so severe that one cannot eat. Seeing the hot fire in front the eyes but has to constantly wipe off the cold tears. If leave it untreated, one may be blind. This is liver deficiency.

腎氣若不足，腰胯收攝難。恍惚心少力，重聽不聞言。眼前如艷水，冷氣在腰間。身中悉皆癢，骨痛不能安。坐復身拘急，氣乏咽喉乾。狀似洋膠汁，腰胯強如寒。此為腎不足，於身不自安。

If kidney Qi is deficient, it is difficult to stretch the back and hips. One may feel uneasy and powerless, may have tinnitus or hearing loss. Sparkles dance before the eyes, and there is chilliness in the back. Itchy everywhere, pain in the bone so that one cannot find a comfortable position. The body contracts as soon as one sat down, shortness of breath with dry throat. Body is so weak, soft like gel; but the back and the hips are stiff and cold. This is the kidney deficiency. With this disease, one cannot be at ease.

脾氣若不足，令人面目黃。食即欲嘔逆，脣乾復口瘡。氣脹四支重，意相竝憧惶。不欲聞人語，脾渴即須漿。此為脾臟不足，急療可為良。醫人。

If the spleen Qi is deficient, it will cause yellow eyes and sallow complexion. Feels nauseous right after eating. Lips are dry and sores in the mouth. Bloated with heavy limbs, easy to get worried and terrified. Doesn't want to hear other people's voice, wants to drink as soon as the spleen is thirsty. This is spleen deficiency. The prognosis will be good if treated as soon as possible. The healer.

藥名之部，所出醫王。黃帝造針經曆有千卷。藥姓名品，若匪神仙，何能備著？且神農本草，辯土地而顯君臣，岐伯經方，說酸醎而陳冷熱。雷公妙典，略述炮炙之宜，弘景奇方，備說根莖之用。

Medicine is contributed by the works of (later) various kings of medicine. The Yellow Emperor wrote "The Canon of Acupuncture" that consists of one thousand volumes. The medicines did not only have their names but also the functions. If this were not a celestial being, how could anyone write such a great book? Meanwhile, the "The Divine Farmer's Classic of Materia Medica" (Shen Nong Ben Cao Jing) did not only tell the region/place that produces the medicine/herb but also classified each medicine. The classics written by Qi Bo explained medicine's (properties like) sour and salty and cold or hot nature. Lei Gong's marvelous classic talked in detail about herbal processing. Tao HongJing's miraculous formulas tirelessly discussed the use of stems and roots.

只如犀角觝觸之義，故能逐汪驅邪。牛黃壞鴆之功，是以安魂，藍田玉屑，可以鎮壓精神，中條麝香，堪將辟邪除鬼。河內牛膝，去朔冷而止腰疼。防風除頭風而抽脇痛。半夏有消痰之力，制毒要用生薑；當歸有止痛之能，會須白芷。晉地龍齒偏差顛癇，太山茯苓延年却老。仁參、薯蕷能令耳目聰明，遠志、菖蒲妙能開心益智。甘草安和諸藥，遂得國老之名；大黃宣引眾功，乃得將軍之号。秦膠結羅紋之狀，乾漆作蜂巢之形。丹砂會取光明，升麻破求青綠。秦椒須汗，樸硝、礬石須熬。杜仲削去麄皮，桂心還求肉味。石英須研似麵，杏仁別擣如膏。兔絲得酒乃良，礬石燒之力好。防葵唯輕唯上，狼毒唯重彌佳。黃芩以腐爛為精，閭茹蚛頭為上。石南採葉，甘菊收花。五茄剝取其皮，牡丹要須去骨。鬼箭破血，乃有射鬼之靈，神屋除温，非無保神之驗。嘔吐湯煎乾葛，轉筋酒煮木瓜。目赤宜點黃連，口瘡宜含石膽。木蘭皮能除黠䵟，流黃妙去死痺。欣草殺齒內之虫，藜蘆爛鼻中宿肉。赤油宜塗雞子，白癲偏衣越挑。火燒多估水萍，杖打須加松實。琥珀拾芥乃辯其真，磁石引針將知不謬。石得鴆糞乃爛如泥，漆遇蟹黃便化為水。三稜破癖，本出行從，劉寄奴療瘡起於田獵。牡蠣助栢仁之力，地黃益天門冬之功。斂及反烏頭之精，梔子解躑躅之毒。苦參、酸棗以味為名，白术、黃連，將色為號。蜈蚣、蜀漆，陸地標名，狗脊、狼牙，因形為記。只如八味腎氣，補六極而差五勞；四色神丹，蕩千痾而除萬病。檳榔下蟲除氣，玉壺丸去積冷消堅。李子預有殺鬼之方，劉涓有遺鬼之錄。耆婆童子，妙述千端，喻父醫王，神方萬品。是以有命者必差，虢太子死而更甦；無命者難理，晉公生而致死。此之養病，如積薪投火而薪存，人若有病，去病而人活，不去火而薪被焚，病不除而徒喪命。是以神方千卷，藥名八百。中黃丸能差千痾，底野迦善除萬病。扁鵲秘論乃揔君臣，冷熱不調，酸鹹各異。

Xi Jiao (犀角, rhinoceros horn) has the power to fight against illness, so it can eliminate chronic infectious disease and disperse evil. Niu Huang (牛黃, cattle gallstone) has the function to damage Zhen (a legendary bird with poisonous feathers) so that it can calm the soul (Hun). Yu Xie (玉屑, Jade Chips) from Lan Tian can tranquilize the mind. She Xiang (麝香, musk) from Zhong Tiao can drive out evil. Niu Xi (牛膝, twotoothed achyranthes root) from He Nei treats cold knee and relieves lower back pain. Fang Feng (防風, siler root, or divaricate saposhnikovia root) heals the head wind, also relieves the hypochondriac pain. Ban Xia (半夏, pinellia tuber) dissolves phlegm; Sheng Jiang (生薑, fresh ginger) can counteract its toxicity. Dang Gui (當歸, Chinese angelica root) can stop pain, but it must be combined with Bai Zhi (白芷, Dahurian angelica root). Long Chi (龍齒, fossilized animal teeth) from Shanxi can treat epilepsy; Fu Ling (茯苓, Indian bread, or poria*) from* Taishan can prolong life. Ren Shen (仁参 or 人参, ginseng root) and Shu Yu (薯蕷 or "Shan Yao" 山药, dioscrea rhizome) can make your eyes bright and ears sharp. Yuan Zhi (遠志, Thinleaf milkwort root) and Chang Pu (菖蒲 or "Shi Chang Pu" 石菖蒲, grass-leaf sweetflag rhizome) can clear the brain and improve the intelligence. Gan Cao (甘草, licorice root) has the function of harmonizing; thus, it has been called the "Guo Lao," a respected elder in the kingdom. Da Huang (大黄, rhubarb root) has the function of opening and inducing the elimination. That's why it was called the "Marshall General." Qin Jiao (秦膠 or 秦艽, largeleaf gentian root) pertains spiral shape; Gan Qi 乾漆, dried lacquer) looks like honeycomb. Dan Sha (丹砂 or "Zhu Sha" 朱砂, cinnabar) should be shiny; Sheng Ma (升麻, largetrifoliolious bugbane Rhizome) should be blue and green. Qin Jiao (秦椒, prickly ash peel) needs to be steamed; Pu Xiao (樸硝, a crude form of sodium sulfate) and Fan Shi (礬石 or "Ming Fan" 明矾, a sulfate of alum-stone, or white alum-stone) should be roasted; Du Zhong (杜仲, eucommia bark) must peel off the outer skin; Gui Xin (桂心 or "Rou Gui" 肉桂, cinnamon bark) must have meaty fragrance. Shi Ying (石英, Cristobalite) must be powdered; Xing Ren (杏仁, apricot seed) should be grinded until gets creamy. Tu Si (菟丝, Chinese dodder seed) must be soaked with alcohol; Fan Shi (礬石 or "Ming Fan" 明矾, a sulfate of alum-stone, or white alum-stone) must be calcinated. Fang Kui (防葵, white flower hog fennel root) the lighter the better; Lang Du (狼毒, Bracteole-lacked Euphorbia root) the heavier the better. Good Huang Qin (黄芩, Baical skullcap root) looks like rotten intestine; only use Lin Ru's (閭茹, Euphorbia Lanru root) top part. Shi Nan (石南, Chinese photinia Leaf) should pick its leaves; Gan Ju (甘菊, sweet chrysanthemum flower) uses its flower. Wu Jia (五茄, slenderstyle acanthopanax Bark) only uses the bark; Mu Dan (牡丹, tree peony bark), need to take the bone out. Gui Jian (鬼箭 or "Gui Jian Yu" 鬼箭羽, winged branches) can break up the blood stasis thus to kill ghost toxins. Shen Wu (神屋 or 龟板, tortoise carapace and plastron) clears the heat and has magical effect. Decoct Gan Ge (乾葛 or "Ge Geng" 葛根, dried pueraria root) to treat vomiting; use alcohol to decoct Mu Gua (木瓜, Chinese quince fruit) for muscle spasm. Use Huang Lian (黄連, yellow coptis root) to make eye drops for red eyes. Hold Shi Dan (石膽 or "Dan Fan" 膽矾, chalcanthite) in the mouth for mouth ulcer. Mu Lan (木蘭, lily magnolia bark) can remove dead skin; Liu Huang (流黄 or 硫磺, yellow Sulfur) is to treat gangrene. Wang Cao (茵草, leaf of poisonous eightangle tree) treats cavity inside the teeth; Li Lu (藜蘆, veratrum root and rhizome) can dissolve polyps in the nose. Red ulcer should apply Ji Zi (雞子, chicken eggs); tuberculoid leprosy needs to use Yue Tao (越桃 or "Zhi Zi" 梔子, gardenia fruit); burns to be treated by applying Shui Ping (水萍 or "Fu Ping" 浮萍, floating duckweed) topically; wounds from caning can use Song Shi (松實or "Song Zhi" 松脂, pine resin). Real Hu Po (琥珀, amber) can pick up tiny things; if the Ci Shi (磁石, magnetite) can attract needles, which means it is not fake. Zhen Fen (鴆糞, the excrement of a legendary poisonous bird) can make stones melt like mud; Xie Huang (蟹黄, crab yolk) can make paint melt like water. San Leng (三棱, common burred tuber) can break the nodule; this comes from Xing Cong's story; Liu Ji Nu (劉寄奴, diverse wormwood herb) heals the wound. This function was discovered from field hunting. Mu Li (牡蠣, oyster shell) can help the function of Bo Ren (柏仁, Oriental arborvitae seed kernel); Di Huang (地黄, rehmannia root) can benefit the function of Tian Men Dong (天門冬, Cochinchinese asparagus root). Bai Lian (白蔹, Japanese ampelopsis root) is incompatible with Wu Tou (烏頭, Sichuan aconite root); Zhi Zi (梔子, gardenia fruit) is the antidote of Zhi Zhu (躑躅, Chinese azalea flower). Ku Shen (苦参, light-yellow sophora root) and Suan Zao (酸棗, Chinese sour jujube) are named after their taste; Bai Zhu (白术, white atractylodes tuber) and Huang Lian (黄連, yellow coptis root) are named after their colors; Wu Gong (蜈蚣, centipede) and Shu Qi (蜀漆, Sichuan dichroa leaf) are named after their place of origin; Gou Ji (狗脊, cibot rhizome) and Lang Ya (狼牙, the underground winter bud of Agrimonia root) are named after their shapes. Just like Ba Wei Shen Qi (八味腎氣, Eight-Ingredient Kidney Qi Pills), it nourishes the six exhaustions and cures the five strains; Si Se Shen Dan (四色神丹, Four-Color Magic Pills) eliminates thousands of diseases and cures 10,000 illnesses. Bing Lang (檳榔, betel nut) eliminates parasites and relieve bloating; Yu Hu Wan (玉壺丸, Jade Pot Pills) expels coldness and dissolves hardness. Li Ziyu was known to kill ghosts; Liu Juan has a record of expelling ghosts. Jivaka understood medical theory profoundly. He was known as the king of medicine; he had many magical formulas. Those destined to live will recover from illness. Like the Prince of Guo ("Guo" is one of the ancient feudal states), he was resurrected, even though he was considered dead already. Those destined to die are difficult to save. Like the death of the Duke of Jin. Treating an illness is like a fire within a pile of firewood; removing the fire keeps the firewood intact, removing the illness allows the person to live. If the firewood is not removed from the fire, it will be burned in vain; if a person's illness is not treated, they will lose their life in vain. There are thousands of good formulas and 800 names of medicines in the world. Zhong Huang Wan (中黄丸, Central Yellow Pills) can treat thousands of illnesses, and Di Ye Jia (底野迦, Theriac) can cure tens of thousands of diseases. The secret in Bian Que's talk about medicine is that the medicines are categorized into Kings and Ministers. They have cold or hot natures. Their tastes are different as well.

夫五常之體，因暑濕而結百疾。頭風目眩須好菊花，脚弱行遲多添石斛。卒中霍亂宜服茅香之湯，久患脊痾急內蚺蛇之膽。痺濕攣痛須用茵芋，皮膚瘙癢宜加蒴藋。傷寒發汗要用麻黄，壯熱不調宜加竹葉。恒山、鱉甲療瘧之功，枳實、芎藭善除心家之悶。卒患鬼注須用雄黃，忽爾驚邪時須龍齒。當歸、芍藥去肚痛之痾，款冬、紫菀除穎嗽之疾。檳榔、白术理宿食不消，硇硝、大黄瀉癥瘕之病。黄連、阿膠善能止痢，通草有發聲之能。水蛭、虻虫善能破血。蕤仁明目，秦皮、决明去瞖，牛膝止膝痛風冷，鵜脂善治耳聾，蜂房能消毒腫，蟹黄善去漆瘡，蕪夷、狼牙殺白虫，桔梗、蘘荷善除蠱毒，亂髮灰能止血汗，滑石通淋瀝之疾。茵草定其牙疼，海藻能除癭氣。知母、栝樓止渴，麥門冬、石膏除溫。署預補骨，澤瀉能治膀胱，遠志、菖蒲聰明益智。脇中乏痛宜用防風、當歸。艾葉、阿膠善治動，連翹止癧，礬石療耳內之膿，小便不利宜服亭歷，杏人益氣身體輕肥。婦人產後羸弱宜服黄精、酸棗、紫花、白微、生葛。人參治五藏虛熱，麥門、鍾乳補肺安心，紫菀、柴胡療人上氣，雄黄、薤白能止狂風，犀角、升麻、烏梅偏醫熱腫，獨活理人面上游風，茵芋、閭茹治人髭落。天行溫病宜服芍藥、生薑，壯熱口乾宜下大青、知母。甘草宜補五藏，人參好定精神。丹參養魂安魄，地黄能通血脉，黄精定長肌膚。

Human beings as an integral part of nature will get hundreds of diseases due to heat and dampness. Head wind with dizziness must use Ju Hua (菊花, chrysanthemum flower). Weakness of limbs caused difficult walking will be benefit from Shi Hu (石斛, dendrobium stem). Suffering from acute gastroenteritis should take Mao Xiang (茅香 or "Mao Gen" 茅根, imperata rhizome) decoction. Long-term suffering from spinal disease requires immediate use of Ran She Dan (蚺蛇膽, python gallbladder). Painful arthritis uses Yin Yu (茵芋, Japanese skimmia stem and leaf); severe skin itch uses Shuo Huo (蒴藋, Chinese elder). Promote sweat during Shang Han, exogenous pathogenic cold-induced diseases, uses Ma Huang (麻黄, ephedra stem). Constant high fever can benefit from Zhu Ye (竹葉, bamboo leaves). Heng Shan (恒山 or "Chang Shan" 常山, dichroa root) and Bie Jia (鱉甲, Chinese soft-shelled turtle shell) have great function to relieve malaria. Zhi Shi (枳實, immature range fruit) and Xiong Qiong (芎藭 or "Chuan Xiong" 川芎, Sichuan lovage rhizome) are good at treating oppression in the heart. Pestilential illness uses Xiong Huang (雄黄, realgar) immediately. Sudden frightening should ask for Long Chi

(龍齒, fossilized animal teeth) in no time. Dang Gui (當歸, Chinese angelica root) and Shao Yao (芍藥, white peony root) can heal the disease in the abdomen; Kuan Dong (款冬, Common coltsfoot flower) and Zi Wan (紫菀, Tatarian aster root) are good to eliminate cough. Bing Lang (檳榔, betel nut) and Bai Zhu (白朮, white atractylodes tuber) can treat food stagnation; Nao Xiao (硇硝 or "Mang Xiao" 芒硝, Nitrate from saline alkali land) and Da Huang (大黄, rhubarb root) can eliminate abdominal mass. Huang Lian (黄連, yellow coptis root) and E Jiao (阿膠, donkey-hide glue) are good at stopping dysentery disease; Tong Cao (通草, rice paper plant pith) helps to open up voice. Shui Zhi (水蛭, leech) and Mang Chong (虻虫, horse fly) are to break blood stasis; Rui Ren (蕤仁, hedge prinsepia nut) can brighten the eyes; Qin Pi (秦皮, fraxinus bark) and Jue Ming (决明, cassia seeds) can treat cataract. Niu Xi (牛膝, twotoothed achyranthes root) stops knee pains due to wind cold; E Zhi (鵝脂, goose fat) treats deafness; Feng Fang (蜂房, honeycomb) reduces swelling due to toxin; Xie Huang (蟹黄, crab yolk) can heal lacquer dermatitis; Wu Yi (蕪荑, large-fruited elm seed) and Lang Ya (狼牙, the underground winter bud of Agrimonia root) can kill parasites; Jie Geng (桔梗, platycodon root) and Rang He (蘘荷, Mioga ginger rhizome) can treat insect poison; Luan Fa Hui (亂髮灰, human hair ash) can stop bleeding. Hua Shi (滑石, talc) can treat Lin syndrome. Wang Cao (菵草, leaf of poisonous eightangle tree) stops toothache; Hai Zao (海藻, seaweed) reduces goiter. Zhi Mu (知母, common anemarrhena rhizome) and Gua Lou (栝樓 or "Tian Hua Fen" 天花粉, trichosanthes root) quenches thirst; Mai Men Dong (麦門冬, dwarf lilyturf tuber) and Shi Gao (石膏, gypsum) clears heat. Shu Yu (署預 or "Shan Yao" 山药, dioscrea rhizome) can strengthen bones; Ze Xie (澤瀉, alisma tuber) can regulate the bladder function. Yuan Zhi (遠志, Thinleaf milkwort root) and Chang Pu (菖蒲 or "Shi Chang Pu" 石菖蒲, grassleaf sweetflag rhizome) can improve a person's intelligence. Fang Feng (防風, siler root) can treat hypochondriac pain; Dang Gui (當歸, Chinese angelica root); Ai Ye (艾葉, argy wormwood leaf) and E Jiao (阿膠, donkey-hide glue) can calm the fetus; Lian Qiao (连翘, weeping forsythia Capsule) can eliminate scrofula; Fan Shi (礬石, "Ming Fan" 明矾, a sulfate of alum-stone) can treat pus in the ear; difficult urination should take Ting Li (葶歷 or "Ting Li Zi" 葶歷子, tansymustard seed). Xing Ren (杏人 or 杏仁, apricot seed) can supplement qi and help to lose weight. Postpartum women should take Huang Jing (黄精, solomonseal Rhizome) for weakness after childbirth. Suan Zao (酸棗, Chinese sour jujube seed), Zi Hua (紫花 or "Zi Hua Di Ding" 紫花地丁, Tokyo violet herb), Bai Wei (白薇, blackened white swallowwort root), Sheng Ge (生葛 or "Ge Gen" 葛根, dried pueraria root), and Ren Shen (人参, ginseng root) can treat deficiency heat in five zang. Mai Men (麥門 or "Mai Men Dong" 麥門冬, dwarf lilyturf tuber) and Zong Ru (鍾乳 or "Zhong Ru Shi" 鍾乳石, stalactite) can tonify lung and calm the mind; Zi Wan (紫菀, tatarian aster root) and Chai Hu (柴胡, Chinese thorowax root) can treat rebellious Qi; Xiong Huang (雄黄, realgar) and Xie Bai (薤白, long-stamen onion bulb) can stop maniac; Xi Jiao (犀角, rhinoceros horn), Sheng Ma (升麻, largetrifoliolious bugbane Rhizome), and Wu Mei (烏梅, smoked plum) tend to treat swelling and pain due to heat toxin; Du Huo (獨活, doubleteeth pubescent angelica root) can take care of wandering wind on face; Yin Yu (茵芋, Japanese skimmia stem and leaf) and Lü Ru (閭茹, Euphorbia Lanru root) can treat hair loss. If there is a contagious warm disease, take Shao Yao (芍藥, white peony root) and Sheng Jiang (生薑, fresh ginger); if there is high fever and dry mouth, take Da Qing (大青 or "Da Qing Ye", 大青叶, Isatis leaf) and Zhi Mu (知母, common anemarrhena rhizome). Gan Cao (甘草, licorice root) nourishes five zang; Ren Shen (人参, ginseng root) replenishes the vital energy. Dan Shen (丹参, salvia root) calms the Hun and Po; Di Huang (地黄, rehmannia root) unblocks the blood vessels. Huang Jing (黄精, solomonseal Rhizome) helps to grow muscles and skin.

夫以三焦為性，處用不同；五昧酸鹹，其根各異。只如天有五星，地有五岳，而運五藏。所以肺為丞相，肝為尚書，心為帝王，脾為大夫，腎為列女。肝與膽合，脾與胃通，小腸連心，大腸連肺，膀胱合腎。是以肝藏盛則目赤，心熱即舌乾，腎虛即耳鳴，肺風即鼻塞。目是肝候，舌是心官，耳作腎司，鼻為肺應。心主血，肺主皮膚，肝主於筋，腎主於骨。骨假筋立，筋籍肉行，肉假皮存，皮因骨長。故骨患從腎，筋患出肝，肉患傷脾，皮患由肺。只如十二經脉，上下巡還；八八脉冀傾，内外流轉。三焦六腑，四海七神，胷膈咽喉，唇齒臂肋，股肱腴胯，指腕爪甲，九竅八扇，三陰五會，小腸胃口，臍脇脊膂，項頰曲鬚，頜額鼻柱，唇齗牙齒，掌腋髮，已上但有患處，皆有所因，莫不内積虛勞，外緣風濕。察其顏色，即辯寒溫；聽聲音，便知損益。只如戲驚者心疾，多笑者腎邪，呻吟者患脾，啼哭者損肺。聲細者是冷，聲絕者患風，聲輕者患虛，聲麄者患熱。膚白是冷，皮青是風，顏黑者是溫，面黃即熱。心虛忘，脾虛患飢，腎冷腰疼，肝實多怒。視毛知血，見爪知筋，看目知肝，舉齒知骨。骨傷齒黑，損燋筋絕爪乾，氣少聲短，聲聲氣促。髮是血餘，是患之意，原見之可作醫療，即如此委細，乃是良醫。又須用醫方，妙閑藥性，應病與藥性，不羌者是以代無良醫，枉死者半。天地之内，以人為貴，頭圓象天，足方象地。天有四時，人有四支；天有五行，人有五藏；天有六律，人有六腑；天有九星，人有九竅；天有八風，人有八節；天有十二時，人有十二經脉；天有二十四氣，人有二十四俞；天有三百六十五度，人有三百六十五骨；天有日月，人有眼目；天有晝夜，人有寐寤；天有雷電，人有喜怒；天有雨露，人有啼泣；天有陰陽，人有寒暑。地有九州，人有九竅；地有泉水，人有血脉；地有草木，人有毛髮；地有金石，人有牙齒。是以經云皆禀四大五常，假合成身。夫陰陽之氣，情有喜怒哀樂之性，人有禮義智信。故天圓地方，四時八節，五藏六腑，榮衛之氣，九竅呼吸，寒暑皮毛骨齒，經脉表裏虛實。男子陰陽相繫，為之五勞；冷熱相衝，遂為七傷之疾。厥氣入膀脫，夢遊走。陰氣沉而夢大水，兼之恐懼；陽氣發上，夢見大火而煩。上盛則夢飛空，下盛夢見沉水。中渴，渴即是熱也。

San Jiao (triple burner) has different functions based on the locations. Foods have different tastes because they grow up from different plants and places. The heaven has five stars, the earth has five mountains, and the human body has five Zang-organ. So that the lung is like the Cheng Xiang (prime minister), the liver is like the Shang Shu (minister), the heart is like the Emperor, the spleen is like a senior official, and the kidney is like a woman with moral integrity. The liver works with the gallbladder, the spleen connects the stomach, the small intestine links to the heart, the large intestine coordinates with the lung, and the urinary bladder connects the kidney. Therefore, liver excess causes red eyes, heart heat causes dry mouth, kidney deficiency causes tinnitus, and lung wind causes sinus blockage. The liver manifests on eyes, heart manifests on the tongue, kidney manifests on ears, and lung manifests on the nose. The heart rules the blood vessels, the lung rules the skin, the liver rules the tendons, and the kidney rules the bones. Bones depend on tendons to stand straight, tendons make use of muscles so that one can walk, muscle depends on skin to exist, and skin depends on bones to grow. Therefore, the bone disorders are related to the kidney, the tendon disorders are related to the liver, the muscle disorders will damage the spleen, and the skin disorders are related to the lung. There are 12 meridians that circulate upward and downward and eight extraordinary meridians that flow in the human body internally and externally. There are also triple burners and six Fu-organs; four seas and seven spirits; chest, diaphragm, pharynx, and throat; lips, teeth, arms, and ribs; thighs, forearms, and pelvis; fingers, wrists, and fingernails; nine orifices (for human) and eight holes (for animals other than human), three Yin (channels) and five (Zang-organs and six Fu-organs) meeting points, and small intestine and stomach; navel, hypochondriac area, and spine; neck, cheeks, and mustache (bended knees); chin, forehead, and nose; lips cover the teeth; palms, armpit, and hair, all the aforementioned places could suffer from illness, and the illness must have their causes, which are either internal deficiency and impairment or external caught wind damp. By looking at the facial color, you will be able to tell if it is cold syndrome or warm syndrome. By listening to the voice, you will know if the person has excess or deficiency. Someone easy to be frightened could have heart sickness; laughing too much means there is evil in the kidney; moaning and groaning are because of the illnesses of the spleen; and crying and sobbing are due to the illnesses of the lung. A soft voice indicates suffering from cold, no voice indicates suffering from wind, a weak voice indicates suffering from deficiency, and a rough voice indicates suffering from heat. Pale skin indicates cold in the body, blue skin tone indicates wind invasion, dark facial color indicates warmth in the body, and sallow face indicates the heat in the body. Heart deficiency causes forgetfulness, spleen deficiency causes hunger, kidney cold causes the lumbar pain, and liver excess causes anger. Looking at hair can know about the blood, looking at nails can know about tendons, looking at eyes can know about the liver, and looking at the teeth can know about bones. The bone injury causes the teeth to turn into a dark color, the blood injury causes the hair to look burned, the tendon damage causes the nail to be dried, and deficient Qi causes shortness of breath and shallow breathing. Hair is the residual of blood. According to the clinical manifestations of these diseases to determine the root cause for treatment. If it can be investigated in such detail, this is a good doctor. When prescribing herbal formulas, (a good doctor) needs to know each medicine well and prescribe the medicine according to the illness. (If do so), no disease cannot be cured! But there is no good doctor now. Half of the patients died due to improper treatments. Between the heaven and earth, the human being is the most valued. The head is round shaped that imitates the heaven; the feet are square shaped that imitates the earth. (On the analogy concept), the heaven has four seasons, correspondingly, human has four limbs; the heaven has five elements, so does human has five Zang-organs; the heaven has six rhyms, so does human has six Fu-organs; the heaven has nine stars, so does human has nine orifices; the heaven has eight kinds of winds, so does human has eight (big) joints; the heaven has 12 two-hour periods, so does human has 12 meridians; the heaven has 24 divisions of the solar year, so does human has 24 acupuncture shu points. The heaven has 365 days, so does human has 365 bones; the heaven has sun and moon, so does human has eyes; the heaven has days and nights, so does human knows when to sleep; the heaven has thunder and lightning, so does human has joy and anger; the heaven has rains and dews, so does human has cry and weep; the heaven has Yin and Yang, so does human has cold and heat; the earth has nine states, so does human has nine orifices. The earth has spring water, so does human has blood vessels. The earth has trees and grass, so does human has hair. The earth has metals and rocks, so does human has teeth. So theoretically speaking, it is all the human body formed by the aforementioned reasons due to the "four major and five constants." Qi has Yin and Yang; temperament has happiness, anger, sorrow, and joy; and people have (constant virtues of) propriety, righteousness, wisdom, and fidelity. So the sky is round; the earth is square; four seasons and eight solar terms; five Zang-organs and six Fu-organs; ying Qi and wei Qi; nine orifices to breathe; skin and hair, bones and teeth to withstand the cold and heat; through the meridian pulse to indicate whether the disease is internal or external and deficiency or excess. Too much sex for men will cause five strains; the imbalance between heat and cold will cause seven impairments. Rebellious qi that enters the urinary bladder will cause sleepwalks. When Yin Qi is sinking, one will dream of flooding and having nightmares. If Yang Qi rises upward, one will dream of catching fire and get irritated. When the upper part of the body is full, one will dream of flying in the sky, and when the lower part of the body is full, one will dream of sinking into the water. Feeling thirsty is caused by heat.

夫五藏重斤两

The weight of five Zang-organs

心為帝王，監領四方，重十二兩，中有七孔，孔有三毛，盛精汁三合，主藏神。肝為尚書，有五葉，應五常，重三斤十兩。膽為將軍決曹吏，在肝短葉下，重九兩，精汁四合。脾為諫議大夫，重二斤三兩，闊三寸，長五寸，有膏半斤，主囊濕血溫，主藏意，在胃下，助胃氣，主化穀食也。胃重二斤十四兩，盛穀三斗五升。肺為丞相，有四葉，應四時，重二斤十二兩，主藏魄，出音聲。腎臟為列女，在後宮，有兩枚，重二斤一兩。主藏末，灌注諸脉也。

The heart is like an emperor, who monitors and controls all four directions. (The heart) weighs 12 liang (a unit of weight). There are seven holes inside the heart. The hole has three hairs. (The heart) contains 3 he of essence liquid ["he" is a unit of dry measure for grain (= 1 decilitre)] and houses Shen (mind). The liver is like a minister, who has five leaves, corresponding to the five elements, and the weight is 3 jin [a catty (approximately 500 g)] and 10 liang. The gallbladder is like a general or a clerk in the Bureau of Decision. Below the short lobe of the liver, which weighs 9 liang, contains 4 he of essence liquid. The spleen is like an imperial advisor. It weighs 2 jin and 3 liang. It is 3 inches wide, 5 inches long, with a half a catty gao ("gao" is a kind of tissue has the texture of fat). It mainly stores warm blood. It houses Yi (will). It is located under the stomach and helps the stomach to digest food. The stomach weighs 2 jin and 14 liang. It can hold 3 buckets and 5 liters of grain. The lung is like a prime minister, with four leaves, corresponding to four seasons, weighing 2 jin and 12 liang. It houses Po (the corporeal soul) and is in charge of making voices. The kidney is like an upright woman with moral integrity and lives in the harem. It has 2 pieces, weighing 2 jin and 1 liang, and mainly collects the essence, then infuses the essence into the blood vessels.

REFERENCES

1. 世宗御，*医方类聚：第4卷 [M]* (北京：九州出版社, 2002), 41–55.
2. 宮下三郎，“敦煌本張仲景《五藏論》校譯注[J].” *東方學報（京都）*, Vol. 35, No. 3 (1964): 289–330.
3. 张弦，“朝鲜《医方类聚》研究[D].” 博士论文 北京中医药大学 (2013), 14.
4. 张弛，“论宋与高丽间的商贸往来[D].” 硕士论文 延边大学 (2008), 25.
5. 郑麟趾，*高丽史：卷八* [M] (朝鲜: 太白山史库本, 1613), 11.
6. 洪凤汉，增补文献备考：第242卷[M] (朝鲜：洪文馆, 1908), 17.
7. 成建军，“《灵枢经》的文献研究[D].” 博士论文，山东中医药大学 (2005), 65.
8. 崔秀汉，“朝鲜医书《医方类聚》考[J].” *延边医学院学报*, No. 3 (1985): 185–193.
9. 盛增秀等，“医方类聚（重校本）[M].” (北京：人民卫生出版社, 2006), 87–91.
10. 李倩，“《医方类聚》所引中国古代医籍研究[D].” 硕士论文，*北京中医药大学* (2006), 36.

9 This Cross-Century Zhang Zhongjing *Wu Zang Lun* – P. 2115V Housed in France

"The single volume of 'Wu Zang Lun' on the reverse side, due to the overlapping of characters, is easily overlooked and at risk of being lost."

– Zhu Dinghua

Pelliot chinois Dunhuang 2115V (abbreviated as P. 2115 V)[1] is currently housed at the National Library of France in Paris. This historical document features text on both sides. The front side contains the latter part of the Buddhist scripture *Debates on Alarm and Confusion* (Dá Jǐng Mí Lùn, 答警迷论) from the *Discourse on the Elucidation of the Deceptive and Confused* (Qióng Zhà Biàn Huò Lùn, 穷诈辩惑论), while the reverse side meticulously transcribes two medical works: Zhang Zhongjing's *Five Viscera Theory* (Wǔ Zàng Lùn, 五藏论) and *Simplified Examples of Pulse Diagnosis* (Píng Mài Lüè Lì, 平脉略例) totaling 174 lines, all written in ink.

The transcription on the reverse side of Zhang Zhongjing's *Five Viscera Theory* (Wǔ Zàng Lùn, 五藏论) is complete, starting with "Wu Zang Lun, one volume by Zhang Zhongjing" clearly marking the title and author's name, and ending with "Wu Zang Lun, one volume," corresponding to lines 1 to 108 on the reverse side of the original volume. Among the five versions of Zhang Zhongjing's *Five Viscera Theory* (Wǔ Zàng Lùn, 五藏论) unearthed in Dunhuang, this volume ranks first in terms of the amount of text preserved. Due to the manuscript being written on both sides, the ink has bled through, causing some of the content to become blurred and indistinct due to saturation. During the transcription process, some errors and omissions occurred in the text.

In his records on March 14, 1908, Paul Pelliot only mentioned the front side of the scroll, *Debates on Alarm and Confusion* (Dá Jǐng Mí Lùn, 答警迷论) from the *Discourse on the Elucidation of the Deceptive and Confused* (Qióng Zhà Biàn Huò Lùn, 穷诈辩惑论), without mentioning the medical works by Zhang Zhongjing, *Five Viscera Theory* (Wǔ Zàng Lùn, 五藏论), transcribed on the back. As a result, later references to P. 2115 V typically only acknowledge it as *Debates on Alarm and Confusion* (Dá Jǐng Mí Lùn, 答警迷论) from the *Discourse on the Elucidation of the Deceptive and Confused* (Qióng Zhà Biàn Huò Lùn, 穷诈辩惑论), overlooking the content on the reverse side.[2]

DOI: 10.1201/9781032698205-9

In 1985, Zhu Dinghua, a young scholar from the Institute of Medical History Literature at the China Academy of Chinese Medical Sciences, was researching Zhang Zhongjing's *Five Viscera Theory* (Wǔ Zàng Lùn, 五藏论). Guided by Ma Jixing, he consulted the *Comprehensive Index of Dunhuang Manuscripts* (Dūn Huáng Yí Shū Zǒng Mù Suǒ Yǐn, 敦煌遗书总目索引) edited by Wang Chongmin in 1962. Unexpectedly, he discovered a record labeled "Pelliot Chinese 2115V *Discourse on the Elucidation of the Deceptive and Confused*, one volume," with a small note underneath stating, "reverse side is one volume of *Wu Zang Lun*, written by Zhang Zhongjing."[3] The volume had text transcribed on both sides. Upon closer examination, he found that despite some minor damage and unclear characters, the reverse side's *Five Viscera Theory* (Wǔ Zàng Lùn, 五藏论) was a complete manuscript, an especially exhilarating discovery. It was clear that previous researchers had overlooked the *Five Viscera Theory* (Wǔ Zàng Lùn, 五藏论) because the cataloging focused primarily on the *Discourse on the Elucidation of the Deceptive and Confused* (Qióng Zhà Biàn Huò Lùn, 穷诈辩惑论), and the *Five Viscera Theory* (Wǔ Zàng Lùn, 五藏论) was only mentioned as a "note." This fortuitous finding illuminated the significance of Zhang Zhongjing's *Five Viscera Theory* (Wǔ Zàng Lùn, 五藏论) P. 2115V, rescuing a valuable manuscript from the brink of obscurity.

The Pelliot Chinese P. 2115V, as the most completely preserved version of Zhang Zhongjing's *Five Viscera Theory* (Wǔ Zàng Lùn, 五藏论) among the Dunhuang fragments discovered to date, was recognized relatively late compared to other versions such as Pelliot Chinese P. 2755, Pelliot Chinese P. 2378, and Stein Collection S. 5614. The identities of the actual copyists of these Zhang Zhongjing's *Five Viscera Theory* (Wǔ Zàng Lùn, 五藏论) manuscripts, as well as the initial collectors of these precious documents, remain unsolved mysteries that have greatly intrigued the academic community. These questions are not only related to the historical context of the documents but also represent an exploration into the depth and breadth of Dunhuang studies.

Since the discovery of the Dunhuang Mogao Caves by Taoist monk Wang Yuanlu in 1900, scholars and experts from around the world have devoted immense effort to studying the vast collection of manuscripts unearthed there. This has led to the emergence of Dunhuang studies as a profound discipline, encompassing both the art of the Dunhuang grottoes and the manuscripts found within the Hidden Library. While the world marvels at Dunhuang's art and scriptures, there remain stories from Dunhuang that, even decades after the discovery of the Hidden Library, have gone unnoticed.

Between the second and third layers of the caves above the Hidden Library, there is a small Zen cave with plain walls devoid of paintings. Inside, there is a monk statue as tall as a real person placed on the south side of the cave, not directly facing the entrance. This statue of the high monk, unlike other sculptures, is exceptionally realistic and lifelike. Positioned within this simple and cramped cave, it seems out of place to those who view it later, as if it does not belong there. This leads to the question: Where did it originally come from?

In 1965, during a reinforcement project north of the Dunhuang Mogao Caves, scaffolding was erected for the construction work. Chang Shuhong, known as the guardian deity of Dunhuang, was inspecting the progress of the project. As he walked across the scaffold planks, he, too, noticed that the lifelike statue of a monk did not match the simplicity and narrowness of the cave it was placed in. The back of the statue was plain clay, uncolored, with a circular seam about seven to eight centimeters in diameter at the center of the back, presumably a hole left during the sculpting process and later carefully sealed with clay after placing objects inside. There was speculation among those present that the statue might contain something inside, perhaps documents that could shed light on the identity of the statue. Chang Shuhong decided to open the cavity on the spot to discover its contents. After removing the sealing clay, a paper package was retrieved from the hole. The paper was white and sturdy, not appearing very old. Unwrapping the paper revealed several bone relics, or śarīra, sacred in Buddhism, white and hard. The paper was inscribed with inked Chinese characters, but there was nothing about the statue's identity, and the writing was not systematic. Seemingly, the paper was used for calligraphy practice. Later, the package of śarīra was placed back in its original location and resealed with clay.[4]

So who exactly is this statue? Coincidentally, near Cave 17 (the Hidden Library), embedded in the western wall, there is a large stone stele inscribed with the name Hongbian. Hongbian was a high monk during the mid to late Tang Dynasty. This confirms that Cave 17 is undoubtedly Hongbian's Image Hall (Yingtang). An "Image Hall" is a memorial hall built after the death of a revered monk, a practice that was popular during the Tang Dynasty. In Japan, the Tang Dynasty monk Jianzhen's Image Hall still exists in the Toshodai-ji Temple for posterity's commemoration. Building an Image Hall for Monk Hongbian was meant to serve as a memorial for future generations. Logically, a statue of the high monk should be enshrined within the Image Hall, but aside from some murals, no statue of Hongbian was found in Cave 17. Chang Shuhong immediately realized that the statue, squeezed into the small interlayer, was likely the true likeness of the high monk Hongbian. Moreover, the package of śarīra (relics) found within the statue further indicates that it represents the true likeness of Hongbian. Another particularly important point is that among the numerous caves to the north and south of Cave 17, there is no other Image Hall similar to Cave 17. This suggests that the statue of Hongbian was originally meant to be in Cave 17, but why was it placed in this interlayer? Let us travel back nearly 1,200 years to the Tang Dynasty to find out.

In 847 AD, the waning Tibetan Empire faced a significant setback, defeated by the Tang army in the Battle of Yanzhou (present-day Yanchi County in Ningxia). This defeat, amplified by enduring political turmoil, widespread famine, and a gradual relinquishment of their border towns, marked a critical point in their decline. Seizing the opportunity, Zhang Yichao, a prominent local figure in Shazhou (modern-day Dunhuang in Gansu), with the support of local elites and monks, launched a rebellion in 848 AD. He defeated the Tibetan forces and swiftly took control of the city of Shazhou, establishing the famous Guiyi Army. From this point, the Hexi Corridor, which had been under Tibetan control for nearly a century, except for Liangzhou, was reclaimed by the Tang Dynasty.

Monk Hongbian was a leading figure among the monks of Shazhou and the highest ecclesiastical official in the Dunhuang area, with the secular surname Wu.[5] He was also known as Monk Wu or Monk Wu Sengtong. During the Tibetan period, he was appointed to oversee the Buddhist laws and teachings in Shazhou. He played a significant role in supporting the Guiyi Army uprising led by Zhang Yichao, contributing to the defeat of the Tibetan forces. In recognition of his contributions, the Tang Dynasty honored him with the title of "Supreme Monk Official overseeing Buddhist affairs, laws, and teachings in Hexi, including Shazhou," awarded him the title of "Great Virtue who presides over ceremonies both inside and outside the capital," and granted him the privilege of wearing a purple robe. Over the years, Monk Hongbian initiated the excavation of several caves in the Mogao Grottoes, located southeast of Shazhou, where he also established his Image Hall.

Hongbian's Image Hall spans approximately 7.5 square meters, with a dome-shaped ceiling. Excluding some annexes, the usable space is just over 19 cubic meters. Upon receiving the imperial edict from the Tang Dynasty of conferring the head of monks in Shazhou on him, Hongbian immediately commissioned someone to carve this decree into a stone stele and embed it into the alcove of the western wall of his Image Hall.

After Monk Hongbian passed away, his disciples cremated his body and wrapped the remaining dozen or so śarīra (relics) in white silk cotton and white linen paper, placing them into an ash bag that had been prepared in advance. The outer layer of the ash bag was made of fine white silk, while the inner layer was of fine purple silk. The mouth of the bag was tied with white silk thread, then wrapped again with the linen paper that Hongbian favored for calligraphy practice. This package was then inserted through the back into the previously crafted statue representing his true likeness. It was carefully sealed with fine clay, smoothed over, left to dry, and finally, the true likeness statue was moved into the Image Hall for veneration.

Since it was intended as a place for future generations to worship and mourn, there was naturally no need to keep this Image Hall closed. Therefore, for many years afterwards, it remained open. Monk Hongbian's statue thus sat serenely in his modest Image Hall, receiving the offerings of his disciples and their successors.

As dawn gave way to dusk and seasons transitioned from spring to winter, time appeared to halt in this remote, exotic locale. Roughly two centuries after Monk Hongbian's passing, the serene silence of the Mogao Caves was broken by a group of frazzled monks. In a flurry of activity, they brought an array of items from unknown origins – books, scrolls, manuscripts, and silk paintings, all intended for storage in the compact Image Hall. Faced with an abundance of artifacts and limited space, the once spacious sanctuary could hardly contain the new influx. In a desperate bid to accommodate everything, Hongbian's statue was hastily relocated from its place of honor in the Image Hall to a nondescript, small Zen cave. With a sense of urgency, the monks mixed Hongbian's personal relics, sacred texts, and writings indiscriminately with the other items, cluttering the sacred space. This disruption of a revered monk's peaceful afterlife was a grave misstep, yet it seemed driven by an unavoidable necessity.

The entrance to the cave was quickly walled off and the surface meticulously smoothed, before being covered with vibrant Xixia-style frescoes, masterfully hiding any signs of the sealed space. Hidden behind this facade were treasures of untold value, their presence unbeknownst to onlookers. The precise moment of this event is lost to time, leaving us only with conjectures. The motives behind concealing these treasures in such a manner are shrouded in mystery. Was it an attempt to leave a legacy for future generations, a thousand years hence? However, the relentless desert winds soon cloaked these efforts under layers of sand, and the flowing waters of the Dang River washed away any remaining traces, rendering their intentions invisible to the world.

Day by day, year by year, emperors of the Central Plains came and went in succession, and the great Tang Dynasty eventually fell. The capital of the Chinese empire moved from the Guanzhong region to the Central Plains, relocating from Luoyang to Kaifeng, finally settling on the banks of the Grand Canal. From then on, the regions of Guanzhong and Luoyang, despite their natural fortifications, never again served as the center of a unified empire. The warlords of the turbulent times focused their efforts on the Central Plains, with none sparing a thought for the West. Dunhuang, located in the Shazhou region, although still maintaining a Han Chinese regime, was regarded by the central dynasties as a land utterly foreign.

As time progressed, a diverse procession of peoples – Dangxiang, Mongols, Turfan, Manchus, and Dongxiang – traversed this land, transient voyagers with varied religious faiths. Their dealings with the Buddhist relics alternated between attempts at restoration and instances of abandonment, yet their efforts were invariably incomplete. Amidst this transient custodianship, the deep sands and slender ancient walls steadfastly preserved the secret within.

The statue of Monk Hongbian was left forsaken in a Zen cave so diminutive that rotation was impossible, where it sat in silence for centuries. It bore witness to the vast tapestry of the mortal world while maintaining a profound silence.

For countless days and years, Monk Hongbian's statue remained in quiet contemplation within his dimly lit cave, dedicating himself to Zen meditation, believing the world outside would always stay peaceful. Yet the tranquility that had endured for ages was abruptly shattered. A figure, short in stature and dressed in Taoist garb with a pickaxe in hand, accompanied by a scholar holding an oil lamp, approached the cave where scriptures were kept. Suddenly, the sound of breaking stone filled the air as they broke through the wall of what was not only the scripture cave but also Monk Hongbian's Image Hall. Inside, the cave was packed from floor to ceiling with manuscripts, vibrant banners, and holy vessels; scrolls even buried his throne, while cobwebs stretched across the room. By some divine luck, these hidden gems were untouched by the decay typically wrought by insects and rodents. Hidden within what came to be known as the Hidden Library, this vast collection of ancient texts had miraculously survived natural disasters, human conflicts, and the wear of time untouched. Its discovery offered the modern world a glimpse into a thousand years past, opening a remarkable window into the cultural and historical fabric of that distant age.

Let us return to the year 1965, on the day Chang Shuhong was inspecting the reinforcement work. Following Chang Shuhong's instructions, the workers relocated the statue from the small Zen cave back to the Hidden Library. Monk Hongbian, a sage who had attained enlightenment, was finally returned to his Image Hall. If he is aware in the Pure Land, he should now be at peace.

The manuscripts found within this Image Hall have weathered their share of tumultuous fates. As research into these texts deepens, several phenomena observed during their organization and excavation merit discussion.

First of all, among the tens of thousands of manuscripts from the scripture cave, a significant number consist of drafts, handwritten notes, practice books, and assorted sketches and doodles, many of which are fragments or partially complete. Often, these documents feature writing on both sides, with Buddhist scriptures on one side and texts related to social, economic, or medical topics on the other, clearly indicating the repeated use of paper. This suggests that, at that time, paper was an extremely valuable commodity. Consequently, a vast array of outdated official documents unearthed from the cave, such as local registers, neighborhood registers, and tax ledgers, were repurposed as scrap paper. Their reverse sides were then utilized for copying Buddhist scriptures, practicing medicine, calligraphy, and more.

Secondly, among over 50,000 Dunhuang artifacts, only a few dozen are fragments of medical texts, representing an exceedingly small proportion. Today, these medical fragments are housed in European libraries in countries like England, France, and Russia, while the collections of Dunhuang manuscripts in China and Japan contain almost no medical documents. Interestingly, within these few medical fragments, the name of Zhang Zhongjing appears most frequently. His works, such as *Treatise on Cold Damage Disorders* (Shāng Hán Lùn, 伤寒论) or related writings, are the most prevalent. Notably, Zhang Zhongjing's *Five Viscera Theory* (Wǔ Zàng Lùn, 五藏论), a work lost to Chinese history for a thousand years, is the most frequently occurring text among the Dunhuang medical manuscripts, with five versions identified so far. The fact that P. 2115V has been preserved so completely is almost miraculous.

Lastly, the five versions of Zhang Zhongjing's *Five Viscera Theory* (Wǔ Zàng Lùn, 五藏论) discovered to date are not formally produced collectibles. Instead, they were transcribed on the reverse sides of other Buddhist scriptures, casually written in cursive script and all bear corrections, resembling notes taken during the study of medical texts or for practice and review. These five versions of Zhang Zhongjing's *Five Viscera Theory* (Wǔ Zàng Lùn, 五藏论) are distributed across libraries in three different countries, yet the handwriting is strikingly similar, suggesting they could all be the work of a single individual.

These three phenomena indicate that a significant portion of the Dunhuang manuscripts was used for copying and reviewing during the study of Buddhist scriptures and medical texts. At that time, the teachings of medicine often utilized Zhang Zhongjing's medical works as textbooks, which were widely circulated. Why, then, did the locals have such a strong preference for Zhang Zhongjing's writings? What reasons might underlie this favoritism?

This brings us back to the Hidden Library in Dunhuang, also known as Monk Hongbian's Image Hall. Hongbian, who became a monk in his youth, was talented in debate, fluent in Tibetan, translated Buddhist scriptures, and deeply studied the Yogachara. His father, Xu Zhi, and his mother, Madam Zhang, hailed from the distinguished and noble family of Nanyang. The "Monk Wu Sengtong Stele" mentions, "including his compassionate mother, who was of the esteemed lineage from Nanyang."[6] The Dunhuang inscriptions "Genealogy of Surnames and Clans" and

"New Collection of Genealogies of Surnames and Clans" record that this Nanyang refers to Nanyang in Dengzhou.[7] As is widely recognized, Zhang Zhongjing was from Deng County, Henan, which was known as Nanyang Commandery during the Qin Dynasty, became part of Jingzhou during the Han Dynasty, and was renamed Dengzhou during the Sui dynasty, later alternating between Nanyang and Dengzhou. Zhang Zhongjing mentioned in his work *Treatise on Cold Damage and Miscellaneous Disorders* (Shāng Hán Zá Bìng Lùn, 伤寒杂病论) that his "family was large, extending back two hundred members," also considered to be of notable status in Nanyang. By this reasoning, Monk Wu Hongbian's mother, Madam Zhang, could likely be a descendant of the Zhang Zhongjing lineage. Sun Simiao once said, "Doctors in the south of the Yangtze keep Zhang Zhongjing's essential formulas secret." The reason there are so many documents related to Zhang Zhongjing among the Dunhuang medical manuscripts could well be that people from Nanyang in Dunhuang, like Madam Zhang, secretly kept these texts, bringing them to Dunhuang when they moved.

From a young age, Wu Hongbian was deeply influenced by his parents' education, becoming well-versed in the classics. Whether Madam Zhang passed down medical texts to her son remains to be verified. However, Wu Hongbian revered the Medicine Buddha, as noted in the "Monk Wu Sengtong Stele" with the mention of "establishing a hall for the seven Medicine Buddhas and building a stupa for the Lotus Sutra and the Stainless One." The Medicine Buddha, known for removing all beings' suffering, illness, and the cycle of life and death, is typically depicted holding a medicine jar in the left hand and making the three realms gesture with the right, seated in full lotus position on a lotus pedestal.

In the Hidden Library, the colored statue of Wu Hongbian, dressed in monk's robes and emulating the Medicine Buddha as featured on the cover of this book, sits in full lotus position on a rectangular meditation platform. Behind the statue, a mural depicts a woman dressed in men's clothing holding a staff and a cloth on the right and a bhikkhuni holding a fine fan on the left, with a robust tree featuring hanging vines between them, adding a decorative flair. A scripture bag hangs from a branch on the left side of the wall and a medicine bottle on the right, suggesting Wu Hongbian's frequent teachings on Buddhism and medicine to monks.

Wu Hongbian's two successors, one known as the "Medicine King of Dunhuang," Zhai Farong,[8] a renowned monk physician active in the northwest frontier, and the other, the "Medicine King" Suo Chong'en,[9] author of many medical texts likely penned in Dunhuang, owed their medical expertise to Wu Hongbian's tutelage. With their esteemed backgrounds, only Wu Hongbian could have been qualified to teach them medical skills. Neither Zhai nor Suo would have placed their personal medical texts in Wu Hongbian's Image Hall, suggesting that the medical works found in the scripture cave were reflections of Wu Hongbian's life and professional needs.

In the ancient world, where the notions of original editions or copyrights were absent, the utility of texts took precedence for collectors. Consequently, the Dunhuang manuscripts of Zhang Zhongjing's *Five Viscera Theory* (Wǔ Zàng Lùn, 五藏论) incorporate Buddhist thought alongside insights and titles from medical authorities of the Later Han era, reflecting a pragmatic approach to education and learning. It's probable that the medical manuscripts found in the Dunhuang Hidden Library were transcribed with educational aims in mind. In this context, local monks and scholars diligently reproduced medical treatises, including *Five Viscera Theory* (Wǔ Zàng Lùn, 五藏论), both to disseminate knowledge and for their own scholarly pursuits.

Monk Hongbian, as a distinguished high monk in the Dunhuang region during the Tang Dynasty, held an important position not only within the religious community but also as a well-known figure in society. The potential familial connection with Zhang Zhongjing further enhances the likelihood of his involvement in protecting and disseminating literature related to Zhang Zhongjing. Monk Hongbian's profound expertise in both Buddhism and medicine fueled his special interest in significant medical texts like the *Five Viscera Theory* (Wǔ Zàng Lùn, 五藏论), likely facilitating the copying and preservation of these documents.

Just as Wang Shuhe made contributions to the *Treatise on Cold Damage Disorders* (Shāng Hán Lùn, 伤寒论) and Wang Zhu discovered the *Essential Prescriptions from the Golden Cabinet* (Jīn Guì Yào Lüè, 金匮要略) later organized by Lin Yi, Monk Hongbian was very likely the one who collected and organized Zhang Zhongjing's *Five Viscera Theory* (Wǔ Zàng Lùn, 五藏论) Dunhuang manuscripts. Monk Hongbian may have been directly involved in the copying or collection of some Dunhuang documents, particularly those related to his expertise and interests in medicine and Buddhism. Even if Monk Hongbian did not personally transcribe or collect Zhang Zhongjing's *Five Viscera Theory* (Wǔ Zàng Lùn, 五藏论), his status and influence were sufficient to promote the circulation and preservation of such documents in the Dunhuang region.

In the endeavor to excavate and organize the medical documents of Dunhuang, the contributions of numerous scholars have been noteworthy. Prominently, Ma Jixing's efforts have distinguished him as a standout figure in this scholarly pursuit.[10] Not long ago, Tu Youyou mentioned in her Nobel Prize acceptance speech that the earliest use of Artemisia annua in medicine was recorded in the silk manuscript *Prescriptions for Fifty-Two Ailments* (Wǔ Shí Èr Bìng Fāng, 五十二病方) found in Tomb No. 3 at Mawangdui, and it was the inspiration from this ancient Chinese medical text that led to the extraction of artemisinin. The *Prescriptions for Fifty-Two Ailments* (Wǔ Shí Èr Bìng Fāng, 五十二病方), unearthed from the Mawangdui Han tomb, was initially just a fragmentary silk manuscript. Ma Jixing, who was then a doctoral supervisor and professor at the Institute of Medical History Literature at the China Academy of Chinese Medical Sciences and a leading authority in the field of Chinese medical history, conducted a word-by-word verification of this medical text over 40 years ago. It was his work that finally decoded the *Prescriptions for Fifty-Two Ailments* (Wǔ Shí Èr Bìng Fāng, 五十二病方), allowing future generations to witness its contents.

Ma Jixing spent his life immersed in ancient texts, and even his manner of speaking carried an "ancient style." In the eyes of his family and disciples, Professor Ma's perennial image was that of a man never without a book, always reading wherever he was. "Books were his life." He not only read while eating but also during visits with relatives as others chatted, and even on New Year's Eve gatherings, he would be found reading on the side, a sight his family had long since grown accustomed to.

However, fate played a cruel joke on him; Ma Jixing was labeled a rightist. From being "branded" in 1957 to being rehabilitated in 1984, from the age of 33 to 59, he spent the prime years of an intellectual's life in hardship and humiliation. Despite this, he never gave up reading and researching. If he couldn't read during the day, he would read at night; if it wasn't feasible at his workplace, he would read at home. He even felt fortunate that his work with documents didn't require any equipment – just having books was enough.

The study of the silk manuscripts from the Mawangdui Han tombs captivated Ma Jixing with the world of ancient medical texts unearthed, many of which had only been known by their titles without any surviving content. This potential to uncover clues in unearthed artifacts spurred him to embark on nationwide expeditions. He traversed Gansu's Dunhuang, Hubei's Yunmeng, Sichuan's Mianyang, the Heicheng site in Inner Mongolia, and Xinjiang's Turpan, ancient Loulan, and Hotan . . . leaving his mark in each place. Yet what lingered most in his mind were those Dunhuang medical manuscripts that had been lost overseas.

Since the 1950s, Ma Jixing began to progressively collect photographic films and related materials concerning Dunhuang medical manuscripts. In 1965, he wrote an article titled *Preliminary Organization and Study of Dunhuang Medical Manuscripts* (敦煌医学残卷的初步整理研究) and presented his findings at the Chinese Medical History Society in Beijing. Under his guidance in the 1980s, the Institute of Medical History Literature in China organized young and middle-aged scholars to research and identify 84 types of Dunhuang medical manuscripts. Some materials were sourced from libraries in the United Kingdom, France, Japan, Russia, among others, as well as from private collectors.

After years of dedicated research and meticulous investigation, Ma Jixing authored *Annotations on the Ancient Medical Texts from the Dunhuang Cave Library* (Dūn Huáng Gǔ Yī Jí Kǎo Shì, 敦煌古医籍考释) in 1988, marking the first comprehensive and systematic study of Dunhuang medical manuscripts in the field of Chinese medical literature. The book is rich in material and incisive in its textual criticism, allowing the Dunhuang manuscripts that had drifted overseas to finally return to China in reproduced form. The book catalogs over 80 Dunhuang ancient medical texts in 11 categories, including medical classics, theories on the five zang organs, diagnostic methods, discussions on cold-induced disorders, medical techniques, prescriptions, herbal medicine, acupuncture, fasting and mineral therapy and miscellaneous prohibitions, Buddhist and Daoist medical prescriptions, and medical historical materials. Each text is described through six aspects: "Title," "Summary," "Original Text," "Collation and Annotation," "Commentary," and "Appendix." The introduction systematically presents the preservation of unearthed Chinese medical scrolls, the origin, chronological investigation, compilation and research work, philological characteristics, and academic value of Dunhuang medical manuscripts, establishing a foundational work for modern and contemporary research on Dunhuang medical literature. Ma Jixing's *Annotations on the Ancient Medical Texts from the Dunhuang Cave Library* (Dūn Huáng Gǔ Yī Jí Kǎo Shì, 敦煌古医籍考释) includes collations and commentaries on four different versions of Zhang Zhongjing's *Five*

Viscera Theory (Wǔ Zàng Lùn, 五藏论), hailed as a pinnacle in the study of Zhang Zhongjing's work.

In 1984, Chinese scholars formally introduced the concept of "Dunhuang medicine," thereby establishing its unique academic status within the realm of medical research. Dunhuang medicine is defined as an integral part of Chinese medical science, a key branch of Dunhuang studies, focusing on the organization, research, and application of traditional medical knowledge contained in Dunhuang manuscripts, murals, sculptures, and other cultural relics. Its medical content showcases distinct regional characteristics, covering the development of medicine from the Western Han through the Sui and Tang periods, and even into the Qing dynasty, making it a precious component of the world's cultural and scientific heritage. With the advancement of Dunhuang medicine, Zhang Zhongjing's *Five Viscera Theory* (Wǔ Zàng Lùn, 五藏论) has gained increasing recognition and has been subject to more thorough exploration.

In the research conducted by Ma Jixing and other scholars regarding the transcription and dating of Zhang Zhongjing's *Five Viscera Theory* (Wǔ Zàng Lùn, 五藏论), French catalog number P. 2115V, it was discovered that the manuscript avoids the character "世" (shì) associated with Emperor Taizong of Tang, alters the character "治" (zhì) associated with Emperor Gaozong to "疗" (liáo), and omits the name of Emperor Gaozong's son, Li Hong. However, it does not avoid the names of Emperor Zhongzong Li Xian, Emperor Ruizong Li Dan, or Emperor Muzong Li Heng, leading to the deduction that this copy was likely created in the early 7th century during the early Tang Dynasty. This finding provides crucial insights into the historical context of Dunhuang medicine.

Next is a direct translation of the full text of Zhang Zhongjing's *Five Viscera Theory* (Wǔ Zàng Lùn, 五藏论), cataloged under the French number: P. 2115V. The translation process strictly adheres to the original text, translating word for word and sentence by sentence, to ensure that every character and every sentence remains true to the original manuscript:

《五脏论》一卷 张仲景撰

Wu Zang Lun, One Volume, Author: Zhang Zhongjing

普(藥)名之部，出本於醫王，黄帝與造《针灸经》，曆有一千餘卷。耆婆童子，妙闲藥性，况公私等凡夫，何能備矣。

Medicine is contributed from the works of (later) various kings of medicine. Yellow Emperor made "The Canon of Acupuncture" that consists of 1,000 volumes. Jivaka has a miracle skill to adept the medicinal function of herbs. Moreover, how could someone from an ordinary family have mastered that?

天有五星，地有五岳，运有五行，人有五臟。所以肺(肝)为将军，脾为大夫，心为帝王，肺为丞相，肾为列女，肝與胆合，脾以胃通，小肠连心，大肠连肺，膀胱合肾，是以肝盛则目赤，心热则口乾，肾虚则耳聋，肺風则鼻塞，脾病则唇焦。目是肝候，舌是心观，耳作肾思，口是脾主，鼻为肺应。心主血脉，（脾主肌肉），肺主皮肤，肝主于筋，肾主於骨。骨假筋立，(筋籍肉行)，肉假皮存，面肿关脾，皮因骨长。故知骨患由肾，筋患则出肝，肉患则伤心(脾)，皮患则由肺。

The heaven has five stars, the earth has five mountains, the movement has five phases, and the human body has five Zang-organs. So that the lung (liver) is like a general, the spleen is like an officer, the heart is like an emperor, the lung is like a prime minister, and the kidney is like a woman with moral integrity. The liver works with the gallbladder; the spleen connects with the stomach together. The small intestine links to the heart, and the urinary bladder works together with the kidney. Therefore, liver excess causes red eyes, heart heat causes dry mouth, kidney deficiency causes deafness, lung wind causes nose stiffness, and spleen disorder causes lip scorched. The eyes are the gate of the liver, the tongue is the window of the heart, the ears are the thinker for the kidney, and the nose is the reactor of the lung. The heart rules the blood vessels, (the spleen rules muscle), the lung rules the skin, the liver rules the tendons, and the kidney rules the bones. Bones depend on tendon to stand straight (tendons make use of muscles so that one can walk), muscle depends on skin to exist, face swelling is related to spleen, and skin depends on bone to grow. Therefore, the bone disorders are resulted from the kidney, the tendon disorders are resulted from the liver, the muscle disorders will damage the heart (spleen), and the skin disorders are resulted from the lung.

只是十二经上下巡還，八脉寄经，内外流转。三燋六府，四海七神，膲膈咽喉，唇舌牙齿，臂肘指爪，膝胫脚踝，背肋项股，颔额鼻主，鬓眉须发，俱有患处，并有所因。莫不内积虚劳，外缘风袭者也。察其颜色，即辨寒温，听之音声，便知益损。

There are 12 meridians circulate upward and downward, and eight extraordinary meridians flow in the human body internally and externally. There are also triple burners and six Fu-organs; four seas and seven spirits; the space between the flesh, diaphragm, pharynx, and throat; lips, tongue, and teeth; arm, elbows, fingers, and nails; knees, lower leg, feet, and ankles; back, hypochondriac area, and neck; head, chin, forehead, and nose; sideburns, eyebrow, mustache, and hair, all the aforementioned places could suffer from illness, and the illness must have their causes, which are either internal deficiency and impairment or external caught wind. By looking at the facial color, you will be able to tell if it is cold syndrome or warm syndrome. By listening to the voice, you will know the person has excess or deficiency.

喜言者心病，多欠者肾耶。啼哭者患肝，声吟者脾疾。痛白者是冷，皮青者是風，颜黑者是温，面黄者是热。心风者则好妄，脾虚则喜饥，肾冷则腰疼，肺实则多怒，声细者患冷，声沉者患風，声轻者患虚，声粗者患热，视毛则知骨，见爪则知筋，看目则知肝，察齿则知骨，骨伤则齿黑，血伤则皮焦，筋绝则爪乾，声嘶则气少，声赤能发血。餘是患者，植表其原，寻原而作医疗，察外而知臟腑。如此委细，乃是良医。又须巧制医方，妙闲藥性，应病与藥，无病不除。世无良医，枉死者半。

Like to talk a lot could mean heart sickness; yawn too much means there is kidney evil; whimper and cry are due to the illness of liver; moan and groan are because of the illness of spleen. Pale skin indicates cold in the body; blue skin tone indicates wind invasion; dark facial color indicates warmth in the body; sallow face indicates the heat in the body. The heart wind causes preposterous; the spleen deficiency causes hunger; the kidney cold causes the lumbar pain; the lung excess causes anger. A soft voice indicates suffering from cold, a deep voice indicates suffering from wind, a weak voice indicates suffering from deficiency, and a rough voice indicates suffering from heat. Looking at hair can know about the bone, looking at nail can know about tendons, looking at eyes can know about the liver, and looking at the teeth can know about bone. The bone injury causes the teeth to turn dark color; the blood injury causes the skin looks burned; the tendon damage causes the nail to be dried; hoarse voice indicates insufficient Qi; the shouting voice produces swift blood flow. Therefore, the patient has external manifestation and internal causes. To find the causes to treat the illness, to see outside to investigate the inside zang fu organ; if do so, you are a good doctor. (A good doctor) also needs to come up with medical formula carefully. You must prescribe the medicine according to the illness. (If do so), no disease can't be cured! But there is no good doctor now. Half of the patients died due to improper treatments.

天地之内，人最为贵。头圆法天，足方法地。天有四时，人有四肢，天有五行，人有五臟。天有六律，人有六腑。天有七星，人有七孔。天有八风，人有八節。天有十二时，人有十二經。天有二十四氣，人有二十四俞。天有三百六十五日，人有三百六十骨節。天有晝夜，人有睡眠。天有雷电，人有嗔怒。天有日月，人有眼目。地有泉水，人有血脉。地有九州，人有九窍。地有山石，人有骨齿。地有草木，人有毛发。四大五蔭，假合成身，一大不調，百病俱起。

Between the heaven and the earth, the human being is the most valued. The head is round shaped that imitates the heaven; the feet are square shaped that imitates the earth. (On the analogy concept), the heaven has four seasons, correspondingly, human has four limbs; the heaven has five elements, so does human has five Zang-organs; the heaven has six rhyms, so does human has six Fu-organs; the heaven has seven stars, so does human has seven orifices; the heaven has eight kinds of winds, so does human has eight (big) joints; the heaven has 12 two-hour periods, so does human has 12 meridians; the heaven has 24 divisions of the solar year, so does human has 24 acupuncture shu points. The heaven has 360 days, so does human has 360 joints; the heaven has day and night, so does human knows when to sleep; the heaven has thunder and lightning, so does human has anger. The heaven has sun and moon, so does human has eyes; the earth has spring water, so does human has blood vessels. The earth has nine states, so does human has nine orifices. The earth has mountains and rocks, so does human has bones and teeth. The earth has grass and trees, so does human has hair. The human body is created by four greats and five ordinalities. If one does not balance, it will cause hundreds of illnesses.

经曰：神农本草辨土地显君臣；陶景注经，说酸咸而陈冷热，雷公妙典，咸述炮炙之宜；仲景其方，委说根茎之用；周公药对，虚谈犯触之能，宋侠正方，直说五风之妙；扁鹊能回丧车，起死人，昧后并是神方；华佗割骨除根，患者悉得瘳愈；刘涓子秘述，学在鬼边；徐百一之丹方，偏疗小儿之效；淮南葛氏之法，秘要不传；集验之方，人间行用。药疗也，疗人万病，服用俱解，子孙昌盛，众从爱敬，皆由药性。

Medical classic canon indicated: *Shennong's Classic of Materia Medica* (Shén Nóng Běn Cǎo Jīng, 神农本草经) differentiated the earth to manifest as King and Minister. In "Variorum of the Classic of Materia Medica," Tao Hongjing explained sour and salty, discussed cold and hot nature (of the herbs). Lei Gong's marvelous classic talked in detail about herbal processing. Zhang ZhongJing's formulas tirelessly discussed the use of stems and roots. "Zhou Gong's pair herbs" concisely talked about the contraindications. "Song Xia Zheng Fang" directly discusses the wonder of the five winds. Bian Que can call back the funeral canopy and rescue the people back to life from death. All rely on magical formulas. Hua Tuo scratched the bones to eliminate the root of poison. That's why patients can get fully recovered.

Liu Juanzi's secret talk was from his learning by the side of the ghost. Xu Baiyi's pill formulas specialized in children's illness. Scholar Ge, who came from south of Huai River, kept his formulas secret. Formulas from "The Collection of Clinical Effective Formulas" (Jí Yàn, 集验) were used widely. The effect of the herbs and formulas can treat many human illnesses. People recover from taking the medicine. The descendants can be prosperous. They can respect and love each other all because of the effect of the medicine.

只如八味肾气，补六极而差五劳；四色神丹，荡千疴而除万病。有命者差必，虢太子死苏生；无命者难为，秦景公于焉致死。人之养病，如火积薪中，去火如薪得全，去病人皆得活。薪不去火，虚被焚烧；有病不医，徒劳丧命。贵人之所贵，贱人之所贱，昔季康子馈药，夫子拜而受之。上古圣贤，犹敬其药。是以上、中、下药，所疗不同；甘苦酸咸，随其本性。若能君臣行用，玄疾能瘳；倘若参差，损他身命。

For example, Ba Wei Shen Qi (八味肾气, Eight-Ingredient Kidney Qi Pills) tonifies six types of extreme deficiencies to recover from five exhaustions. Si Se Shen Dan (四色神丹, Four-Color Magic Pills) cleans up thousands of illnesses to eliminate tens of thousands of diseases. If the person is meant to live, (with medical treatment), that person will live. That is why Prince Guo was revived from death. If the person is meant to die, (without medical treatment), that person will die. That is the reason why Qin Jing Gong died. A person taking care of his illness is like fire accumulating in the wood. The wood will survive if the fire has been extinguished. Same thing, the patient could recover if he takes care of the illness. Wood would be burned if the fire cannot be put out. If a patient leaves illness untreated, he will suffer and die. One should treat valuable things as being precious and treat valueless things as being worthless. In ancient times, Ji Kangzi gave medicines to Confucius. Confucius bowed and received the medicine with respect. Since ancient times, the saints and intelligence all respected medicine. The plants were divided into upper, middle, and lower classes. Each class treats different conditions; sweet, bitter, sour, and salty, follows the plant's nature. If one could also use the principle of King and Minister in a formula, even some very difficult diseases could be cured. If prescribed wrong medicine, people's life could be impaired.

故本草云：灵端之草，然则长先生；钟乳饵之，令人悦愈。犀角有抵触之义，故能趁疰驱邪；牛黄怀沉香之功，是以安魂定魄；蓝田玉屑，镇压精神；中台射香，差(瘥)除妖魅。河内牛膝，疗膝冷而去腰疼；上蔡防风，愈头风而瘳胁痛。晋地龙骨，绝甘利（疳痢）而去头疼；泰山茯苓，发阴阳而延年益寿。片草有安和之性，故受国老之名；大黄宣引众公，乃得将军之号。半夏有消痰之力，制毒要藉生姜；当归有止痛之能，相使还须白芷。泽泻、茱萸，能使耳目聪明；远志、人参，巧含开心益智。

Thus, in "Materia Medica," it said: Ling Rui Zhi Cao (灵瑞之草 or "Ling Zhi" 灵芝, lucid ganoderma) could make people live forever. Taking Zhong Ru (钟乳, stalactite) could make people happier. Xi Jiao (犀角, rhinoceros horn) has the power to fight against illness, so it can eliminate chronic infectious disease and disperse evil. Niu Huang (牛黄, cattle gallstone) has the function like Chen Xiang (沉香, Chinese eaglewood) to calm the Hun (ethereal soul) and the Po (corporeal soul). Yu Xie (玉屑, Jade Chips) from Lan Tian can tranquilize the mind. She Xiang (麝香, musk) from Zhong Tai can drive out evil. Niu Xi (牛膝, two-toothed achyranthes root) from He Nei treats cold knee and relieves lower back pain. Fang Feng (防风, siler root) from Shang Cai heals the head wind, also relieves the hypochondriac pain. Long Gu (龙骨, dragon bone fossil, or fossilized animal bone) from Jin Di can stop greediness so to relieve headache. Fu Ling (茯苓, Indian bread or poria) from Tai Shan Mountain balances yin and yang to achieve longevity. Gan Cao (甘草, licorice root) has the function of harmonizing; thus, it has been called the "Guo Lao," a respected elder in the kingdom. Da Huang (大黄, rhubarb root) has the function of opening and inducing the elimination. That's why it was called the "Marshall General." Ban Xia (半夏, pinellia tuber) dissolves phlegm; raw ginger can counteract its toxicity. Dang Gui (当归, Chinese angelica root) can stop pain, but it must be combined with Bai Zhi (白芷, Dahurian angelica root). Ze Xie (泽泻, alisma tuber) and Zhu Yu (茱萸, or "Shan Zhu Yu" 山茱萸, cornus fruit) can benefit hearing and vision. Yuan Zhi (远志, Thinleaf milkwort root) and Ren Shen (人参, ginseng root) magically open the heart to make people smart.

赤疮宜涂鸡子，白癞须附越桃。火烧宜贴水萍，杖打稍加营实。飞屍走疰，速用雄黄；忽而惊邪，急求龙齿。头风眩闷，须访菊花。脚弱行迟，宜求石斛。欲令见鬼，久服麻花。拟去白虫，漆和鸡子。蔷薇却其疥癣，蟹黄嗜去漆疮。通草巧疗耳聋，胆石唯除眼膜。

Red ulcer should apply Ji Zi (鸡子, chicken eggs); tuberculoid leprosy needs to use Yue Tao (越桃 or "Zhi Zi" 栀子, gardenia fruit); burns to be treated by applying Shui Ping (水萍 or "Fu Ping" 浮萍, floating duckweed) topically; wounds from caning can use Ying Shi (营实 or "Qiang Wei Zi" 蔷薇子, multiflora Rose Fruit). Pestilential illness uses Xiong Huang (雄黄, realgar) immediately. Sudden frightening should ask for Long Chi (龙齿, fossilized animal teeth) immediately. Head wind with dizziness must use Ju Hua (菊花, chrysanthemum flower). Weakness of limbs caused difficult walking will be benefit from Shi Hu (石斛, dendrobium stem). If see ghost, consume Ma Hua (麻花, cannabis bud) long-term. If you want to eliminate white parasite, use Qi (漆, lacquer) and Ji Zi (鸡子, chicken eggs). Qiang Wei (蔷薇, multiflora Rose) can get rid of fungal infection; Xie Huang (蟹黄, crab yolk) can eliminate eczema. Tong Cao (通草, rice paper plant pith) can magically treat deafness; Shi Dan (石胆, chalcanthite) eliminates cataract.

秦艽有结罗纹之状，干漆作蜂巢之形。丹砂会取光明，升麻只求青绿。秦膠须汗，矾石须炮。杜仲削去腴(酸)皮，桂心取其有味。石英研之似粉，杏仁别捣如膏。菟丝酒渗乃良，朴硝火烧方好。防葵为轻唯上，狼毒为重唯佳。黄芩以附肠为精，蘭茹漆头为用。石南采叶，甘菊收花。五加割取其皮，牡丹槌其去骨。鬼箭破血，仍有射鬼之灵。神屋除温，非带报神之验。

Qin Jiao (秦艽, largeleaf gentian root) pertains spiral shape; Gan Qi (干漆, dried lacquer) looks like honeycomb. Dan Sha (丹砂 or "Zhu Sha" 朱砂, cinnabar) should be shiny; Sheng Ma (升麻, largetrifoliolious bugbane Rhizome) should be blue and green. Qin Jiao (秦椒, prickly ash peel) needs to be steamed; Fan Shi (矾石 or "Ming Fan" 明矾, a sulfate of alum-stone, or white alum-stone) should be roasted; Du Zhong (杜仲, eucommia bark) must peel off the outer skin; Gui Xin (桂心 or 肉桂, cinnamon bark) must have intense fragrance. Shi Ying (石英, Cristobalite) must be powdered; Xing Ren (杏仁, apricot seed) should be grinded until gets creamy. Tu Si (菟丝, Chinese dodder seed) must be soaked with alcohol; Pu Xiao (朴硝, a crude form of sodium sulfate) must be calcinated. Fang Kui (防葵, white flower hog fennel root) the lighter the better; Lang Du (狼毒, Bracteole-lacked Euphorbia root) the heavier the better. Good Huang Qin (黄芩, Baical skullcap root) looks like rotten intestine; only use Lin Ru's (藺茹, Euphorbia Lanru root) top part. Shi Nan (石南, Chinese photinia Leaf) should pick its leaves; Gan Ju (甘菊, sweet chrysanthemum flower) uses its flower. Wu Jia (五加, Slenderstyle Acanthopanax Bark) only uses the bark; Mu Dan (牡丹, tree peony bark), hammer its stem and take the bone out. Gui Jian (鬼箭 or "Gui Jian Yu" 鬼箭羽, winged branches) break up the blood stasis thus to kill ghost toxins. Shen Wu (神屋 or 龟板, tortoise carapace and plastron) clears the heat and has magical effect.

喷吐汤煎干葛，筋转酒煮木瓜。目赤须点黄连，口疮宜含黄柏。痹转应痛，须访茵芋。甚痒皮痛，汤煎蒴藋。伤寒发汗，要用麻黄。壮热不除，宜加竹叶。恒山鳖甲大有差疟之功，蛇蜕绿丹善除癫痫之用。雄黄除黑干，木兰能去死皮。莽草煞齿内之虫，黎芦除烂鼻中宿肉。黄连断痢除疳。子支悦愈面皮。桃花润泽肤体。芎藭、枳实，心急即用加之，紫菀、款冬，气嗽要须當用。虻虫、水蛭，即破血之功。白术、槟榔，有散气消食之效。昌蒲强寄(记)，鳖甲通神。

Decoct Gan Ge (干葛 or "Ge Gen" 葛根, dried pueraria root) to treat vomiting; use alcohol to decoct Mu Gua (木瓜, Chinese quince fruit) for muscle spasm. Use Huang Lian (黄连, yellow coptis root) to make eye drops for red eyes. Hold Huang Bo (黄蘗 or "Huang Bo" 黄柏, phellodendron bark) in the mouth for mouth ulcer. Painful arthritis uses Yin Yu (茵芋, Japanese skimmia stem and leaf); severe skin itch uses Shuo Huo (蒴藋, Chinese elder) decoction. Promote sweat during Shang Han, exogenous pathogenic cold-induced diseases, uses Ma Huang (麻黄, ephedra stem). Constant high fever can benefit from Zhu Ye (竹叶, bamboo leaves). Heng Shan (恒山 or "Chang Shan" 常山, dichroa root) and Bie Jia (鳖甲, Chinese soft-shelled turtle shell) have great function to relieve malaria. She Tui (蛇蜕, snake slough) and Lü Dan (铝丹, aluminum pill) relieve seizure attacks. Xiong Huang (雄黄, realgar) is to treat gangrene; Mu Lan (木兰 or "Hou Po" 厚朴, lily magnolia bark) can remove dead skin. Mang Cao (莽草, leaf of poisonous eightangle tree) treats cavity inside the teeth; Li Lu (藜芦, veratrum root and rhizome) can dissolve polyps in the nose. Huang Lian (黄连, yellow coptis root) stops dysentery disease and eliminates malnutrition; Zhi Zi (支子 or "Zhi Zi" 栀子, gardenia fruit) benefits facial skin; Tao Hua (桃花, peach blossom) can moisten body skin. Xiong Qiong (芎藭 or "Chuan Xiong" 川芎, Sichuan lovage rhizome) and Zhi Shi (枳实, immature range fruit) treat anxiety; Zi Wan (紫菀, Tatarian aster root) and Kuan Dong (款冬, Common coltsfoot flower) are used for asthma and cough. Mang Chong (虻虫, horse fly) and Shui Zhi (水蛭, leech) are to break up blood stasis. Bai Zhu (白术, white atractylodes tuber) and Bing Lang (槟榔, areca nut) relieve bloating and promote digestion. Chang Pu (菖蒲 or "Shi Chang Pu" 石菖蒲, grass-leaf sweetflag rhizome) enhances memory; Bie Jia (鳖甲, Chinese soft-shelled turtle shell) promotes spiritual function.

阴阳疮汤煎蛇床，淋涩须加滑石。仙零脾(仙灵脾)草能去腰疼，然则忘杖归家；天鼠煎膏巧疗耳聋，得莀麻而加妙；蛇咬宜封人粪，蜂螫荜菝妙除。零(羚)羊角通噎驱邪，青羊肝疗疳明目。石脂加颜发色，白芨卷面除皮。知母通痢开胸。空青消徵(癥)止泪。孔公孽消食肥泽，密陀僧去疥癞人，压石寄假蜂房，水肿惟须仗大戟。肠结通惟甘遂，患眼宜取蕤仁。安胎必藉紫威(薇)，伤身要须地髓。恼心闷偏加木笔，血闭急觅蒲黄。连翘却瘰疬疮痈，地胆破癥瘕息肉。斑蝥能除鼠漏，松脂瘆恶刺風疽。牵牛泻水排脓，葶苈大枣除水。桃仁绝其鬼气，石南复去诸风。瘿气昆布妙除。肠痈必须硝石，脱肛宜取鳖头。下贱虽曰地浆，天行病飲者皆愈；黄龙汤出其厕内，时气病者能除。贫者虽号小方，不及君臣，取写有处，出处有灵有验，有贵有贱，有高有下，净秽亢草山中药。

Vaginal discharge, exterior vaginal itching, and redness, use She Chuang (蛇床, common cnidium fruit) to decoct. Urgent or hesitate urination, add Hua Shi (滑石, talc). Xian Lin Pi (仙灵脾 or "Yin Yang Huo" 淫羊藿, horny goat weed or epimedium) relieves lower back pain so that the patient can walk back home without the crutches. Syrup made from Tian Shu (天鼠 or "Bian Fu" 蝙蝠, bat) treats deafness, to add Bi Ma (蓖麻, castor leaf or bean) for better results. Topically cover with Ren Fen (人粪 or "Ren Zhong Huang" 人中黄, human feces) for snake bite; bee sting can be treated by Bi Ba (荜茇, piper longum). Ling Yang Jiao (零羊角 or 羚羊角, antelope's horn) is for esophageal obstruction and to eliminate evil. Qing Yang Gan (青羊肝, goral liver) treats malnutrition (anemia) and brightens vision. Shi Zhi (石脂, halloysite) darkens hair; Bai Ji (白芨, bletilla tuber) removes dead skin and regenerates new skin. Zhi Mu (知母, common anemarrhena rhizome) treats dysentery and opens chest; Kong Qing (空青, azurite) eliminates abdominal lump and stops tearing. Kong Gong Nie (孔公孽, Calcite) helps digest food and gains weight. Mi Tuo Seng (密陀僧, lithargite) treats eczema and skin infection. Feng Fang (蜂房, honeycomb) used to calm down the rebellious Qi caused by taking Ru Shi (乳石, stalactite). Edema can use Da Ji (大戟, Peking spurge root). Intestinal obstruction uses Gan Sui (甘遂, gansui root). Eye disease uses Rui Ren (蕤仁, hedge prinsepia nut). Calm down fetus must use Zi Wei (紫威 or 紫薇, Chinese Trumpetcreeper Flower); Di Sui (地髓 or "Gan Di Huang" 干地黄, drying rehmannia root) is for physical exhaustion. Mentally depress use Mu Bi (木笔 or "Xin Yi Hua" 辛夷花, magnolia flower); amenorrhea uses Pu Huang (蒲黄, cat-tail pollen) immediately. Scrofula and boils use Lian Qiao (连翘, weeping forsythia Capsule); Di Dan (地胆, a kind of blister beetles) treats mass, nodules, and polyps. Ban Mao (斑猫, mylabris) can treat chronic skin abscess; Song Zhi (松脂, pine resin) is anti-infection. It can promote discharge of pus. Qian Niu (牵牛, morning glory) is a strong diuretic to reduce swelling. It also helps discharge pus; Ting Li (葶苈 or "Ting Li Zi" 葶苈子, tansymustard seed) and Da Zao (大枣, Chinese date) eliminate edema. Tao Ren (桃人 or 桃仁, peach kernel) stops evil energy; Shi Nan (石南, Chinese photinia Leaf) to eliminate all kinds of internal wind. Kun Bu (昆布, kombu) relieves goiter; Xiao Shi (硝石or "Mang Xiao" 芒硝, nitrate from saline alkali land) treats intestinal abscess; Bie Tou (鳖头, soft-shell turtle head) treats rectal prolapse. Regardless of the degrading name of "Di Jiang" (地浆, Earth Slurry), Tian Xing Bing, epidemic diseases caused by natural factors, gets healed by taking Di Jiang (地浆, Earth Slurry). Although Huang Long Tang (黄龙汤, Yellow Dragon Decoction) came from toilet, it can treat infectious disease.

《五脏论》一卷

"Wu Zang Lun," one volume.

REFERENCES

1. Shanghai Chinese Classics Publishing House and Bibliotheque Nationale de France, *Dunhuang and Other Central Asian Manuscripts in the Bibliotheque Nationale de France: Volume 6 Fonds Pelliot chinois 2114–2141* (Shanghai: Shanghai Chinese Classics Publishing House, 1998), 13–32.
2. [法] 保罗・伯希和，*伯希和西域探险日记[M]*. （*1906–1908*）[M]，耿昇译（北京：中国藏学出版社, 2014), 491.
3. 朱定华，"敦煌残卷医籍张仲景《五藏论》辨析[J]."*上海中医药杂志*,No.10(1985): 6–9.
4. 孙儒僩，"莫高轶事我的敦煌生涯（七）– 千相塔残塑的整理及第 17 窟洪辩像的迁移[J]." *敦煌研究*, No. 6 (2015): 122–125.
5. 彭建兵，"归义军首任河西都僧统吴洪辩生平事迹述评[J]." *敦煌学辑刊*, No. 2 (2005): 157–163.
6. 郑炳林，*敦煌碑铭赞辑释[M]* ((兰州：甘肃教育出版社，1992), 63.
7. 唐耕耦，*敦煌四件唐写本姓望氏族谱残卷研究[A]*. 见：*敦煌吐鲁番文献研究论集（第二辑）[C]* (北京：北京大学出版, 1983), 211–280.
8. 党新玲，"唐代敦煌医王翟法荣[J]." *甘肃中医学院学报*, Vol. 10, No. 3 (1993): 8–59.
9. 新玲，"唐敦煌药王索崇恩[J]." *甘肃中医学院学报*, Vol. 10, No. 1 (1993): 61–62.
10. 王国平，"马继兴：住在书袋里" *光明日报[N]*. April 4 (2013): 1–6.

10 Feared to Be Deemed a Forgery – Zhejiang Edition

> "If this item had fallen into the hands of past 'authenticity verifiers,' it would have been labeled as a 'forgery.'"
>
> **– Geng Jianting**

Compared to other versions of Zhang Zhongjing's *Five Viscera Theory'* (Wǔ Zàng Lùn, 五藏论), the Zhejiang edition stands out for its completeness, readability, and extensive inclusion of medicinal varieties. Its preface, penned by Zhang Yunsu, a highly esteemed traditional Chinese medicine (TCM) physician from the Jin Dynasty, adds its historical significance.

In Ma Jixing's *Annotations on the Ancient Medical Texts from the Dunhuang Cave Library* (Dūn Huáng Gǔ Yī Jí Kǎo Shì, 敦煌古医籍考释), he particularly mentioned this Zhejiang edition. He named it as "an old block-printed edition":

> which circulating among the populace (the publication year remains unspecified), featuring a preface wrote by Zhang Yuansu of the Jin Dynasty. However, this particular reprint has been lost to time, leaving only the version transcribed during the Qing Dynasty by Zhang Yicheng, a renowned Zhejiang doctor, still extant.[1]

Zhang Yuansu stated in the preface that he edited the book based on familial transmissions yet maintained the original's core ideas and sentence structures. Consequently, this edition bears the editorial mark of Zhang Yuansu, though the extent of alterations to the content remains uncertain.

Two individuals have reported the discovery of the Zhejiang edition. The first is Chen Yongzhi from the Dama Township Medical Center in Tongxiang County, Zhejiang Province. In 1979, he published an article titled *Manuscript Copies of "Zhang Zhongjing's Five Viscera Theory" and Their Comparison with Foreign Collections* (传抄本<张仲景五藏论>及其与国外藏本的比较) in issue 2 of the *Jiangsu Journal of Traditional Chinese Medicine* [江苏医药 (中医分册)]. In this article, he noted that the Zhejiang edition he unearthed was a hand-copied version by the late renowned Zhejiang physician Zhang Yicheng (1879–1954), featuring a preface written by Zhang Yuansu of the Jin Dynasty.[2]

Another individual who reported the discovery of the Zhejiang edition is Chu Jinxiang, also affiliated with the Dama Township Medical Center in Tongxiang County, Zhejiang Province. In 1983, Chu Jinxiang published an article titled

DOI: 10.1201/9781032698205-10

Discussion on the Authenticity of Zhang Zhongjing's "Wu Zang Lun" (张仲景<五藏论>真伪问题的探讨) in the *Chinese Journal of Medical History* (中华医史杂志). In the article, he mentioned:

> Years ago, I acquired a volume of the Zhang Zhongjing *Wu Zang Lun* manuscript from a friend. It is said that this book was transcribed from the *Family Tree of Qinghe* (Qīng Hé Pǔ Dié, 清河谱牒) by a renowned physician in western Zhejiang Province during the late Qing Dynasty, with a preface by Zhang Yuansu attached at the beginning.[3]

The content of the *Five Viscera Theory* (Wǔ Zàng Lùn, 五藏论) referenced in these two articles remains consistent, with both attributing the manuscript to the renowned Zhejiang physician Zhang Yicheng. The only discrepancy lies in the latter's assertion that this version of the *Five Viscera Theory* (Wǔ Zàng Lùn, 五藏论) was hand-copied from the *Family Qinghe Genealogy* (Qīng Hé Pǔ Dié, 清河谱牒). Regarding the question of whether it was discovered by Chen Yongzhi or Chu Jinxiang, we will refrain from further discussion.

Both discoverers, Chen Yongzhi and Chu Jinxiang, shared the belief that the Zhejiang edition, rather than being authored by Zhang Zhongjing himself, was attributed to him posthumously. They argued that it likely originated after the Six Dynasties or the Tang Dynasty, considerably later than Zhang Zhongjing's lifetime during the Eastern Han Dynasty.

At the conclusion of Chen Yongzhi's article in the *Jiangsu Journal of Traditional Chinese Medicine* [江苏医药(中医分册)], an appended postscript by editor Geng Jianting offers further insight. Geng remarked:

> The Zhejiang edition presented here has undoubtedly undergone revisions and enhancements by later generations. The individual who supplemented *Wu Zang Lun* appears to have possessed considerable talent, evident in the seamless unity and coherence of the writing. However, verifying whether this was the work of Zhang Yuansu or another individual remains challenging. Nevertheless, the acknowledgment of some additions to the original text is undeniable. Should this manuscript fall into the hands of those discerning forgeries, it might be dismissed as such once more. Yet, I am inclined to believe otherwise.

Geng's stance suggests a leaning towards the possibility that this edition of the *Five Viscera Theory* (Wǔ Zàng Lùn, 五藏论) was augmented by Zhang Yuansu rather than by subsequent generations. Nonetheless, lacking definitive evidence, it's understandable why some scholars later questioned its authenticity through their writings.

Indeed, 38 years after the initial publication of the Zhejiang edition in 2017, Chinese scholar Hui Yongyan and colleagues raised doubts about this version of Zhang Zhongjing's *Five Viscera Theory* (Wǔ Zàng Lùn, 五藏论).[4] Upon comparing it with Dunhuang manuscripts and the Korean version, Hui Yongyan et al. concluded that the Zhejiang edition was derived from Zhao Youchen's *An Introduction of Zhang Zhongjing "Wu Zang Lun"* (介绍张仲景五藏论), which was published in the fifth issue of the *Jiangsu Journal of Traditional Chinese Medicine* (江苏中医) in 1963.[5] They further posited that modifications and supplements to parts of the text were made with reference to the Korean edition and Miyazaki Saburo's *About*

Zhang Zhongjing Wu Zang Lun (張仲景五蔵論について), published in the *Journal of Kampo Medicine* (漢方の臨床) in 1959.[6]

In their article, Hui Yongyan et al. addressed three key points:

> Firstly, they noted the striking similarity between the Zhejiang version and the compilation by Zhao Youchen in terms of structure and medicinal content. Given that Zhao's version was published in 1963 and the Zhejiang edition in 1979, there arises the possibility that the latter was revised based on Zhao's compilation.

Secondly, upon comparison, Hui Yongyan et al. observed remnants of the Korean edition and Miyazaki Saburo's compiled version within the Zhejiang edition. However, they found no discernible link between the Zhejiang edition and the Dunhuang manuscript P. 2115, which was published later in 1985. This discrepancy suggests that the Zhejiang edition might be a contemporary creation dating between the 1960s and 1970s.

Lastly, the scholars highlighted extensive revisions and additions made to the Zhejiang edition when compared with the Dunhuang manuscripts. Despite Zhang Yuansu's mention in the preface of "making some corrections," this statement sparked controversy as the substantial alterations in the Zhejiang edition raised suspicions of forgery.

Let's set aside for now the doubts about whether the Zhejiang edition is authentic or fake and treat it as another version of Zhang Zhongjing's *Five Viscera Theory* (Wǔ Zàng Lùn, 五藏论) for discussion. Here raises one question. Zhang Zhongjing hailed from Nanyang, Henan. Why would his work appear in Zhejiang?

There could be two possibilities. Firstly, based on certain research findings, it is known that in addition to Nanyang, Henan, descendants of Zhang Zhongjing also had a branch that migrated to Qiantang, present-day Hangzhou. Therefore, it is plausible that the *Five Viscera Theory* (Wǔ Zàng Lùn, 五藏论) could have been brought to Hangzhou by one of Zhongjing's descendants. Secondly, during the Southern Song Dynasty, the royal family relocated to Hangzhou, and along with them, the imperial collection of books likely also moved to Hangzhou. In this context, Zhang Zhongjing's *Five Viscera Theory* (Wǔ Zàng Lùn, 五藏论) could have been among the books transported to Hangzhou during this period.

Now, let's delve into the first hypothesis. The emergence of Zhang Zhongjing's work in Zhejiang Province might be attributed to the migration of the Zhang clan's descendants. We may uncover relevant records within Zhang Zhongjing's family history or genealogy to support this notion.

"Pu Die" (谱牒) refers to ancient books that record the genealogy of a clan. It is a form of literature that emerged alongside the family system, documenting familial blood relations. The surname "Zhang" originated in the vicinity of Qinghe in present-day Hebei Province.[7] During the Sui and Tang dynasties, the "Qinghe Zhang clan" was a prestigious and influential family. The origin of this surname can be traced back to the Neolithic period of primitive society, spanning approximately 5,000 years of history.

During the reign of Emperor Taizong of the Tang Dynasty, after conducting a comprehensive survey of surnames and clans across China along with their genealogies, ten surnames were officially recognized as "Guozhu" (National Surnames, 国柱). Among these, the Zhang clan, led by the "Qinghe Zhang" branch, was appointed as the foremost "Guozhu." According to the *Great Song Dynasty revised and expanded rhymes* (Dà Sòng Chóng Xiū Guǎng Yùn, 大宋重修广韵), the lineage of the Zhang clan can be traced back to Hui (挥), the fifth son of the Yellow Emperor. Hui was credited with inventing the bow and arrow and overseeing its production, leading to the grant of the Zhang surname. The Zhang clan flourished in 14 prominent regions, including Qinghe, Nanyang, Haojun, Anding, Dunhuang, Wuwei, Fanyang, Jianwei, Peiguo, Liangguo, Zhongshan, Jijun, Henei, and Gaoping. This narrative underscores the prominence of the Zhang family, particularly in areas like Nanyang, which ranked second only to Qinghe as a hub for the Zhang clan.

Zhang Zhongjing, originally named ZhangJi, hailed from Jiyang, Nanyang County, during the Eastern Han Dynasty, situated in what is now Zhangciyuan Village, Guanzhuang Township, Henan Province.[8] While historical records provide some information about Zhang Zhongjing, they lack comprehensive details, particularly concerning his life story, a subject that many scholars have endeavored to uncover. Even today, in Zhangciyuan Village, a ballad persists among the local populace in remembrance of Zhongjing. The ballad recounts:

> The old man bore a child in his twilight years, bringing joy to thousands of households in Changsha upon hearing the news. If this child proves promising, he may one day become the prefect of Changsha, presiding over the court.

Over the course of millennia, variations and alterations in wording are inevitable in oral traditions. Nonetheless, this folk song provides valuable insights, revealing the following:

1. In his later years, Zhongjing still had descendants in the south, or Zhang Zhongjing was born to his father in his later years.
2. Zhongjing's dual role as an official and a physician garnered strong support from the people of Changsha, who also held lofty expectations for his descendants.
3. Originating from the Eastern Han Dynasty, the ballad's tone permeated among the descendants of the Zhang family. It stands to reason that only Zhongjing's progeny would feel fervently inclined to recite this ballad.

According to the Zhang family genealogy, the Zhang lineage has branches in Jiangyou and Qiantang.[9] Jiangyou is situated in present-day Jiangxi, while Qiantang corresponds to modern-day Hangzhou. In the preface of *Shang Han Lun Zong Yin* (伤寒论宗印) authored by Zhang Zhicong during the Qing Dynasty, it is noted: "Originally, my family hailed from Nanyang but later settled in Jiangyou during the Han Dynasty's rebellion. The 11th generation of our lineage relocated to Bozhu Lake in Qiantang. It has been 43 generations since our ancestor Zhongjing." Zhang Zhicong explicitly states in his preface that he is a descendant of Zhongjing. Subsequently, the family moved to Jiangyou before ultimately settling in Qiantang. Sun Simiao of the Tang Dynasty mentioned in *Supplement to the Formulas of a Thousand Gold*

Worth (Qiān Jīn Yì Fāng, 千金翼方) that "Masters in Jiangnan (regions south of the Yangtze River) would not pass on the secret of Zhongjing's formulas." This indicates that Zhang Zhongjing's works had already been studied by local doctors in Jiangnan during the Tang Dynasty or even earlier.

Throughout history, a town named Wuzhen in Zhejiang Province has been renowned for nurturing numerous eminent physicians. This reputation can be attributed to the presence of the Grand Canal, which facilitated bustling commercial activities and provided convenient access to medical care seekers. Since the Song Dynasty, Wuzhen has served as a hub for Chinese medicine practitioners. By the early 1950s, shortly after the establishment of the People's Republic of China, Wuzhen boasted a remarkable count of 40 Chinese medicine doctors despite its modest size of only 3.5 square kilometers. This concentration of medical expertise was unparalleled in China at that time. Intense competition among practitioners necessitated the demonstration of reliable curative effects to earn patient trust. Consequently, patients from across the nation flocked to Wuzhen seeking treatment, earning the town the moniker of the "wharf of doctors."

Over time, Wuzhen developed its own distinctive medical tradition, eventually termed the "Wuzhen School" by Qing Dynasty scholar Lu Yiwan in his *Lenglu Medical Talk* (Lěng Lú Yī Huà, 冷庐医话). The hallmark of this school lies in its approach of assimilating strengths from various medical traditions while addressing their shortcomings. Consequently, succeeding generations were able to inherit the essence of the Wuzhen School and innovate upon it, further advancing the field of medicine.

Among the numerous doctors in Wuzhen, one figure stood out prominently: a monk physician known as Yuelin, or Yiling. Having entered monastic life during childhood, Yuelin eventually ascended to the position of abbot at the "Xianjing Temple" in Xizha, Wuzhen. Renowned for his multifaceted talents, Yuelin possessed expertise in poetry, painting, musical instruments, and the game of Go. As a physician, he excelled in the field of medicine, particularly renowned for his prowess in treating internal and women's ailments. His compilation of medical cases, titled *Yiling's Medical Case* (Yì Líng Yī Àn, 逸龄医案), was meticulously studied and passed down through generations. Among his many disciples, Zhang Yicheng stood out as the foremost. Zhang Yicheng practiced medicine in both Shanghai and Hangzhou, and it was said that his reputation even eclipsed that of his esteemed teacher, Yuelin.

Being a descendant of the Zhang family, Zhang Yicheng likely had access to a copy of the *Qinghe Genealogy* (Qīng Hé Pǔ Dié, 清河谱牒). While it remains uncertain whether Zhang Zhongjing's *Five Viscera Theory* (Wǔ Zàng Lùn, 五藏论) was explicitly documented in the *Qinghe Genealogy* (Qīng Hé Pǔ Dié, 清河谱牒), we cannot dismiss the possibility that the text was passed down to Zhang Yicheng as a cherished heirloom within the family lineage. This historical connection may have contributed to Zhang Yicheng's elevated reputation, potentially surpassing even that of his esteemed teacher.

Another plausible reason for the presence of Zhang Zhongjing's *Five Viscera Theory* (Wǔ Zàng Lùn, 五藏论) in Zhejiang could be attributed to the southward relocation of the Song Dynasty's royal family to Hangzhou. This migration likely entailed the transfer of the royal collection of books to Hangzhou as well.

Recall that in our discussion of the P. 2378 edition, we conducted a thorough investigation into the records of Zhang Zhongjing's *Five Viscera Theory* (Wǔ Zàng Lùn, 五藏论) within the *Records of Arts and Literature* (Yì Wén Zhì, 艺文志) of the Song Dynasty and earlier dynasties. Our findings revealed that the earliest documented mention of Zhang Zhongjing's *Five Viscera Theory* (Wǔ Zàng Lùn, 五藏论) can be traced back to the *Comprehensive Catalogue of Literature During the Song Dynasty* (Chóng Wén Zǒng Mù, 崇文总目), compiled and printed during the Northern Song Dynasty. Before delving into the details of the *Comprehensive Catalogue of Literature During the Song Dynasty* (Chóng Wén Zǒng Mù, 崇文总目), let us briefly revisit the historical context of the Song Dynasty.

The Song Dynasty (960–1279) was distinguished by two significant eras: the Northern Song (960–1127) and the Southern Song (1127–1279). Spanning a duration of 319 years, the dynasty was characterized by the reign of 18 emperors. The Northern Song period commenced in 960 AD following Zhao Kuangyin's ascent to power through the overthrow of the Later Zhou dynasty. Proclaimed Emperor Taizu of Song, Zhao established the Northern Song Dynasty and designated Dongjing (now Kaifeng, Henan) as its capital. However, the Northern Song Dynasty faced a formidable challenge in 1125 when the Jurchen launched aggressive invasions from the north, ultimately leading to the demise of the Northern Song era. Subsequently, in 1127, the Song Dynasty lost control of North China, prompting a southward retreat to Lin'an (present-day Hangzhou) to establish the Southern Song Dynasty. This relocation marked the onset of the Southern Song period.

The Northern Song Dynasty commenced in 960 AD, putting an end to the turbulent era of the Five Dynasties and Ten Kingdoms. Influenced by Neo-Confucian political ideology, the early rulers of the Song Dynasty were determined to rejuvenate China culturally and intellectually. However, the prolonged turmoil within the nation resulted in the loss of a significant number of books, severely impeding progress in culture and education.

During this period, three imperial archives played pivotal roles in the preservation and revision of documents and books: the Shi Guan (Historiography Institute, 史馆), the Zhao Wen Guan (Institute for the Glorification of Literature, 昭文馆), and the Ji Xian Yuan (Academy of Scholarly Worthies, 集贤院). In 978 AD, the Chong Wen Yuan (崇文院) was established as the leading institution among the imperial archives. Simultaneously, the fourth library of the imperial archives, known as the Mi Ge (秘阁), was founded. Housing over 10,000 volumes of documents and books compiled from the other three libraries, the Mi Ge was accessible exclusively to personnel within the inner palace. Collectively, the Shi Guan, the Zhao Wen Guan, the Ji Xian Yuan, and the Mi Ge were known as the "Four Libraries," serving as the central repositories for imperial archives.

During the early Song Dynasty, the combined collection of documents and books from the Zhao Wen Guan, Shi Guan, and Ji Xian Yuan amounted to just over 13,000 volumes. In response, the court initiated several measures aimed at augmenting the book collection.

Firstly, efforts were made to collect books from preceding dynasties. Secondly, individuals from the populace were encouraged to contribute books, with generous rewards offered to those who did so. Rewards ranged from golden tripods to official government titles. Lastly, court officials were dispatched to locate, copy, and engrave print books that were scattered among the populace.

Furthermore, government agencies persisted in printing books, facilitating a rapid expansion of the national book collection. By 978 AD, a mere two decades into the Song Dynasty, the national book collection had surged from slightly over 13,000 volumes to surpass 80,000 volumes.

In 1015 AD, a devastating fire ravaged Rongwang Palace, resulting in significant damage to the Chong Wen Yuan and a catastrophic loss to the book collection. Numerous historical texts were tragically consumed by the flames. In response, Emperor Renzong issued a decree to re-catalog the surviving books within the imperial archives. Subsequently, Wang Yaochen, a scholar from the Hanlin Academy, meticulously compiled a comprehensive bibliography with annotations for each book. Impressed by Wang's scholarly endeavor, Emperor Renzong bestowed upon the compilation the title of *Comprehensive Catalogue of Literature During the Song Dynasty* (Chóng Wén Zǒng Mù, 崇文总目).

Comprehensive Catalogue of Literature During the Song Dynasty (Chóng Wén Zǒng Mù, 崇文总目), serving as the official bibliography of the Northern Song Dynasty, meticulously cataloged 3,445 books, marking the earliest extant nationwide bibliography in China. Comprising 66 volumes, it was organized into the traditional four categories of literature – Confucian classics, history, philosophy, and literature – further subdivided into 45 sub-categories. Subsequently, *Comprehensive Catalogue of Literature During the Song Dynasty* (Chóng Wén Zǒng Mù, 崇文总目) garnered immense acclaim among scholars for its comprehensive scope and meticulous organization.

The inclusion of Zhang Zhongjing's *Five Viscera Theory* (Wǔ Zàng Lùn, 五藏论) in the *Comprehensive Catalogue of Literature During the Song Dynasty* (Chóng Wén Zǒng Mù, 崇文总目) serves as concrete evidence of its existence during the Northern Song Dynasty. More specifically, this indicates that a copy of the *Five Viscera Theory* (Wǔ Zàng Lùn, 五藏论) was indeed housed within the imperial archives of Dongjing, the capital city of the Northern Song Dynasty (now Kaifeng, Henan).

Furthermore, as discussed in the preceding chapter, during the third year of Renzong Jiayou in the Northern Song Dynasty (1058), Goryeo received engravings of seven new Chinese medical classics. These included the following: *Yellow Emperor's Canon of 81 Difficult Issues* (Huáng Dì Bā Shí Yī Nàn Jīng, 黄帝八十一难经); *Chuan Yu Ji* (川玉集); *Treatise on Cold Damage Disorders* (Shāng Hán Lùn, 伤寒论); *Summarization of the Essentials of Materia Medica* (Běn Cǎo Kuò Yào, 本草括要); *Chao's Etiology of Children's Diseases* (Xiǎo'ér Cháo Shì Bìng Yuán, 小儿巢氏病源); *Eighteen Discussions of the Medications, Symptoms, and Causes of Pediatric Diseases* (Xiǎo'ér Yào Zhèng Bìng Yuán Yī Shí Bā Lùn, 小儿药证病源一十八论); and *Zhang Zhongjing's Five Viscera Theory* (Zhāng Zhòng Jǐng Wǔ Zàng

Lùn, 张仲景五脏论). In total, 99 engravings from the Song Dynasty were acquired, all of which were received by the Mi Ge (imperial archives).

Let us delve into the heart of book printing during the Northern Song Dynasty: Kaifeng, the illustrious capital. Kaifeng served not only as the seat of the imperial archives but also as the political, commercial, and cultural hub of the era. Alongside the Imperial College and other official institutions, numerous bookshops dotted the city, engaged in both printing and selling books. The transmission of these engravings of medical literature to Korea during the Northern Song Dynasty once again attests to the existence of Zhang Zhongjing's *Five Viscera Theory* (Wǔ Zàng Lùn, 五藏论) during this period. Given Kaifeng's status as the epicenter of book printing and publishing in the Northern Song Dynasty, coupled with its role as the location of the imperial archives, it is entirely plausible that copies of Zhang Zhongjing's *Five Viscera Theory* (Wǔ Zàng Lùn, 五藏论) were present in Kaifeng.

Following the Song Empire's relocation to Lin'an in 1127, a portion of the imperial archives was also transferred southward. Emperor Gaozong of Song initiated efforts to gather books from various sources. In 1131, the Song government established the Department of the Palace Library (Mi Shu Shen) in Lin'an to house books transported from the north. By 1143, the Palace Library was fully operational, with one of its key responsibilities being the reconstruction of the *Comprehensive Catalogue of Literature During the Song Dynasty* (Chóng Wén Zǒng Mù, 崇文总目). However, the invasion of the Jin Dynasty led to the plundering of many engraved woodblocks used for book printing as war spoils. Additionally, during the capital's relocation to Lin'an, numerous books were lost during transit.

In response, the imperial court tasked the Department of the Palace Library with organizing the imperial archives and revising the *Comprehensive Catalogue of Literature During the Song Dynasty* (Chóng Wén Zǒng Mù, 崇文总目). The revised version, an abridged edition, omitted prefaces, commentaries, and detailed book descriptions, retaining only the titles, number of volumes, and authors. Books lost over the years were marked with the character "阙" (quē, missing) following their titles. Consequently, two versions of the *Comprehensive Catalogue of Literature During the Song Dynasty* (Chóng Wén Zǒng Mù, 崇文总目) circulated in China: the complete edition and the abridged edition. Emperor Gaozong of Song dispatched the abridged version to magistrates of states and counties to aid in the search for lost books. Both editions continued to circulate during the Song and Yuan dynasties, but by the end of the Song Dynasty and the early Yuan Dynasty, complete copies of either edition were rare.

In subsequent Ming and Qing dynasties, the original edition gradually vanished. However, a fortunate preservation occurred at the Tianyige Library in Ningbo, Zhejiang Province, which retained a copy of the abridged version transcribed during the Ming Dynasty.

The *Comprehensive Catalogue of Literature During the Song Dynasty* (Chóng Wén Zǒng Mù, 崇文总目) stands as the earliest extant bibliography compiled by the government, wielding significant influence in the Song Dynasty for locating lost books, confirming their existence, and verifying their authenticity. Upon perusing the abridged edition of this catalog, the character "阙" (quē, missing) was appended to nearly all entries for works titled "Wu Zang Lun," except for Zhang Zhongjing's *Five Viscera Theory* (Wǔ Zàng Lùn, 五藏论). This suggests that Zhang Zhongjing's *Five Viscera Theory* (Wǔ Zàng Lùn, 五藏论) remained within the imperial archives in Lin'an during the Southern Song Dynasty.

This preservation could be attributed to Emperor Gaozong of Song's relocation of the capital southward, which likely facilitated the transfer of numerous imperial archives, including Zhang Zhongjing's *Five Viscera Theory* (Wǔ Zàng Lùn, 五藏论), to Lin'an. Consequently, this seminal work managed to evade destruction and find a new home in Zhejiang Province. While it remains challenging to definitively ascertain whether the Zhejiang edition of Zhang Zhongjing's *Five Viscera Theory* (Wǔ Zàng Lùn, 五藏论) was copied from the imperial archives in Lin'an at that time, its geographic presence aligns logically with this hypothesis.

During the mid-reign of Emperor Qianlong in the Qing Dynasty, the empire entered a period of unprecedented prosperity after more than a century of astute governance. This era marked the culmination of nearly two millennia of Chinese intellectual and cultural development, spanning from the Classical Studies of the Han Dynasty to the Neo-Confucianism of the Song and Ming dynasties. Under Emperor Qianlong's patronage and amidst a stable political and economic environment, there arose a resounding call from the scholarly community to embark on a grand intellectual endeavor.

The confluence of these factors presented an opportune moment to undertake a large-scale compilation project, thereby enriching the grandeur of the flourishing age. The Qing government, cognizant of its responsibility to fulfill the aspirations of the epoch, embraced this initiative with zeal.

Under the auspices of Emperor Qianlong during the Qing Dynasty, the monumental *Complete Library in Four Sections* (Sì Kù Quán Shū, 四库全书) was meticulously compiled by over 360 esteemed officials and scholars, with Ji Yun and Lu Xixiong serving as chief editors. More than 3,800 individuals were tasked with hand-copying every word of this comprehensive work. The exhaustive effort spanned an arduous 13 years before the encyclopedia was finally completed.

The *Complete Library in Four Sections* (Sì Kù Quán Shū, 四库全书) was meticulously organized into four main sections: jing (classics), shi (histories), zi (philosophies), and ji (literature), hence, the name "Si Ku" which translates to "four sections."

By 1782, the monumental task of compiling the *Complete Library in Four Sections* (Sì Kù Quán Shū, 四库全书) was nearing completion, alongside the initial draft of the *Annotated Catalog of the Complete Library in Four Sections* (Sì Kù Quán Shū Zǒng Mù Tí Yào, 四库全书总目提要). Following numerous revisions, the final version of the *Annotated Catalog of the Complete Library in Four Sections* (Sì Kù Quán Shū Zǒng Mù Tí Yào, 四库全书总目提要) was sent for printing in 1789 and ultimately published in 1793. Renowned as the largest book catalog in ancient China, the *Annotated Catalog of the Complete Library in Four Sections* (Sì Kù Quán Shū Zǒng Mù Tí Yào, 四库全书总目提要) provided comprehensive bibliographic entries for all 3,461 works featured in the *Complete Library in Four Sections* (Sì Kù Quán Shū, 四库全书). Additionally, it included concise notes on 6,793 additional works, which were solely listed by title (Cunmu 存目). Each listed book was meticulously annotated, earning the catalog its title of *Annotated Catalog of the Complete Library in Four Sections* (Sì Kù Quán Shū Zǒng Mù Tí Yào, 四库全书总目提要), commonly abbreviated as *Siku Zongmu* (四库总目).

In 1773, Fan Maozhu, the eighth-generation descendant of Fan Qin, who oversaw the Tianyige Library in Ningbo, Zhejiang Province, answered Emperor Qianlong's call to gather books nationwide for the compilation of the *Complete Library in Four Sections* (Sì Kù Quán Shū, 四库全书). He contributed 641 different titles from the Tianyige Library, ranking second in the country in terms of quantity. Notably, the collection also boasted the highest quality, as most volumes were rare and scarce. Of the submitted works, 377 titles were included in the *Annotated Catalog of the Complete Library in Four Sections* (Sì Kù Quán Shū Zǒng Mù Tí Yào, 四库全书总目提要), and 96 made it into the final *Complete Library in Four Sections* (Sì Kù Quán Shū, 四库全书) compilation. Regrettably, not all the books from the collection were returned to the Tianyige Library, resulting in a reduction of its holdings to 4,819 titles.

The *Comprehensive Catalogue of Literature During the Song Dynasty* (Chóng Wén Zǒng Mù, 崇文总目) compiled during the Northern Song Dynasty stands as the earliest circulated official bibliography, serving as a fundamental source for subsequent historical compilations. Notably, it was ranked at the pinnacle under the "shi" (histories) category in the *Annotated Catalog of the Complete Library in Four Sections* (Sì Kù Quán Shū Zǒng Mù Tí Yào, 四库全书总目提要). But where did this foundational text originate? Surprisingly, it was indeed from the collection of the Tianyige Library in Ningbo, Zhejiang Province, part of the extensive offerings made by Fan Maozhu for the compilation of the *Complete Library in Four Sections* (Sì Kù Quán Shū, 四库全书). This particular edition of the *Comprehensive Catalogue of Literature During the Song Dynasty* (Chóng Wén Zǒng Mù, 崇文总目) was an abridged version published during the Southern Song Dynasty, painstakingly hand-copied by Zhu Yizun during the Qing Dynasty. Subsequently, it was refined and expanded based on references from the *Comprehensive Catalogue of Literature During the Song Dynasty* (Chóng Wén Zǒng Mù, 崇文总目) cited in the *Yongle Encyclopedia* (Yǒng Lè Dà Diǎn, 永乐大典), culminating in a 12-volume masterpiece.

Within the *Annotated Catalog of the Complete Library in Four Sections* (Sì Kù Quán Shū Zǒng Mù Tí Yào, 四库全书总目提要), under the subsection dedicated to "zi" (philosophies), there were detailed bibliographic entries for 97 medical texts, along with succinct notes on an additional 92 medical works. Furthermore, an appendix featured six veterinary texts, totaling 195 entries related to medicine related works. Surprisingly, amidst these meticulously cataloged medical texts, there was no mention of *Five Viscera Theory* (Wǔ Zàng Lùn, 五藏论). This absence indicates that by the time Emperor Qianlong undertook the compilation of the *Annotated Catalog of the Complete Library in Four Sections* (Sì Kù Quán Shū Zǒng Mù Tí Yào, 四库全书总目提要), the imperial archives had already lost any records of Zhang Zhongjing's *Five Viscera Theory* (Wǔ Zàng Lùn, 五藏论). Nevertheless, within the *Comprehensive Catalogue of Literature During the Song Dynasty* (Chóng Wén Zǒng Mù, 崇文总目) included in the *Complete Library in Four Sections* (Sì Kù Quán Shū, 四库全书), Zhang Zhongjing's *Five Viscera Theory* (Wǔ Zàng Lùn, 五藏论)

still found its place. This signifies a significant shift, marking the disappearance of Zhang Zhongjing's *Five Viscera Theory* (Wǔ Zàng Lùn, 五藏论) from the imperial archives, leaving scholars to rely solely on references within the *Comprehensive Catalogue of Literature During the Song Dynasty* (Chóng Wén Zǒng Mù, 崇文总目) to affirm its historical existence.

The significance of the *Comprehensive Catalogue of Literature During the Song Dynasty* (Chóng Wén Zǒng Mù, 崇文总目) manuscript being housed in the Tianyige Library stems from its pivotal role in the history of China's private-owned libraries.[10] Situated on Tianyi Street, west of Yuehu Lake, in Ningbo City, Zhejiang Province, the Tianyige Library stands as not only the oldest private library in China but also in the world.

Established in 1561 under the supervision of Fan Qin, a distinguished Co-Minister of Wars,[11] the Tianyige Library stands as a testament to his lifelong passion for literature. Fan Qin's love for reading began in his youth, and after successfully passing the Jinshi examination, he embarked on a career in government service. Throughout his extensive travels, he made it a priority to collect books from every place he visited. Upon retiring from public office, Fan Qin devoted himself wholeheartedly to expanding his collection. Recognizing the need for a dedicated space to house his ever-growing repository of books, he made the decision to construct the Tianyige Library.

Fan Qin spared no expense in ensuring that the Tianyige Library boasted both a meticulously designed interior and an impressive exterior. The entire structure was painted black, a color symbolizing "water" in the five elements. The library's name, Tianyige, is derived from the phrase "Tian Yi Sheng Shui" (The universe generates water first). This name was chosen with great care, as it embodies the idea of using water to counteract the destructive force of fire, thus safeguarding the precious collection within. A prominent feature of the library is the "Tianyi Pond" situated in front of the main building. This pond serves as a reservoir for water used in fire prevention measures. In 1665 AD (the fourth year of Kangxi), Fan Wenguang, Fan Qin's great-grandson, further enhanced the surroundings by constructing rockeries, pavilions, and bridges around the pond. He also adorned the area with lush vegetation, creating an ambiance reminiscent of a tranquil garden in Jiangnan, south of the Yangtze River.

Later, Emperor Qianlong decreed the construction of seven grand libraries across the country, namely, the Wenyuange, Wenyuange, Wenjinge, Wensuge, Wenlange, Wenhuige, and Wenzongge Libraries. Each of these libraries housed one of the seven copies of the *Complete Library in Four Sections* (Sì Kù Quán Shū, 四库全书) and replicated the design of Tianyige Library's main buildings and bookcases. This initiative further elevated Tianyige Library's reputation nationwide. Since the Ming and Qing dynasties, gaining access to this prestigious library became a source of pride for literati and scholars.

For over 400 years spanning 13 generations, the collection of Tianyige Library has been meticulously preserved. While many collectors' holdings often dissipate within a century, Fan Qin's collection has endured through the ages. This longevity can be attributed to Fan Qin's meticulous management system. He established stringent family rules to safeguard the collection, which successive generations of his descendants have faithfully adhered to. Here are some examples:

- Consumption of tobacco and alcohol is strictly prohibited within the premises.
- None of the inheritors are permitted to separate the books or remove them from the library.
- The keys to the storage must be collectively held by several designated family members. The door can only be unlocked in the presence of all key holders.
- Individuals with foreign surnames are not granted entry to the library.
- Bringing relatives or friends into the library without prior permission is forbidden.
- Entry into the library without a valid reason is prohibited.
- Books are not to be lent to individuals with foreign surnames.

Violators will face severe penalties, and comprehensive measures including fire prevention, waterproofing, pest control, rodent prevention, and theft prevention have been implemented.

As a result of these strict rules, the Tianyige Library's collection has remained intact to the present day. The restriction that "individuals with foreign surnames are not allowed to enter the library" kept the treasures of the Tianyige Library shrouded in secrecy, unknown to outsiders. It wasn't until 1673, during the twelfth year of Emperor Kangxi's reign in the Qing Dynasty, that Huang Zongxi, a distinguished thinker and historian from the late Ming and early Qing dynasties, had the unique opportunity to become the first outsider to step foot inside the library. This rare privilege was granted by Fan Guangxie, the great-grandson (fourth generation) of Fan Qin. Subsequently, the Tianyige Library began to gradually open its doors to select prominent scholars, albeit sparingly. Huang Zongxi was afforded the extraordinary privilege of perusing the entirety of the library's collection, enabling him to compile a bibliography of the lesser-known works titled *Records of the Collections of the Tianyige Library* (Tiān Yī Gé Cáng Shū Jì, 天一阁藏书记).

Throughout its 400-year history, the Tianyige Library has faced numerous challenges resulting in the loss of many valuable books. Despite occasional major thefts, the Fan family was determined to recover these losses at any cost. In 1808, the library boasted 4,094 types of books comprising over 53,000 volumes. However, during the chaos of the Opium War, British invaders pillaged numerous ancient texts, including *Comprehensive Records* (Yī Tǒng Zhì, 一统志). Subsequently, during the Xianfeng period (1851–1861), thieves infiltrated the library, stealing a considerable number of books that were then sold to French missionaries and paper mills. The turmoil continued in 1861 when the Taiping Army attacked Ningbo, leading to further thefts of the library's collections. Fortunately, some of the stolen books were eventually repurchased by Fan Bangsui, a descendant from the tenth generation of the Fan family.

Over time, the library faced various setbacks and transformations. By 1940, its collection had dwindled to just 1,591 types of books, totaling 13,038 volumes.

Following the establishment of a designated management agency by the local government in 1949, efforts were made to protect and restore the library. Extensive searches were conducted, resulting in the recovery of over 3,000 volumes of lost books. Additionally, numerous ancient texts were generously donated by local collectors, bolstering the library's collection to over 80,000 volumes in the present day.

Since the Qing Dynasty, several notable bibliographies have documented the collection of the Tianyige Library, including the *Si Ming Tianyige Collection Catalog* (四明天一阁藏书目录) by an anonymous author, the *Bibliography on Tianyige Library Collection* (天一阁书目) compiled by Ruan Yuan and Fan Bangdian, the *Bibliography of the Existing Books of Tianyige Library* (天一阁见存书目) by Xue Fucheng et al., and others.[12] Despite extensive records, none of these sources mention Zhang Zhongjing's *Five Viscera Theory* (Wǔ Zàng Lùn, 五藏论). This absence suggests that the oldest private library in Chinese history, Tianyige Library, may not have possessed this particular book. However, the library's most cherished treasure, the *Comprehensive Catalogue of Literature During the Song Dynasty* (Chóng Wén Zǒng Mù, 崇文总目), does record: "*Wu Zang Lun*, one volume, original annotation, written by Zhang Zhongjing. (See the manuscript collected in Tianyige Library.)"

The notation "See the manuscript collected in Tianyige Library" refers to this particular copy of *Comprehensive Catalogue of Literature During the Song Dynasty* (Chóng Wén Zǒng Mù, 崇文总目) that is collected in Tianyige, rather than to Zhang Zhongjing's *Five Viscera Theory* (Wǔ Zàng Lùn, 五藏论). Despite Tianyige Library's nearly 500-year history and its status as a venerable institution in Zhejiang Province, it remains unclear whether the library ever possessed manuscripts of Zhang Zhongjing's *Five Viscera Theory* (Wǔ Zàng Lùn, 五藏论) in the past.

In summary, we have explored the authenticity of the Zhejiang edition of Zhang Zhongjing's *Five Viscera Theory* (Wǔ Zàng Lùn, 五藏论) and examined two potential reasons for its presence in Zhejiang. Furthermore, an examination was conducted into whether Zhang Zhongjing's *Five Viscera Theory* (Wǔ Zàng Lùn, 五藏论) is included in the *Annotated Catalog of the Complete Library in Four Sections* (Sì Kù Quán Shū Zǒng Mù Tí Yào, 四库全书总目提要) and the collection catalog of Tianyige Library. From our investigation, it is evident that Zhang Zhongjing's *Five Viscera Theory* (Wǔ Zàng Lùn, 五藏论) indeed existed in the imperial archive during both the Northern and Southern Song dynasties. However, after the Song Dynasty, it vanished from the imperial records, only to resurface in Zhejiang. The emergence of the Zhejiang edition raises questions about how it came to be in the possession of local residents. Possible explanations include meticulous preservation by Zhang Zhongjing's descendants or the unauthorized copying or theft of the book from the imperial archive, making it accessible to the community. Further research is required to ascertain the precise circumstances surrounding its circulation in Zhejiang.

Here is the direct translation of the full text of Zhang Zhongjing's *Five Viscera Theory* (Wǔ Zàng Lùn, 五藏论), Zhejiang edition. The translation process strictly adheres to the original text, translating word for word and sentence by sentence, ensuring that every word and every sentence remains faithful to the original text.

金·张元素序文张仲景《五藏论》
Zhang Zhongjing *Wu Zang Lun* with the preface by Zhang Yuansu, Jin Dynasty:

世传本金·张元素《五藏论》序

The Preface of "Wu Zang Lun" by Zhang Yuansu, Jin Dynasty:

唐故散骑侍郎许胤宗云：医者意也。在人思虑，脉候幽微，口莫能宣。古之上医，要在辨药、别脉、识病。病与药值，唯用一物，药力既纯，病即立愈。今人既不辨药，别脉，又不识病，以情臆度，多安药味，譬之猎兔，未探其窟，广发人马，空地遮围，犹冀万一，如此疗疾，不亦疏乎？假令一药偶当，都与他药相共，君臣交制，气势不行，欲病之瘥，岂可得耶？吾家仲景，学究素灵，术精歧黄，悯举世昏迷，不自爱惜己身，遇灾值晦，只知钦望巫祝，委付凡医，咄嗟呜呼！束手无策，告穷归天，饮恨幽泉，故发天人之秘，阐医药之理，撰此《五脏论》一卷，法简意深，普告世人，按病寻源，依症服药，虽约而未赅，亦足资儒门之参悟，与夫初学之指津也。盖明此一论，不必明医，可以察疾；不别君臣，可以施药，且所举皆乡闾之通病，所取多山野蔬供，即为石药，亦值贱而易致。是以李唐以来，传诵市井，几为家户所共喻。惜夫数百年来，转辗摹写，颠乱错谬，其与经语相悖，乖失医理，只是贻笑方家，至如药性违碍，讵免残害之惨。爰就家乘秘传，重加厘正，但于论义迭句，悉仍原文。良以此论病该众药，语多简要，愿世之览者，勤加冥索，推原病之所自，瞭其一物之用，药病相当，必得灾消祸灭，共跻仁寿之域，将使此论广为流布，家有明医，则仲景之德，溥利万世，亦余仁心之所寄尔。

The late Policy Advisor in Tang Dynasty Xu Yinzong once said: medicine is beyond technique. The information delivered by pulse palpation is very subtle and minute, and it is hard to describe by language. By studying those great doctors in antient times, the most important quality is the ability to distinguish medicines, differentiate pulses, and diagnose diseases. When the medicine matches with the disease, only use this one medicine, the power of the medicine is pure, then the disease will be cured immediately. Doctors today do not know how to distinguish medicines, or differentiate pulses, or diagnose diseases. Only to guess subjectively, and use multiple medicines, like hunting the rabbit without searching for its nest, instead of dispatching a big troop to cover all the grounds in order to not miss any chance. If treating patient like this, isn't it inattentive? If one of the medicines happened to be against other medicines, the chief (herbs) and the deputy (herbs) would fight with each other, then the entire formula won't be as effective, so how could the disease be cured? Zhongjing from my family thoroughly studied *Yellow Emperor's Classic of Internal Medicine* (Huáng Dì Nèi Jīng, 黄帝内经), mastered the skills passed down from Qibo and the Yellow Emperor. He was worried about the ignorance of the people nowadays. People now do not take care of themselves. Whenever there is disaster or any bad thing happens, they only look for the help from shaman or go to see some mediocre doctors. How sad! (At the end, those people), they do not know what to do. They tried everything but are still dying, with deep regret. Therefore, Zhongjing revealed the secrets taught by the celestial beings, trying to explain the law of medicine, thus, to have written *Five Viscera Theory* (Wǔ Zàng Lùn, 五藏论), one volume. (The book) contained a profound truth in simple language so that this book can reach large amount of population. (It teaches people how to) search for the cause of the disease based on the symptoms and take medicines according to the diseases. Although (the content) is concise, not in detail, still, it is enough for those who reads this book to learn from. (This book) provided guidance and pointed out the right path for beginners. That is why by understanding this book, even if the person does not understand thoroughly about medicine, he/she can still distinguish the diseases; without differentiating the chief (herbs) from the deputy (herbs), he/she can still give medicines. Moreover, (in the book), the diseases mentioned are all common ones we usually see around the village. The medicine used are mostly wild plants and vegetables to make as herbs, not only inexpensive but also easy to obtain. Since the Tang Dynasty, this book was widely read by ordinary townsfolk and was known to almost every household. Unfortunately, after hundreds of years, it has been passed through many hands and had been copied by many people. (Some of the contents) were misplaced or replaced with nonsense, which made it to be conflict to the classic teaching and was different from the principles of medicine. This will leave a handle for ridicule. Even worse, what if the property of the medicine was against the treatment? That would even cause the tragedy of harming the patients. I edited this book based on the one passed down in my family, but the main idea and the structure of the sentences were still the same as the original one. Using this book to study diseases and to give medicines, the language is mostly concise. Hope those who read the book can take time to study it, try to figure out the real cause of the disease, and find the one medicine they can use so that the medicine can match with the disease, then any calamity would be over and people would all be happy and healthy. If this book can be circulated widely, every household can have a good doctor, then the contribution of Zhongjing would benefit future generations. This is also my kind wish.

大金大定二十二年岁次壬寅中秋日易水后裔元素拜撰

Written by Zhang Yuansu, the descendant of the Yishui school of medicine, in the 22nd year of Dading in Jin Dynasty (year 1182) on a mid-autumn day.

传本《张仲景五脏论》全文

Full text of the inherited “Zhang Zhongjing Wu Zang Lun.”

药名之部，出本岐黄，黄帝造有二十余卷，若非妙娴，何能备著。

Medicine is contributed by the works of Qibo and the Yellow Emperor. The Yellow Emperor wrote more than 20 volumes (of books). If this were not a celestial being, how could anyone write such a great book?

夫天有五星，地有五岳，运有五行，人有五脏；故肝为将军，脾为大夫，心为帝王，肺为丞相，肾为内官，肝与胆合，脾与胃通，小肠连心，大肠连肺，膀胱合肾。是以肝盛则目赤，心热则舌干，肾虚则耳鸣，肺风则鼻塞，脾病则唇焦。目为肝候，舌是心官，耳作肾司，口是脾主，鼻为肺应。心主血脉，脾主肌肉，肺主皮肤，肝主于筋，肾主于骨。骨假肾立，肉假脾存，面肿关肺，皮因肺长，血因心荣。故知血患由心，骨患由肾，筋患由肝，肉患则由脾，皮患则由肺。

The heaven has five stars, the earth has five mountains, the movement has five elements, and the human body has five zang. So that the liver is the general, the spleen is like a senior official, the heart is like the emperor, the lung is like the prime minister, and the kidney is like the inner court official. The liver works with the gallbladder, the spleen connects the stomach, the small intestine links to the heart, the large intestine coordinates with the lung, and the urinary bladder connects the kidney. Therefore, liver excess causes red eyes, heart heat causes dry mouth, kidney deficiency causes tinnitus, lung wind causes sinus blockage, and spleen disease causes scorched lips. The liver manifests on eyes, heart manifests on the tongue, kidney manifests on ears, spleen manifests on mouth, and lung manifests on the nose. The heart rules the blood vessels, the spleen rules the muscles, the lung rules the skin, the liver rules the tendons, and the kidney rules the bones. Bones depend on the kidney to stand straight, muscles depend on the spleen to exist, face swelling relates to the lung, the growth of the skin depends on the lung, and the blood get nourished because of the heart. Therefore, we know the blood disorders are related to the heart, the bone disorders are related to the kidney, the tendon disorders are related to the liver, the muscle disorders are related to the spleen, and the skin disorders are related to the lung.

只是十二经脉，上下巡还；八脉奇经，内外流转，三焦六腑，四海七冲，胸膈咽喉，唇舌牙齿，臂肘股肱，膝胫脚踝，脐胁脊膂，鼻柱额颔，髭发须眉，指腕爪甲，俱有患处，并有所因，莫不内积虚劳，外缘风湿者也。察其颜色，即辨寒温，听之音声，便知损益。

There are 12 meridians that circulate upward and downward, and eight extraordinary meridians flow in the human body internally and externally. There are also triple burners and six Fu-organs; four seas and seven spirits; chest, diaphragm, pharynx, and throat; lips, tongue, and teeth; arms, elbows, thighs, and forearms; knees, lower leg, feet, and ankles; umbilicus, flanks, and backbones; nose, forehead, and chin; mustache, hair, and eyebrow; fingers, wrists, and finger nails, all the aforementioned places could suffer from illness, and the illness must have their causes, which are either internal deficiency and impairment or external caught wind damp. By looking at the facial color, you will be able to tell if it is cold syndrome or warm syndrome. By listening to the voice, you will know the person has excess or deficiency.

盖喜惊者心疾，多欠者肾邪，呻吟者患脾，啼哭者损肺，叫呼者伤肝，肤白者是冷，皮青者是风，颜黑者是湿，面赤者是火，唇黄者是热。心虚则善忘，脾虚则善饥，肝实则多怒，肺实则喘咳，肾冷则腰痛。声细者患冷，声沉者患虚，声绝者患风，声麁者患热。视毛则知肺，见爪则知肝，望唇则知脾，候脉则知心，举齿则知肾，肾热则齿黑，血伤则发枯，筋绝则爪干，声嘶则息短，善饥则肉痿；齿为骨馀，发是血余。是患者，推远其原，寻原脏腑。如此委细，乃是良医，须用医方，妙娴药性，应病与药，无病不除。世无良医，枉死者半，释邪攻正，绝人长命。

Someone easy to be frightened could have heart sickness, yawning too much means there is kidney evil, moaning and groaning are because of the illness of spleen, crying and sobbing are due to the illness of lung, and screaming and yelling are because of the injury of liver. Pale skin indicates cold in the body, blue skin tone indicates wind invasion, dark facial color indicates warmth in the body, and yellow lips indicate the heat in the body. Heart deficiency causes forgetfulness, spleen deficiency causes hunger, liver excess causes anger, lung excess causes breathing heavily and coughing, and kidney cold causes lumbar pain. A soft voice indicates suffering from cold, a deep voice indicates suffering from deficiency, no voice indicates suffering from wind, and a rough voice indicates suffering from heat. Looking at hair can know about the lung, looking at nails can know about the liver, looking at lips can know about spleen, looking at blood vessels can know about heart, and looking at the teeth can know about the kidney. Heat in kidney will cause teeth to darken, loss of blood (quantity/quality) will cause hair withered, exhaustion in tendon will cause nails dry, people with hoarse voice (usually) have shallow breath, and people easy to get hungry (usually) have muscle atrophy. Teeth are the surplus of bones; hair is the surplus of blood. Based on the symptoms, from the outside can see the real cause inside, then to look for the related Zang Fu (internal organs). If it can be investigated in such detail, this is a good doctor. When prescribing herbal formulas, (a good doctor) needs to know each medicine well and prescribe the medicine according to the illness. (If do so), no disease cannot be cured! But there is no good doctor now. Half of the patients died due to improper treatments. They attack the healthy Qi and encourage the evil Qi, thus shortening people's life.

天地之内，以人为贵，头园法天，足方法地。天有四时，人有四肢；天有五行，人有五脏；天有六律，人有六腑；天有七星，人有七窍；天有八风，人有八节；天有十二时，人有十二经；天有二十四气，人有二十四俞；天有三百六十五日，人有三百六十五骨；天有日月，人有眼目；天有昼夜，人有寤寐；天有雷电，人有喜怒；天有雨露，人有涕泣；天有阴阳，人有寒热。地有泉水，人有血脉；地有九野，人有九藏；地有金石，人有骨齿；地有草木，人有毛发。四大五常，假合成身，若有不调，百病俱起。

Between heaven and earth, the human being is the most valued. The head is round shaped that imitates the heaven; the feet are square shaped that imitates the earth. (On the analogy concept), the heaven has four seasons, correspondingly, human has four limbs; the heaven has five elements, so does human has five Zang-organs; the heaven has six rhyms, so does human has six Fu-organs; the heaven has seven stars, so does human has seven orifices; the heaven has eight kinds of winds, so does human has eight (big) joints; the heaven has 12 two-hour periods, so does human has 12 meridians; the heaven has 24 divisions of the solar year, so does human has 24 acupuncture shu points. The heaven has 365 days so does human has 365 bones; the heaven has sun and moon so does human has eyes; the heaven has days and nights, so does human knows when to sleep; the heaven has thunder and lightning, so does human has joy and anger; the heaven has rains and dews, so does human has cry and weep; the heaven has Yin and Yang, so does human has cold and heat; the earth has spring water, so does human has blood vessels. The earth has nine states, so does human have nine Zang. The earth has metals and rocks, so does human have bones and teeth. The earth has trees and grass, so does human has hair. It is all the human body formed by the aforementioned reasons due to the "four major and five constants." If there is disharmony, hundreds of diseases will arise.

经曰：神农本草，辨百药而制君臣；歧伯注经，说酸碱而陈冷热。雷公妙典，咸述炮炙之宜；弘景别录，委说根茎之用；徐王药对，侈谈犯触之忌；桐君药录，直接五风之妙。扁鹊能迴丧车，起死人；文挚使背明立，见心孔。徒痈留树，封骨除根，患者悉得抽愈。刘涓子秘述，学在鬼遗。徐百一丹方，偏疗小儿。淮南葛氏之法，秘要不传；僧垣集验之方，人间行用；药疗备急，疗人万病，服用俱解，子孙昌盛，众人爱敬，皆由药性。

The classic says: *Shennong's Classic of Materia Medica* (Shén Nóng Běn Cǎo Jīng, 神农本草经) distinguishes hundreds of medicines/herbs so thus to classify each medicine. The classics written by Qi Bo, explained medicine's (properties like) sour and salty and cold or hot nature. Lei Gong's marvelous classic talked in detail about herbal processing. Tao HongJing's miraculous formulas tirelessly discussed the use of stems and roots. "Xu Wang's pair herbs" talked extensively about the contraindications. *Record of Herb Collecting by Tong Jun* (Tóng Jūn Yào Lù, 桐君药录) directly discusses the wonder of the five winds. Bian Que can call back the funeral canopy and rescue the people back to life from death. Wen Zhi asked (Long Shu) to stand with his back towards the bright side to see the orifices in the heart. (Hua Tuo) scratched the bones to eliminate the root of poison. That's why patients can get fully recovered. Liu Juanzi's secret talk was from his learning by the side of the ghost. Xu Baiyi's pill formulas specialized in children's illness. Scholar Ge, who came from south of Huai River, kept his formulas secret. Formulas from *The Collection of Clinical Effective Formulas* (Jí Yàn, 集验) by Yao Sengyuan were used widely. The effect of the herbs and formulas can treat many human illnesses. People recover from taking the medicine. The descendants can be prosperous. They can respect and love each other all because of the effect of the medicine.

只如八味肾气，补六极而差五劳；四色神丹，荡千疴而除万病。有命必差，虢太子死而甦生；无命难理，晋景公于焉致死。

For example, Ba Wei Shen Qi (八味肾气丸, Eight-Ingredient Kidney Qi Pills) tonifies six types of extreme deficiencies to recover from five exhaustions. Si Se Shen Dan (四色神丹, Four-Color Magic Pills) cleans up thousands of illnesses to eliminate tens of thousands of diseases. Those destined to live will recover from illness. That is why Prince Guo was revived from death. Those destined to die are difficult to save. That is the reason why Jin Jing Gong died.

人之养病，如火积薪中，去火则薪得全，去病则人皆得活。薪不去火，虚被焚烧，有病不医，徒劳丧命。贵人之所贵，贱人之所贱；昔季康子馈药，夫子拜而受之。上古贤圣，犹敬其药，惟以上中下品别不同，甘苦酸咸，各随本性；若能君臣行用，六疾能差，气血正平，长有天命。故本草云：灵瑞之草，久服延年，然则长生钟乳，俗以丧身，必辨精麄，方致遐龄，岂但充体愈疾而已哉。

Treating an illness is like a fire within a pile of firewood; removing the fire keeps the firewood intact, removing the illness allows the person to live. If the firewood is not removed from the fire, it will be burned in vain; if a person's illness is not treated, they will lose their life in vain. One should treat valuable things as being precious and treat valueless things as being worthless. In ancient times, Ji Kangzi gave medicines to Confucius. Confucius bowed and received the medicine with respect. Since ancient times, the saints and intelligence all respected medicine. The plants were divided into upper, middle, and lower classes. Sweet, bitter, sour, and salty, follows the plant's nature. If one could also use the principle of King and Minister in a formula, six diseases (means many diseases) could be cured. Qi and blood can be balanced, then one can live to his/her natural death. Thus, "The Divine Farmer's Classic of Materia Medica" says: "Long term taking Ling Rui Zhi Cao (灵瑞之草 or 灵芝, lucid ganoderma) can pronlong life." But instead of taking Zhong Ru (钟乳, stalactite) to reach eternal life, people usually lose their lives because of this. One should distinguish the fine from coarse, then can reach their designated age, it is more than just cure all the diseases.

犀角有抵触之义，故能逐疰驱邪。牛黄愈惊痫之疴，更得安魂定魄。兰田玉屑，可以镇厌精神。中台麝香，堪将辟除梦魇。河内牛膝，去膝冷而止腰疼。上蔡防风，除头风而抽胁痛。晋地龙齿，偏差癫痫。太山茯苓，服治恚满。甘草安和诸药，故得国老之名。大黄宣引众功，乃有将军之号。半夏善消痰饮，制毒要用生姜。当归能止疼痛，相使还须白芷。泽泻薯蓣，能令耳目聪明。远志菖蒲，巧合开心益智。赤油宜涂茆蒜，白癞当服越桃。火烧水萍贴肉，杖打山棘生肌。伏暑霍乱，急求藿香。走疰飞尸，速用雄黄。头风目眩，须访薄荷。脚弱行迟，当求石斛。欲令见鬼，配入麻花。拟去回虫。漆和鸡子。蜂蜜妙止瘙痒。蟹黄善去漆疮。通草通利血脉，石胆唯除眼膜。秦胶结罗纹之状，血痔疝瘕可行。丹砂会取光明，功镇惊风。升麻只术青绿，妙解肿毒。秦椒宣汗，可除风邪。矾石当炮，能止衄血。杜仲削去麄皮，主治腰痛。桂心还求肉厚，堪镇胁风。石英须研如面，攻疗风热。杏人必捣如膏，消散嗽咳。菟丝酒渗乃良，功补劳伤。扑消火烧方好，耑消肿痛。防葵汤可迷心，狼毒气能伤人，并消疝瘕。黄芩烂腹是用，閭茹漆头为上，俱主疮痈。石南采叶，去风养肾。甘菊收花，乌发延年。五加封皮，益精强骨。牡丹去骨，降火除烦。鬼箭破血，仍有射鬼之灵。神屋除温，非无保神之验。呕吐汤煎干葛。转筋酒煮木瓜。目赤可点黄连。口疮宜含蘖木。瘴湿挛痛，酒渍茵芋。皮肤瘙痒，汤煎蒴藋。伤寒发汗，要用麻黄。壮热不除，宜加竹沥。恒山鳖甲，大有疗疟之功。蛇蜕铝丹，亦除癫痫之效。雄黄傅除鼻齇。木兰能去面皯。茧草杀齿内蚛痛。藜芦吐膈上风涎。支子悦愈面皮，桃花润泽肤体。芎藭枳实，胸膈噎满加用。紫苑款冬，胃脏咳逆可除。水蛭蝱虫，善能破血逐瘀。槟榔白术，俱理宿食不消。龙眼归脾强记。虎骨养血愈风。湿痒阴痿，汤煎蛇床。淋沥便止，水捣滑石。仙灵脾草，能愈腰痛，拌羊脂以入配。天鼠煎膏．巧疗耳聋，得蓖麻而加妙。蛇咬宜封人粪。蜂螫急擦芋茎。紫苏子消膈止咳，青羊肝疗瘠明目。赤脂发颜加色。白芨卷面除皮。知母利肠开胸，空青去翳止泪。孔公孽消食肥泽。密陀僧香口去瘢。厌石可假蜂房。水肿须杖大戟。腹饮结满，唯须甘遂。火赤羞明，宣取蕤人。安胎必藉紫威。伤中要须地髓。头脑风痛，偏加木笔。妇人崩中，急觅蒲黄。连翘却瘰疬恶疮。地胆破症瘕息肉。槐子疗五痔疮瘘。斑猫治九漏脓疡。松脂抽风治疽。鹤虱杀虫止疟。牵牛子泻水利便。苦楝根驱蛔消渴。鸡矢妙愈臌胀。蚕砂功疗瘾疹。葶苈伐脾泄水。茺蔚益母调经。桃人绝其鬼气，得免传尸。茅根消化肺痰，兼收客热。桑白皮疗治百损。鹿角胶滋补元阳。瘿气昆布妙除。肠风鳢肠焙研。痈肿硇砂食却。膝疼狗脊修治。脱肛宜取鳖头，反胃煮饮马苋。亡阳厥冷，救治急熨葱白。壮骨益精，延年蒸服首乌。诸般虫痞，榧实频啖。一切毒气，食盐万治。下贱纵为人溺，饮之扑损可消。卑微乃至地浆，服之天行皆愈。猥论虽缀小方，不及君臣，取写出本经传，有灵有验，有贵有贱；盖净秽百草，山中玉石，俱为青囊妙药也。

Xi Jiao (犀角, rhinoceros horn) has the power to fight against illness, so it can eliminate chronic infectious disease and disperse evil. Niu Huang (牛黄, cattle gallstone) has the function to heal the epilepsy due to fright, thus, to calm the Hun (ethereal soul) and the Po (corporeal soul). Yu Xie (玉屑, Jade Chips) from Lan Tian can tranquilize the mind. She Xiang (麝香, musk) from Zhong Tai can drive out evil. Niu Xi (牛膝, twotoothed achyranthes root) from He Nei treats cold knee and relieves lower back pain. Fang Feng (防风, siler root) from Shang Cai heals the head wind, also relieves the hypochondriac pain. Long Chi (龙齿, fossilized animal teeth) from Shanxi can treat epilepsy. Take Fu Ling (茯苓, Indian bread or poria) from Taishan to treat the fullness due to anger. Gan Cao (甘草, licorice root) has the function of harmonizing; thus, it has been called the "Guo Lao," a respected elder in the kingdom. Da Huang (大黄, rhubarb root) has the function of opening and inducing the elimination. That's why it was called the "Marshall General." Ban Xia (半夏, pinellia tuber) dissolves phlegm; raw ginger can counteract its toxicity. Dang Gui (当归, Chinese angelica root) can stop pain, but it must be combined with Bai Zhi (白芷, Dahurian angelica root). Ze Xie (泽泻, alisma tuber) and Shu Yu (薯蓣 or "Shan Yao" 山药, dioscrea rhizome) can benefit hearing and vision. Yuan Zhi (远志, Thinleaf milkwort root) and Chang Pu (菖蒲 or "Shi Chang Pu" 石菖蒲, grassleaf sweetflag rhizome) magically open the heart to make people smart. Red ulcer should apply Mao Suan (茆蒜, sand leek) tuberculoid leprosy needs to use Yue Tao (越桃 or "Zhi Zi" 栀子, gardenia fruit); burns to be treated by applying Shui Ping (水萍 or "Fu Ping" 浮萍, floating duckweed) topically; wounds from caning can use Shan Ji (山棘 or "Qiang Wei Zi" 蔷薇子, multiflora Rose Fruit) to generate new tissues. Acute gastroenteritis due to latent summer heat need to take Huo Xiang (藿香, Korean mint or agastache rugosa) as soon as possible. Pestilential illness uses Xiong Huang (雄黄, realgar) immediately. Head wind with dizziness must use Bo He (薄荷, peppermint). Weakness of limbs caused difficult walking will be benefit from Shi Hu (石斛, dendrobium stem). If see ghost, add Ma Hua (麻花, cannabis bud). If you want to eliminate white parasite, use Qi (漆, lacquer) and Ji Zi (鸡子, chicken eggs). Feng Mi (蜂蜜, honey) can effectively stop itching. Xie Huang (蟹黄, crab yolk) can eliminate eczema. Tong Cao (通草, rice paper plant pith) can unblock the blood vessels. Shi Dan (石胆, chalcanthite) eliminates cataract. Qin Jiao (秦胶 or 秦艽, largeleaf gentian root) pertains spiral shape; it can treat bleeding internal hemorrhoids and abdominal hernia. Dan Sha (丹砂 or "Zhu Sha" 朱砂, cinnabar) should be shiny; it can tranquilize convulsive disease. Sheng Ma (升麻, largetrifoliolious bugbane Rhizome) should be blue and green; it can treat toxic swelling. Qin Jiao (秦椒, prickly ash peel) need to be steamed; it can expel evil wind. Fan Shi (矾石 or "Ming Fan" 明矾, a sulfate of alum-stone, or white alum-stone) should be roasted; it can stop hemorrhage. Du Zhong (杜仲, eucommia bark) must peel off the outer skin; it mainly treats back pain. Gui Xin (桂心 or 肉桂, cinnamon bark) must be meaty; it can calm down intercostal pain due to the wind. Shi Ying (石英, Cristobalite) must be powdered to fight with wind heat. Xing Ren (杏人 or 杏仁, apricot seed) should be grinded until gets creamy; it can dissipate cough. Tu Si (菟丝, Chinese dodder seed) must be soaked with alcohol; it can help with overexertion. Pu Xiao (朴硝, a crude form of sodium sulfate) must be calcinated; it is specialized in swelling and pain. Fang Kui (防葵, white flower hog fennel root) decoction can confuse the mind. Lang Du's (狼毒, Bracteole-lacked Euphorbia root) property can hurt people; both can diminish abdominal hernia. Good Huang Qin (黄芩, Baical skullcap root) looks like rotten intestine; only use Lin Ru's (藺茹, Euphorbia Lanru root) top part. Both can treat ulcerative carbuncle. Shi Nan (石南, Chinese photinia Leaf) should pick its leaves; it can expel wind and nourish the kidney. Gan Ju (甘菊, sweet chrysanthemum flower) uses its flower; it can darken hair and prolong life. Wu Jia (五加, slenderstyle acanthopanax Bark), slice off its bark; it can nourish the essence and strengthen the bone. Mu Dan (牡丹, tree peony bark), hammer its stem and take the bone out. It can purge the fire and relieve restlessness. Gui Jian (鬼箭 or "Gui Jian Yu" 鬼箭羽, winged branches) can break up the blood stasis thus to kill ghost toxins. Shen Wu (神屋 or 龟板, tortoise carapace and plastron) clears the heat and has magical effect. Decoct Gan Ge (干葛 or "Ge Geng" 葛根, dried pueraria root) to treat vomiting; use alcohol to decoct Mu Gua (木瓜, Chinese quince fruit) for muscle spasm. Use Huang Lian (黄连, yellow coptis root) to make eye drops for red eyes. Hold Bo Mu (蘗木 or "Huang Bo" 黄柏, phellodendron bark) in the mouth for mouth ulcer. Painful arthritis uses alcohol-soaked Yin Yu (茵芋, Japanese skimmia stem and leaf); severe skin itch uses Shuo Huo (蒴藋, Chinese elder) decoction. Promote sweat during Shang Han, exogenous pathogenic cold-induced diseases, uses Ma Huang (麻黄, ephedra stem). Constant high fever can benefit from Zhu Li (竹沥, bamboo juice). Heng Shan (恒山 or "Chang Shan" 常山, dichroa root) and Bie Jia (鳖甲, Chinese soft-shelled turtle shell) have great function to relieve malaria. She Tui (蛇蜕, snake slough) and Lü Dan (铝丹, aluminum pill) relieve seizure attacks. Xiong Huang (雄黄, realgar) is to treat pimples on nose; Mu Lan (木兰 or "Hou Po" 厚朴, lily magnolia bark) can remove rough skin on face; Mang Cao (莔草, leaf of poisonous eightangle tree) treat toothache from decaying. Li Lu (藜芦, veratrum root and rhizome) can expel the phlegm above the diaphragm caused by wind. Zhi Zi (支子 or "Zhi Zi" 栀子, gardenia fruit) benefits facial skin; Tao Hua (桃花, peach blossom) can make skin moist and smooth. Xiong Qiong (芎藭 or "Chuan Xiong" 川芎, Sichuan lovage rhizome) and Zhi Shi (枳实, immature range fruit) can be added if has chest and abdominal fullness, difficulty swallowing, and hiccups. Zi Wan (紫菀, Tatarian aster root) and Kuan Dong (款冬, Common coltsfoot flower) can eliminate cough with dyspnea in the stomach. Shui Zhi (水蛭, leech) and Mang Chong (虻虫, horse fly) are good at break up blood stasis. Bing Lang (槟榔, areca nut) and Bai Zhu (白术, white atractylodes tuber) can both help with food stagnation. Long Yan (龙眼 dried longan) goes to spleen and enhances memory. Hu Gu (虎骨, tiger bone) nourishes the blood and heals calms the wind. Vaginal discharge, exterior vaginal itching, and impotence use She Chuang (蛇床, common cnidium fruit) to decoct. Dribbling or hesitate urination, add water to pound Hua Shi (滑石, talc) into powder. Xian Lin Pi (仙灵脾 or "Yin Yang Huo" 淫羊藿, horny goat weed or epimedium) relieves lower back pain, add Yang Zhi (羊脂, suet) as a pair. Syrup made from Tian Shu (天鼠 or "Bian Fu" 蝙蝠, bat) treats deafness, to add Bi Ma (蓖麻, castor leaf or bean) for better results. Topically cover with Ren Fen (人粪 or "Ren Zhong Huang"人中黄, human feces) for snake bite; bee sting should immediately apply Yu Jing (芋茎, petiole of dasheen). Zi Su Zi (紫苏子, perilla fruit) can relieve chest and abdominal fullness and stop coughing. Qing Yang Gan (青羊肝, goral liver) treats malnutrition and brightens vision. Shi Zhi (石脂, halloysite) darkens hair; Bai Ji (白及, bletilla tuber) removes dead skin and regenerates new skin. Zhi Mu (知母, common anemarrhena rhizome) treats intestinal diseases and opens chest; Kong Qing (空青, azurite) eliminates cataract and stops tearing. Kong Gong Nie (孔公孽, Calcite) helps digest food and gains weight. Mi Tuo Seng (密陀僧, lithargite) clears up bad breath and removes scar tissues. Feng Fang (蜂房, honeycomb) used to calm down the rebellious Qi caused by taking Ru Shi (乳石, stalactite). Edema can use Da Ji (大戟, Peking spurge root). Ascites and intestinal obstruction only needed Gan Sui (甘遂, gansui root). Eye redness and sensitive to light, need to use Rui Ren (蕤人, hedge prinsepia nut). Calm down fetus must use Zi Wei (紫葳, Chinese Trumpetcreeper Flower); Di Sui (地髓 or "Gan Di Huang" 干地黄, drying rehmannia root) is for physical exhaustion. Headache from wind needs to add Mu Bi (木笔 or "Xin Yi Hua" 辛夷花, magnolia flower). Women who have metrorrhagia should seek for Pu Huang (蒲黄, cat-tail pollen) immediately. Scrofula and boils use Lian Qiao (连翘, weeping forsythia Capsule); Di Dan (地胆, a kind of blister beetles) treats mass, nodules, and polyps. Huai Zi (槐子, pagodatree pod) can treat hemorrhoid and blood in the stool. Bai Mao (斑猫, mylabris or blister beetle) can treat scrofula and abscess. Song Zhi (松脂, pine resin) can expel wind and treat scabies. He Shi (鹤虱, common carpesium Fruit) kills parasites and stops malaria. Qian Niu (牵牛, morning glory) is a strong diuretic to reduce swelling. Ku Lian Pi (苦楝皮, chinaberry bark) can expel parasites and treat diabetes. Ji Shi (鸡矢, chicken excrement) marvelously cures bloating and fullness. Can Sha (蚕砂, silkworm shit)'s function is to treat urticaria. Ting Li (葶苈 or "Ting Li Zi" 葶苈子, tansymustard seed) can purge the spleen (should be lung) and expel fluid retention. Chong Wei (茺蔚, motherwort herb or fruit) can benefit the mother and regulate menstruation. Tao Ren (桃人 or 桃仁, peach kernel) stops evil energy to avoid tuberculosis. Mao Gen (茅根, imperata rhizome) dissolves phlegm in the lung, also clears the heat. Sang Bai Pi (桑白皮, white mulberry root-bark) treats hundreds of exhaustions. Lu Jiao Jiao (鹿角胶, deer antler glue) tonifies primordial yang. Kun Bu (昆布, kombu) relieves goiter. Hemorrhoidal hemorrhage to roast and grind Li Chang (鳢肠, or "Han Lian Cao" 旱莲草, yerbadetajo herb). Eat Nao Sha (硇砂, sal ammoniac) to get rid of carbuncle. Use Gou Ji (狗脊, cibot rhizome) to treat knee pain. Prolapse of rectum can use Bie Tou (鳖头, soft-shell turtle head). Nauseous can drink Ma (Chi) Xian (马齿苋, purslane) decoction. To treat exhaustion of yang and cold extremities, need to apply Cong Bai (葱白, fistular onion stalk) at once. In order to strengthen the bones, nourish the essence, and prolong the life, one needs to steam and eat Shou Wu (首乌, Fleeceflower Root). All kinds of infantile malnutrition due to intestinal parasites, need to eat Fei Shi (榧实 or "Xiang Fei Zi" 香榧子, torreya seed) often. Taking Shi Yan (食盐, salt) can cure all the toxic qi. As nasty as Ren Ni (人溺 or "Tong Niao" 童尿 boys' urine), to drink it can treat traumatic injury. Regardless of the degrading name of "Di Jiang" (地浆, Earth Slurry), Tian Xing Bing, epidemic diseases caused by natural factors, gets healed by taking Di Jiang (地浆, Earth Slurry). Although small formula was considered lower class, it doesn't even have King and Minister herbs in the formulation (still, you know) where the formula originally come from, and the formula is clinically proven, the medicine could be expensive or cheap, and they could be different kinds of herbs, or they could be jade or stone in the mountain. All can be doctor's miraculous cure.

REFERENCES

1. 马继兴，*敦煌古医籍考释[M]* (南昌：江西科学技术出版社, 1988), 16.
2. 陈永治，"传抄本《张仲景五脏论》及其与国外藏本的比较[J]." *江苏医药（中医分册）*, No. 2 (1979): 44.
3. 褚谨翔，"张仲景《五藏论》真伪问题的探讨[J]." *中华医史杂志*, Vol. 13, No. 4 (1983): 240–242.
4. 田永衍，"张元素修订本《五藏论》辨伪[J]." *敦煌辑刊*，No. 2 (2017): 135–138.
5. 赵有臣，"介紹張仲景五藏論 [J]." 江苏*中医药*, No. 5 (1963): 31–34.
6. 宮下三郎，"張仲景五蔵論について[J]." *漢方の臨床*, Vol. 6, No. 4 (1959): 187–192.
7. 沈世远，*张姓探源：张氏世系源流考[D]*, (河北省清河：清河年鉴, 1996–2000), 557–559.
8. 杜雨茂，"关于张仲景生平一些问题的探讨[J]." *陕西中医学院学报*, No. 5 (1982): 38–42.
9. 张鸿盘，"试谈张仲景后裔去向[J]." *河南中医*, Vol. 15, No. 2 (1995): 60.
10. 邓雪峰，"天一阁藏书的利用及其对《四库全书》的贡献[J]." *图书馆建设*，No. 2 (2002): 111–112.
11. 王敏，"天一阁藏书研究[D]." 硕士学位论文，郑州大学 (2006), 6.
12. 骆兆平，*天一阁藏书史志[M]* (上海: 上海古籍出版社，2005), 80.

11 The Fragment Sealed in Leningrad – The Russian Collection Дx.01325v

"The fragment was not an 'unidentified medical formula' but another manuscript of Zhang Zhongjing's 'Wu Zang Lun.'"

– Li Yingcun

Zhang Zhongjing's *Five Viscera Theory* (Wǔ Zàng Lùn, 五藏论), the Russian collection PДx.01325v, abbreviated as Дx.01325v, is currently held at the Saint Petersburg branch of the Institute of Oriental Studies of the Russian Academy of Sciences.[1]

The Dunhuang manuscript PДx.01325v, a fragment from the Russian collection, features brush writing on both sides. The front side contains "Buddhist Sutra Commentary" written in standard script, with both the beginning and end missing, preserving a total of 14 lines of text. The reverse side is a copy of a medical text written in running script, also missing the beginning and end, with nine lines of text remaining.

Regarding the Russian collection document PДx.01325v, Mi Morong referred to it as a "medical text," while Ma Jixing named it "the fortieth type of unidentified medical formula." The PДx.01325v fragment contains ancient characters, as well as variant characters commonly found in Dunhuang materials. Therefore, in 2006, Chinese scholar Li Yingcun preliminarily identified the PДx.01325v fragment from the Russian collection of Dunhuang manuscripts as a Dunhuang manuscript dating from the Sui, Tang to Five Dynasties period.[2] Upon comparing it with lines 9–15 of the French collection P. 2115 Zhang Zhongjing's *Five Viscera Theory* (Wǔ Zàng Lùn, 五藏论) and lines 8–14 of the British collection S.5614 Zhang Zhongjing's *Five Viscera Theory* (Wǔ Zàng Lùn, 五藏论), Li Yingcun discovered that the fragment was not an "unidentified medical formula" but another manuscript of Zhang Zhongjing's *Five Viscera Theory* (Wǔ Zàng Lùn, 五藏论). To date, five versions of Zhang Zhongjing's *Five Viscera Theory* (Wǔ Zàng Lùn, 五藏论) discovered in Dunhuang are held in the National Library of France in Paris, the British Library in London, and the Saint Petersburg branch of the Institute of Oriental Studies of the Russian Academy of Sciences. Additionally, the *Five Viscera Theory* (Wǔ Zàng Lùn, 五藏论) found in the "Five Zang Organs Category" section of volume 4 of the Korean *Categorized Collection of Medical Formulas* (Yī Fāng Lèi Jù, 医方类聚) and the Zhejiang edition of Zhang Zhongjing's *Five Viscera Theory* (Wǔ Zàng Lùn, 五藏论) share many

DOI: 10.1201/9781032698205-11

similarities with the five Dunhuang versions of Zhang Zhongjing's work, indicating their interconnectedness.

In November 1957, Saint Petersburg was cloaked in winter's serene beauty. Snowflakes danced through the air, dressing the streets, flora, and buildings in a thick white winter coat. The city's vast squares and grand structures, now seemingly in a state of hibernation, radiated tranquility and harmony. Interestingly, the chilly weather seemed to barely register with the city's inhabitants. Dressed warmly, people carried on with their daily lives: workers headed to their jobs, students to their schools, and homemakers bustled about, eager to prepare the evening's meal. In these peaceful times, life flowed comfortably, and the mood was universally upbeat.

At the nearby Leningrad branch of the Institute of Oriental Studies, Zheng Zhenduo,[3] a scholar from China, couldn't spare a moment to admire the beautiful view outside the window. Early in the morning, he had arrived at the Institute, eager to examine the Dunhuang manuscripts stored there. He never anticipated finding so many scrolls that had originated from China. Rapidly browsing through the hundreds of items selected by the staff, he was overwhelmed with excitement, feeling his pulse race at the sight of what were undoubtedly rare treasures. He described the experience as "more than the eye could see or the hand could copy," even encountering the original of the long-lost *Liu Zhiyuan Zhu Gong Diao* (刘知远诸宫调, "Zhu Gong Diao" is a style of songs prevalent in the 11th century). Despite the limited time, which didn't allow for a complete viewing of all the Dunhuang manuscripts, he felt the visit was incredibly worthwhile.

As dusk fell and the city lights started to twinkle, Zheng Zhenduo reluctantly stepped out of the Institute, his heart still racing with excitement from the day's discoveries. The chilly air transformed his breath into swirling mists of white, gently dispersing into the evening. The Neva River lay beneath a blanket of ice and snow, its surface gleaming so brilliantly, it blurred the lines between river and roadway. That night, Saint Petersburg unfurled its beauty like an alluring noblewoman, beckoning with a charm that called for deeper exploration.

Founded in November 1818, the Institute of Oriental Studies is Russia's largest institution for Oriental studies. Along with its Saint Petersburg branch, it is among the oldest Russian institutions dedicated to the study of Chinese affairs. The Institute, together with the British Library in London, the National Library of France in Paris, and the National Library of China, is recognized as one of the four major holders of Dunhuang manuscripts in the world. Its collection boasts 11,014 Dunhuang documents, including 364 manuscript scrolls and 10,650 fragments. The collection encompasses not only texts handpicked from the Hidden Library but also fragments left behind by the Qing government during the transport of Dunhuang manuscripts, documents in Tibetan not taken due to lack of interest, and some Chinese and Uighur scrolls acquired from Wang Tao-shih.

Regrettably, these invaluable cultural treasures have remained hidden within the Institute for many years, never formally made public. Over the past half century, only a handful of foreign scholars have had the privilege of seeing a very limited number of scrolls or obtaining a few photographs of fragments, leaving the comprehensive scope of the manuscripts largely unknown to the outside world.

During his visit and lecture tour in Eastern Europe, Zheng Zhenduo quickly traveled from Moscow to Leningrad by overnight train, following his participation in academic events. In the span of four days in Leningrad, he not only delivered two academic lectures but also devoted all his available time to the meticulous examination and transcription of Dunhuang manuscripts, as well as museum visits. In a whirlwind effort, Zheng managed to review around 500 Dunhuang scrolls in less than a day's total time. This endeavor marked a significant milestone, echoing the scholarly pursuits of predecessors like Xiang Da and Wang Zhongmin, who had explored Dunhuang manuscripts in Europe during the 1930s. Zheng's visit was particularly groundbreaking, as he became the first Chinese scholar to access the Russian-held Dunhuang manuscripts, unraveling the enigma of Russia's collection that had long been shrouded in secrecy.

Zheng Zhenduo was deeply engaged in the modern patriotic movement and gained recognition as a distinguished writer, poet, scholar, literary critic, and translator. He held a profound affection for books, particularly focusing on the collection and study of folk literature, novels, and drama. Notably, he compiled an extensive collection of folk literature materials from Dunhuang. In May 1927, Zheng Zhenduo took a ship to Europe to seek refuge and further his education. While in the libraries of France, England, and other countries, he extensively read books on ancient Chinese novels, dramas, and folk tales (bianwen). Afterwards, he wrote a lengthy article that included a section on "Dunhuang literature," offering a comprehensive summary of nearly 30 years of discoveries and organization of Dunhuang literary materials. In 1929, Zheng Zhenduo published the article *Folk Literature of Dunhuang* (Dūn Huáng De Sú Wén Xué, 敦煌的俗文学), introducing the term "folk literature" (俗文学) to the history of modern Chinese literature for the first time. This had a milestone significance for the study of Dunhuang literature.

Due to his particular affection for Chinese folk literature, Zheng Zhenduo was especially interested in the folk literary work *Liu Zhiyuan Zhu Gong Diao* (刘知远诸宫调), expressing a longing of over 20 years to see the original manuscript. One can only imagine his excitement upon discovering that the Institute of Oriental Studies housed such an extensive collection of Dunhuang manuscripts, particularly the original *Liu Zhiyuan Zhu Gong Diao* (刘知远诸宫调). Recalling this moment, Zheng said:

> It wasn't until the winter of 1957, during our visit to Leningrad with comrades Ayrin and Solokin, that I finally saw it at the Institute of Oriental Studies. What an exhilarating moment it was! My blood raced, my breathing became tense, and my face was alight with joy. The original manuscript was being mounted for preservation. There, at the mounting table, I turned it over and over, looking at it again and again. . . . But as I touched this ancient edition of the Zhugongdiao, carved more than seven hundred years ago and the oldest of its kind from China, my heart was filled with both joy and melancholy.

The joy, of course, came from the fortune of beholding the original in its true form, while the melancholy stemmed from the fact that this original had ended up so far from home.

In April 1958, the Soviet Union's Committee for Cultural Relations with Foreign Countries returned the manuscript of *Liu Zhiyuan Zhu Gong Diao* (刘知远诸宫调) to China. Zheng Zhenduo, representing the Chinese Ministry of Culture, was the one who accepted it and subsequently transferred it to the collection of the Beijing Library. In August of the same year, the Cultural Relics Publishing House issued a facsimile edition of *Liu Zhiyuan Zhu Gong Diao* (刘知远诸宫调), for which Zheng Zhenduo wrote a postscript on July 28, 1958. Tragically, less than three months later, on October 17, 1958, while on his way to Moscow, Zheng Zhenduo died in a plane crash. Although the book had been printed, Zheng never had the chance to see the published work.

The richness of the Dunhuang manuscripts in Russia owes much to a figure named Sergey Fyodorovich Oldenburg.[4] Oldenburg (С.ф.Олъденбург, 1863–1934), an academician of the Russian Academy of Sciences, was renowned for his studies in Sanskrit and Buddhism. Between 1909 and 1910, he led expeditions to Xinjiang for "explorations," acquiring a collection of cultural relics from Kashgar, Turpan, and Kucha among other places. From May 1914 to January 1915, he ventured to Dunhuang, where he mapped the facades of 443 caves, took over 2,000 photographs, and removed many frescoes, cloth paintings, silk paintings, paper paintings, manuscripts, silk textiles, and other items. After these artifacts arrived in Leningrad, they were stored in the Asian Museum. Currently, the physical artifacts are kept in the Hermitage Museum in Saint Petersburg (formerly known as the Winter Palace), while the manuscripts reside at the Saint Petersburg branch of the Institute of Oriental Studies of the Russian Academy of Sciences.

Upon returning to Russia, Oldenburg kept his work diaries and the acquired documents secret, not revealing them to the public for a long time. It wasn't until Zheng Zhenduo's visit to Leningrad that the mystery surrounding the Russian collection of Dunhuang manuscripts began to slowly unravel.

By the year 1960, it was not until the 25th International Congress of Orientalists held in Moscow that the Leningrad branch of the Institute of Oriental Studies finally exhibited several Dunhuang manuscripts. In 1963, the first volume of *Explanatory Catalogue of the Dunhuang Chinese Manuscripts Collection of the Leningrad Branch of the USSR* (苏联科学院亚洲民族研究所藏敦煌汉文写本解说目录) compiled by Menshikov (л.н.Меньшиков) et al. was published, listing 1,707 manuscripts from Dunhuang and Xinjiang. The second volume, published in 1967, included manuscripts numbered 1708 to 2954. In 1964, the French Sinologist Professor Paul Demiéville published an article titled *Chinese Dunhuang Manuscripts in Leningrad* (列宁格勒的中国敦煌手卷) which introduced and researched some of the Soviet-held manuscripts. However, all these developments occurred after Zheng's death. The letters Zheng Zhenduo wrote to his friends during his visit to Leningrad were the first detailed reports about the Russian collection of manuscripts, marking a significant contribution to the field before these later developments.

Following the dissolution of the Soviet Union, the Russian collection of Dunhuang manuscripts was made accessible. In 1990, the Shanghai Classics Publishing House signed an agreement with the Institute of Oriental Studies of the Russian Academy of Sciences to collaborate on compiling and publishing facsimile editions of the entire Russian collection of Dunhuang manuscripts. Starting from 1992, through the efforts of the Shanghai Classics Publishing House and under the editorship of Russian scholar Lev Menshikov and Chinese scholar Qian Bocheng, the series *Russian Collection of Dunhuang Manuscripts* (É Cáng Dūn Huáng Wén Xiàn, 俄藏敦煌文献) had published 17 volumes by the end of 2001. To date, the series has organized and cataloged over 19,000 manuscript numbers from the Russian collection.

Within the Russian collection of Dunhuang manuscripts, a significant number are akin to small scraps of paper. Beyond the previously cited reason, which involves fragments left behind by the Qing government during the transportation of these manuscripts, there's an alternative explanation for the accumulation of such small scraps in the collection. This raises the need for a detailed investigation into the procurement practices behind these artifacts.

As mentioned in the second chapter, during his pursuit of a murderer in southern Xinjiang, British officer Hamilton Bower unexpectedly acquired what appeared to be an ancient manuscript from a local Afghan merchant. The manuscript, written on birch bark and featuring ancient script unrecognizable to him, was eventually deciphered by the German-born British scholar Augustus Rudolf Hoernle. It was discovered to be one of the world's oldest Sanskrit and Prakrit manuscripts, subsequently named the "Bower Manuscript."

The revelation of the "Bower Manuscript" sent shockwaves through the Western Indological community, reshaping the focus of international Central Asian explorations. Western scholars began to realize that in China's Tarim Basin in Xinjiang, thanks to its unique cultural and climatic conditions, one could find the world's oldest documents written in Indian languages and scripts.

To decipher the script of the "Bower Manuscript," from 1893 to 1898, upon the suggestion of the Asiatic Society of Bengal's Secretary, Hoernle, the Indian government instructed British and Indian diplomatic missions in Central Asia to purchase ancient Central Asian manuscripts. They placed particular emphasis on acquiring documents originating from the Taklamakan Desert in China's Xinjiang region.

This initiative undoubtedly unlocked a gateway for the massive acquisition of "ancient manuscripts," setting off a relentless flow of documents akin to the "Bower Manuscript," which emerged like an unending spring in the years that followed.

At that time, the British Consul in Kashgar was George Macartney, a man of no ordinary background.[5] His father, Halliday Macartney, joined the foreign-led Ever Victorious Army under the command of the American Frederick Townsend Ward in 1862, aiding Li Hongzhang's Huai Army against the Taiping Rebellion. During the "Suzhou Massacre," Macartney Sr. married a woman from the household of Gao Yongkuan, one of the leaders of the Taiping Heavenly Kingdom, and George Macartney was born in Nanjing in 1867. Leveraging his mixed British-Chinese heritage, fluency in Chinese, and deep understanding of Chinese culture and customs, Macartney excelled in his role as Consul in Kashgar, often outperforming his counterpart, the Russian Consul General in Kashgar, Nikolai Petrovsky. Macartney was passionately devoted to collecting artifacts from Xinjiang and Central Asia, particularly ancient manuscripts with inscriptions. He amassed a significant collection of precious documents written in Chinese, Brahmi, Turkic, Arabic, Tocharian, and Sogdian languages.

Even with George Macartney's broad experience and expertise in ancient manuscripts, he was unable to decipher the script on the documents sold to him, noting their resemblance to the Brahmi script of the "Bower Manuscript." Furthermore, the layout and binding methods of these manuscripts differed, yet they seemed nearly identical to other ancient texts previously unearthed.

Consequently, George Macartney decided to send these manuscripts to a more specialized scholar for detailed analysis. He chose Augustus Rudolf Hoernle, who had gained considerable fame a few years earlier for decoding the "Bower Manuscript." By this time, Hoernle had moved to Calcutta in British India, continuing his research on ancient scripts at the Asiatic Society of Bengal. Upon receiving the ancient manuscripts from Macartney, Hoernle immediately embarked on the task of deciphering them.

However, by 1897, after nearly three years of strenuous efforts, Hoernle was still at a loss with these ancient manuscripts. They appeared to be parts of a complete ancient text, within which he could identify some characters that might be Brahmi script used for writing the Sogdian language. Despite this, the majority of the text remained undeciphered. Hoernle decided to compile his initial research findings into a report on manuscript interpretation. Apparently, this first phase of interpretation did not yield any useful results. In his report, Hoernle even began to doubt his scholarly abilities, writing despondently:

> The script is quite unknown to me, or perhaps due to my lack of knowledge, I am unable to prepare a thorough interpretation during the scant leisure available from my regular duties. . . . I hope among those experts who specialize in Central Asian languages, perhaps someone may recognize the script and language of these unusual documents.

As Hoernle continued to struggle, more manuscripts inscribed with unknown scripts were sent to him by Macartney from Kashgar, urging him to persevere. Gritting his teeth to carry on, Hoernle finally made some progress. In his second report on manuscript interpretation, published in 1899, Hoernle categorized the manuscripts into nine types based on the scripts he could recognize. These included documents written in symbols resembling Kharosthi, Indian Brahmi, Central Asian Brahmi, Tibetan, Chinese, Uighur, Persian, Arabic, Aramaic, and Greek scripts. However, that was as far as he could go. The texts of these ancient manuscripts, whether handwritten or woodblock printed, still could not be fully deciphered.

Unexpectedly for the British, while Macartney was collecting these ancient manuscripts written in unknown scripts and steadily sending them to Hoernle in India, the Russian Consulate General in Kashgar also began to acquire a significant number of handwritten or printed ancient manuscripts from the local area.

These ancient manuscripts, inscribed with indecipherable script, were similarly sent back to Russia for study and decipherment. Among the most baffling aspects for Russian experts was the frequent appearance of characters resembling Cyrillic letters or inverted Russian letters within these documents. This phenomenon of "temporal disarray" defied any logical explanation.

At the same time, voices questioning the authenticity of these ancient manuscripts began to emerge. Skeptics primarily focused on the manuscripts' cryptic and peculiar text, the large quantity discovered, their unusually well-preserved condition, their abrupt and contextless emergence, and their strange binding methods. Among the many doubters, Swedish missionary Magnus Backlund even wrote to Hoernle expressing his skepticism. In his letter, he mentioned encountering a man named Islām Ākhūn in Kashgar, who offered to sell him ancient manuscripts that were nearly identical.[6]

Another skeptic was Aurel Stein. In the early stages of his explorations in Khotan, Stein had also heard of Islām Ākhūn and his ancient manuscripts and even purchased some from him. Initially, Stein thought he had discovered numerous rare artifacts and ancient texts previously unseen, even acquiring several rough, yellowed, slightly damaged, and scorched copies of ancient Khotanese manuscripts with simple symbols from Islām Ākhūn's accomplices. However, Stein realized that Islām Ākhūn and his associates could continually, and even cater to Stein's specific needs, supply various ancient manuscript copies.

What further aroused Stein's suspicions was his own experience excavating ancient Khotanese manuscripts during his personal exploration of the ruins of ancient Khotan. These manuscripts bore no resemblance to those sold to him by Islām Ākhūn, and the local residents were completely unaware of such items being found at the site. Stein's doubts grew, and at the same time, he heard that the renowned Swedish explorer and archaeologist Sven Hedin had also purchased identical ancient copies from individuals similar to Islām Ākhūn.

At this point, Stein only knew that this elusive figure was a very ordinary local Uighur from Khotan, who made a living by selling artifacts found at ancient sites to Western explorers. The question Stein wanted to ask him was this: Who exactly are you, capable of creating forgeries that have deceived numerous professional scholars and archaeologists? What Stein didn't realize at the time was that the person behind these "ancient manuscripts" was in fact completely illiterate.

On April 25, 1901, Aurel Stein finally located Islām Ākhūn in Khotan and spent several days in deep conversation with him. Islām Ākhūn, who had once traded in antiquities, had by then transformed into a nomadic traditional herbalist. When presented to Stein, alongside Islām Ākhūn were his herbal medicine kit and various old-looking pieces of paper, even including fragments from French novels.

Stein surmised that the pieces of paper inscribed with text unintelligible to the locals were likely used by Islām Ākhūn as talismans or prayers, purported to have magical healing properties, to deceive those seeking cures for their ailments. Islām Ākhūn might even have shredded these inscribed papers to present as divine medicine, tricking patients into ingesting them.

Stein immediately resolved to uncover the truth behind the series of ancient manuscript forgeries from this man. Faced with eyewitnesses brought forth by Stein, along with more detailed textual evidence, the illiterate yet cunning Islām Ākhūn eventually confessed to fabricating the counterfeit ancient manuscripts.

Initially, Islām Ākhūn made his living by selling coins and seals at makeshift stands in villages near Khotan. In 1894, observing that white traders from India paid handsomely for ancient manuscripts inscribed with text, he saw an opportunity and shifted his focus. Ākhūn started crafting counterfeit documents himself to sell to these collectors.

Initially, he meticulously copied the cursive Brahmi script from ancient manuscripts excavated at nearby sites, faithfully replicating each stroke on paper. However, he soon realized that the Westerners purchasing these manuscripts couldn't understand the text at all, making such careful copying unnecessary. Liberating his mind and loosening his hand, he began to write randomly, often engaging in mechanical, repetitive scribbling. Surprisingly, this had no negative impact on his business.

After Hoernle suggested that the "ancient manuscripts" he produced might pertain to ancient Indian Sanskrit religious doctrines, demand surged, leading to a situation where supply could not keep up. Islām Ākhūn found himself compelled to hire assistants and even resort to woodblock printing techniques for mass production on a frenzied scale.

The method for crafting the "ancient paper" used in the forgeries was strikingly simple: willow branches were soaked in water until it turned yellow or light brown. Subsequently, sheets of paper were immersed in this tinted water to fully absorb the color. Once dried, "script" was either inscribed or stamped onto them. To mimic aging, the paper was then subjected to smoke over a fire, creating a crispy, charred effect. The final step involved burying the treated paper in sand. A month or two later, it was retrieved, marking the completion of the aging process.

It's evident that there was a trend of fabricating fake artifacts at the time, with even Stein being deceived. A significant portion of the forged ancient manuscripts sent back to Russia has vanished without a trace. As for whether these forgeries have been included in the collections of the Institute of Oriental Studies remains unknown.

Huang Wenbi, a contemporary Chinese archaeologist and a professor at Peking University at the time, acquired these so-called "ancient manuscripts" in the Hotan market in 1929. He designated them as "Ancient Khotanese Manuscripts" and brought them back to Beijing to study with Ji Xianlin. Ji Xianlin, too, was misled, identifying them as "a form of ancient Khotanese script," though he remarked that "their content could not yet be determined."

It wasn't until 1959 that Ji Xianlin's teacher, the German Indologist Ernst Waldschmidt, saw these "ancient manuscripts" at Ji Xianlin's place and couldn't help but point out to him that they were actually forgeries left by Islām Ākhūn. Only then did Ji Xianlin realize that these "ancient manuscripts" were all fabrications.

Therefore, within the nearly 20,000 Dunhuang manuscripts in the Russian collection, it's challenging to ascertain whether forgeries posing as "ancient manuscripts" are interspersed among them. Despite the vastness of this collection, documents related to Dunhuang medicine are exceedingly rare, with only about 30 scroll numbers identified so far. The majority of these documents were acquired during the second Central Asian expedition led by Sergei Fyodorovich Oldenburg, which took place from August 20, 1914, to January 26, 1915, in Dunhuang.

In 1999, Chinese scholar Ma Jixing published *Unearthed Ancient Chinese Medical Literatures Currently Housed in Russia* (俄国现藏的中国出土古医药文献),[7] focusing on the medical literature among ancient documents excavated by Russian-organized expeditions in the vast northwestern regions of China in the early 20th century, now housed at the Saint Petersburg branch of the Institute of Oriental Studies of the Russian Academy of Sciences. The paper begins by detailing the excavation and collection circumstances of these documents in Russia, followed by a systematic discussion of the contents that have been made public by the country, providing a detailed evaluation of the medical documents unearthed in locations such as Dunhuang, Heicheng (Khara-Khoto), and Khotan, including their catalog numbers, titles, authors, preservation status, and contents.

In 2006, Chinese scholar Li Yingcun published several articles that further researched the Dunhuang manuscript РДх.01325v held in Russia, revealing that this fragment was another copy of Zhang Zhongjing's *Five Viscera Theory* (Wǔ Zàng Lùn, 五藏论). With this discovery, a fifth version of *Five Viscera Theory* (Wǔ Zàng Lùn, 五藏论), identified among the Dunhuang manuscripts, came to light.

In 2008, Li Yingcun compiled and published *A Synopsis of Dunhuang Medical Documents in Russia* (俄罗斯藏敦煌医药文献释要),[8] which is divided into eight chapters. The first chapter provides an overview of the source, preservation, research status, and academic value of the Dunhuang medical documents held in Russia. Chapters 2 through 8 delve into seven aspects: medical theories; diagnostic methods; herbal formulation; acupuncture and moxibustion; Mongolian medical texts and fragments of practice scripts; Buddhist, Daoist, and Confucian medicine; and divination texts related to illnesses, offering synopses of 31 types of medical and medically related documents. Due to its collection of new materials and the precision in text identification and collation, this book has become an influential work in recent Dunhuang medical document research.

Li Yingcun has closely linked the content of herbal formulation, acupuncture, and moxibustion found in Dunhuang medical studies to clinical practice. To date, over 1,240 ancient herbal formulas from Dunhuang medical literature have been discovered, all of which await further clinical research and development. For example, Zhang Zhongjing's *Five Viscera Theory* (Wǔ Zàng Lùn, 五藏论) lists 12 pairs of medicinal ingredients, among which the Angelica-Dahurica (Dang Gui–Bai Zhi) pair is one of the commonly used prescriptions by Professor Li Yingcun in clinical settings, specifically for treating headaches, dysmenorrhea, sciatica, postpartum body pain, rheumatism, and other conditions.[9]

Dunhuang medicine boasts profound content and immense clinical value. These manuscripts have endured over a century of tumultuous changes, witnessing the profound transformations of several countries. Today, most of these documents have been meticulously preserved and have undergone organization, correction, and interpretation, providing a wealth of research material for scholars and medical practitioners alike. They also play a significant role in advancing contemporary medical development.

Next is the direct translation of Zhang Zhongjing's *Five Viscera Theory* (Wǔ Zàng Lùn, 五藏论) from the Russian collection. The translation process adheres strictly to the original text, translating word by word and sentence by sentence to ensure that each word and each sentence remain true to the original manuscript:

(Front missing)

⊠肤

[unrecognizable] (the lung rules the) skin

⊠，实（肉）假皮存，面⊠

[*unrecognizable*] muscle depends on skin to exist, face [*unrecognizable*]

□知骨患由肾，筋患出肝，实□则伤

[*missing*] the bone disorders are resulted from the kidney; the tendon disorders are resulted from the liver; muscle [*missing*] will hurt

心，皮患则由肺，只如十二经脉，上下旬还，

heart; the skin disorders are resulted from the lung. There are 12 meridians circulating superiorly and inferiorly,

八脉几经，内外流转，三焦六腑，四海七

eight extraordinary meridians flow in the human body interiorly and exteriorly. Triple burner, six Fu-organs; four seas and seven spirits.

身，肮膈咽喉，唇舌牙齿，臂肘指□

Huang (which indicates below the heart and above the diaphragm), diaphragm, pharynx, and throat; lips, tongues, and teeth; arm, elbows, fingers [*missing*]

膝胫脚踝，手腕腿股，八节三☒

knees, lower leg, feet, and ankles; hands, wrists, upper leg, and thigh, eight joints and three [*unrecognizable*]

小肠肚口，脐肋脊背，胁项孤☒

lower abdomen, navel, and ribs; spine, back, intestine, and nape; back, hypochondriac area, neck (孤) [*unrecognizable*]

主，鬓眉髭发，俱有患处。

chin, forehead, nose; sideburns, eyebrow, mustache, and hair, all the aforementioned places could suffer from illness.
(Back missing)

REFERENCES

1. St. Petersburg Institute of Oriental Studies of the Academy of Sciences of Russia and The Central Department of Oriental Literature, "NAUKA" Publishing House and Shanghai Chinese Classics Publishing House, *Dunhuang Manuscripts Collected in the St. Petersburg Institute of Oriental Studies of the Academy of Sciences of Russia: Volume 8 Дх01185-Дх02000* (Shanghai: Shanghai Chinese Classics Publishing House and The Central Department of Oriental Literature, "NAUKA" Publishing House, 1997), 91
2. 李应存，"新发现Дx.01325v为敦煌《张仲景五脏论》又一写本[J]." 敦煌研究, Vol. 95, No. 1 (2006): 89–90.
3. 刘进宝、王睿颖，"郑振铎与俄藏敦煌文献[J]." 南京师大学报（社会科学版）No. 3 (2009): 71–76.
4. 刘进宝，"鄂登堡考察团与敦煌遗书的收藏[J]." 中国边疆史地研究, No. 1 (1998): 23–31.
5. 崔延虎，"英国驻喀什噶尔首任总领事乔治・马嘎特尼(马继业)评述." No. 2 (1998): 58–63.
6. 马继兴，"俄国现藏的中国出土古医药文献[J]." *中华医史杂志*, Vol. 9, No. 1 (1999): 10–14.
7. 李应存、李金田、史正刚，*俄罗斯藏敦煌医药文献释要[M]*（兰州： 甘肃科学技术出版社, 2008), 32.
8. 葛政、李应存、李鑫浩，"李应存ff用敦煌张仲景《五脏论》药对当归-白芷经验[J]." *亚太传统医药*, No. 22 (2017): 86–87.
9. Mark Aurel Stein, *Sand-buried ruins of Khotan* (London: Hurst and Blackett, Limited, 1904), 450.

12 Forgotten by History – The Gakkundō Wooden-Movable Type Edition from Japan

"This book is a compilation from the 'Categorized Collection of Medical Formulas,' also transcribed by my younger brother, Yirou."

– Taki Mototane

The Gakkundō wooden-movable type edition of *Five Viscera Theory* (Wǔ Zàng Lùn, 五藏论), a single volume, is currently preserved in the Waseda University Library in Japan.[1]

This volume was compiled by the Japanese scholar Taki Mototane and completed in the fourth year of the Kaei era (1851). It is a compilation derived from the Korean medical masterpiece, *Categorized Collection of Medical Formulas* (Yī Fāng Lèi Jù, 医方类聚). The book measures approximately 26 cm in height and 18 cm in width, representing a thread-bound edition from the early modern period made with wooden movable type. The beginning of the text includes a preface written by Kitamurana Ohira, and the end features an epilogue by Taki Mototane himself. The title page displays phrases such as "Categorized Collection of Medical Formulas: A Compilation," "Wu Zang Lun," and "Xue Xun Tang Ju Zhen Ban" (the Gakkundō wooden-movable type edition). "Xue Xun Tang" (Gakkundō) refers to the name of Kitamura Chokukan's library, while "Ju Zhen" adopts a Chinese-style elegant name for the movable type used.

Regarding the phrase "Categorized Collection of Medical Formulas: A Compilation," it was a monumental project that began in 1443 and was not completed until 1477, taking 34 years to compile, revise, and finally publish. Of the initial 30 volumes printed using movable type, only one volume has been preserved relatively intact, and it was taken to Japan as a trophy by Katō Kiyomasa. It later found its way into the collection of Kyūkei Kudō, a medical professional in Sendai, Japan. According to Junzaburō Mori's *The Achievements of the Tajika Family* (多纪氏の事绩), Kudō mentioned that he owned 430 volumes of the *Categorized Collection of Medical Formulas* (Yī Fāng Lèi Jù, 医方类聚), missing just over ten volumes. Due to the extensive size of the work and the difficulty in preserving it from damage and decay, Kudō expressed a wish to entrust it to the Seijukan library, owned by the Taki family. Subsequently, the Seijukan library acquired this collection.[2]

DOI: 10.1201/9781032698205-12

Seijukan was the only private medical school in Japan during the Edo period of the Tokugawa shogunate. It was founded by Taki Motoyasu, the grandfather of the renowned Japanese textual scholar Taki Mototaka, in the second year of the Meiwa era (1765). Over the generations, the Taki family engaged in various activities, including lecturing on medical texts, conducting examinations, dispensing medicines, and particularly excelling in the editing and printing of medical books. Their contributions have been notably recorded in Japanese history.[3]

The compiler of the Gakkundō wooden-movable type edition of *Five Viscera Theory* (Wǔ Zàng Lùn, 五藏论), Taki Mototane, was a descendant of the Taki family. This family has a distinguished history of serving as imperial physicians, significantly influencing the Japanese royal medical system over the years. Remarkably, their ancestry even traces back to having lineage from the Han Chinese imperial family.

In fact, the profound research into traditional Chinese medicine (TCM) by Japanese scholars can be attributed to the long history of TCM in Japan. The earliest introduction of Chinese medicine to Japan is speculated to have occurred during the reign of Emperor Qin Shi Huang, with Xu Fu's voyage across the sea in search of immortality, supposedly bringing along experts in various crafts, including medical practitioners, though this is based on historical conjecture. According to historical records, TCM was first introduced to Japan via the Korean Peninsula about 1,500 years ago.

In the year 220 AD, during a period of turmoil and decline for the Han Dynasty, Emperor Xian of Han, Liu Xie, was forced to abdicate by Cao Pi. Following his abdication, Liu Xie and the Empress chose to live among the common people, dedicating themselves to the practice of medicine. They traveled to impoverished areas, employing the royal medical techniques of Qihuang to treat the people without seeking any compensation. Their selfless service earned them the local populace's admiration, who revered them as the "Dragon and Phoenix Medical Family." On his deathbed, Liu Xie advised his descendants to stay away from the court, pursue a career in traditional medicine, delve deeply into medical knowledge, and dedicate themselves to the well-being of the common folk.

During the Western Jin dynasty, to escape the chaos of war, Liu Xie's great-great-grandson, Liu Azhi, led his family and over 20,000 members of the Liu clan, along with a collection of medical texts, to cross the sea eastward to Japan. This marked the beginning of the Han lineage in Japan, where it took root and flourished, giving rise to several Japanese noble surnames, such as Sakagami, Uzō, Ōzō, Harada, Akizuki, and Takahashi.

In the year 414 AD, Kim Mu from the Silla Kingdom in Korea brought their medical knowledge to Japan and successfully treated the illness of Emperor Yūryaku, marking the earliest recorded instance of TCM being introduced to Japan.

The formal introduction of TCM to Japan is believed to have occurred during the Sui Dynasty in China. Empress Suiko of Japan, eager to embrace Chinese culture, dispatched envoys to the Sui Dynasty on four occasions. Among these exchanges, in 608 AD, Japanese pharmacists E-Nichi and Wa-Kan Naofuki journeyed to China as part of an envoy led by Ono no Imoko, with the specific purpose of delving into the principles of Chinese medicine. They continued their studies in China until 623 AD, well into the Tang Dynasty, before making their way back to Japan. Their return heralded the official entry of TCM into Japanese medical practice, marking a significant milestone in the cross-cultural exchange between Japan and China.

In 753 AD, the Chinese Tang Dynasty monk Jianzhen successfully traveled eastward to Japan, bringing with him a vast collection of TCM texts and medicinal herbs. He established a platform for teaching Buddhism and medicine at the Tōdai-ji Temple in Nara, Japan. It is said that he cured the illness of Empress Kōmyō of Japan, for which he was awarded the title of "Daisōjō," a high-ranking Buddhist honor. The "Miraculous Pills" he created while practicing medicine at the Tōshōdai-ji Temple are still widely used today.

In 806 AD, during his studies in Tang China, the esteemed Kūkai, better known as Kōbō-Daishi, copied the *Treatise on Cold Damage Disorders* (Shāng Hán Lùn, 伤寒论) and brought it back to Japan, where it became known as the *Kanpyō version of the Treatise on Cold Damage Disorders*. Another high-ranking monk who studied abroad, Saichō, also brought back a copy of the *Treatise on Cold Damage Disorders* (Shāng Hán Lùn, 伤寒论), known as the *Kanjizai version of the Treatise on Cold Damage Disorders*. During this time, TCM in Japan was exclusively utilized by the royal family and nobility, remaining inaccessible to the general populace.

As mentioned earlier, a branch of the family of Liu Xie's great-great-grandson, Liu Azhi, established themselves in Japan through the practice of TCM, dedicating their lives to the welfare of the people. By the time of Liu Azhi's eighth-generation descendant, Tamba Yasuyori, a royal physician, significant strides were made in the field. He compiled the *Ishinpō* (医心方), a monumental work consisting of 30 volumes, written in Chinese. This comprehensive text covered the ethics of medical practice, general medical theory, treatments for various diseases, health and wellness maintenance, and techniques related to sexual health. It is recognized as one of the earliest medical texts in Japanese history and incorporated a vast array of 204 ancient Chinese medical texts from the Tang Dynasty, including notable works such as the *Basic Questions* (Sù Wèn, 素问), *Essential Formulas for Emergencies [Worth] a Thousand Pieces of Gold* (Qiān Jīn Yào Fāng, 千金要方), *Shennong's Classic of Materia Medica* (Shén Nóng Běn Cǎo Jīng, 神农本草经), *Huatuo's Formulations* (Huá Tuó Fāng, 华佗方), *Shen Nong's Materia Dietetica* (Shén Nóng Shí Jīng, 神农食经), and *Taiping Holy Prescriptions for Universal Relief* (Tài Píng Shèng Huì Fāng, 太平圣惠方). Its medical significance is immense, and it served as a foundational work for Kanpō medicine in Japan, establishing Tamba Yasuyori as a pioneering figure in the field. In 984 AD, he presented this invaluable work to the imperial court.

Due to his mastery in medicine, Yasuyori was honored with the title of "Doctor of Acupuncture" by the Japanese government, which also bestowed upon him the surname "Tamba no Sukune" from a place-name. From then on, the Tamba family rose to prominence as a distinguished and respected lineage. Tasked with overseeing the Japanese royal medical institution, the family held a significant position in Japan's medical community for a millennium. By the time of the 30th-generation descendant, Motoyasu, the family name was changed to Taki. Mototaka and his son Motonori founded Seijukan, the only private medical school of the Edo period, pioneering the path for medical education in Japan.

The Tamba family has a long tradition of practicing Kanpō medicine, with the most notable members being Taki Motoyasu and his two sons, Motokata and Mototane. Not only were they highly skilled and beloved by the people for their medical expertise but they also had a passion for writing medical texts to pass down through generations. Together, they compiled the *Chinese Medicine Bibliography Researched* (Zhōng Guó Yī Jí Kǎo, 中国医籍考). After the father passed away, the son continued writing; and when the elder brother died, the younger brother took up the pen. Through their persistent and tireless efforts, they eventually completed the manuscript, which has become an important work for the study of traditional Chinese medicine and Kanpō medicine.

In the late Qing Dynasty, Chinese scholar Yang Shoujing purchased tens of thousands of ancient Chinese texts from Japan, among which were 14 works written by three generations of the Tamba family (nine by the father, Motoyasu; four by Motokata; and one by Mototane). These were compiled and published as the *Yuxiutang Medical Series* (Yù Xiū Táng Yī Xué Cóng Shū, 聿修堂医学丛书). The descendants of the Tamba family have continued to follow in their forebears' footsteps, dedicating themselves to the field of medicine, a commitment that has been revered by subsequent generations. Additionally, these three Tamba medical scholars also had Chinese names: Motoyasu was known as Liu Guishan (桂山), Motokata as Liu Chaiting (Saitei, 茝庭), and Mototane as Liu Liupan (柳泮), never forgetting their ancestor, the illustrious founder of the Han Dynasty, Liu Bang.

Among the 152 Chinese medical texts cited in the *Categorized Collection of Medical Formulas* (Yī Fāng Lèi Jù, 医方类聚), 35 original works have been lost in China, and the status of two works is unknown. Through their research on the *Categorized Collection of Medical Formulas* (Yī Fāng Lèi Jù, 医方类聚), Tamba Motokata and others managed to compile 13 of these lost medical works, allowing the world to glimpse the content of these otherwise lost texts. Among these rediscovered works, *Five Viscera Theory* (Wǔ Zàng Lùn, 五藏论) stands out as a notable example.

In the concluding remarks of the standalone volume *Five Viscera Theory* (Wǔ Zàng Lùn, 五藏论), Taki Mototane recorded, "This book is a compilation from the *Categorized Collection of Medical Formulas* (Yī Fāng Lèi Jù, 医方类聚), also transcribed by my younger brother, Yirou." The mentioned Yirou refers to Taki Mototane's brother, Taki Motokata. His courtesy name is Yirou, with the pseudonyms Saitei and San Song. This indicates that Taki Mototane's brother, Motokata, transcribed the *Five Viscera Theory* (Wǔ Zàng Lùn, 五藏论) from the *Categorized Collection of Medical Formulas* (Yī Fāng Lèi Jù, 医方类聚), and it was edited by Mototane himself. It was through the collaborative effort of the two brothers that later generations were able to gain a complete view of Zhang Zhongjing's *Five Viscera Theory* (Wǔ Zàng Lùn, 五藏论).

As for Kitamura Chokukan, the one who penned the preface at the beginning, who exactly is he?

Kitamura Chokukan (1804–1876),[4] known by his literary name Shilu and commonly referred to as Anzai, and later succeeded his father's title as Ansei, was a giant in the field of Japanese scholarly research. Along with Taki Motokata and Kojima Housu, he was recognized as one of the most erudite and respected figures in medical scholarship during the Bunsei and Tenpō periods (early to mid-19th century) in Japan, revered for his vast knowledge and ability to meet the great expectations of his time. In 1821, Chokukan began his studies at the Edo Medical Institute, quickly rising to prominence by becoming the top scholar a year later, thus taking on the role of a medical educator. By 1841, at 38 years old, he became a medical instructor at the institute, attracting doctors from all over the country who admired his reputation. Later in life, he served as a court physician and was honored with the prestigious title of Hōin. After the Taki family came into possession of the *Categorized Collection of Medical Formulas* (Yī Fāng Lèi Jù, 医方类聚), Chokukan, who was well-versed in the details of the book, was inspired to pursue the reprinting of the original publication.

Starting from the fifth year of the Kaei era (1852), in order to publish this extensive medical text, Kitamura Chokukan received financial support from many colleagues, even borrowing a hundred ryo (a unit of gold currency) from the Japanese shogun of the time. The reprinting work officially commenced in April of the Kaei five year. To address the missing content in the *Categorized Collection of Medical Formulas* (Yī Fāng Lèi Jù, 医方类聚) originally held by the Taki family, Chokukan invited Shibue Chūsai to join the project. Shibue referred to various texts to supplement the missing parts to a certain extent. The entire endeavor took ten years to complete, culminating in the reprinting of the *Categorized Collection of Medical Formulas* (Yī Fāng Lèi Jù, 医方类聚) in the first year of the Bunkyū era (1861), historically known as the Bunkyū first-year edition.

The contributions of the Taki Mototane brothers to the compilation of ancient Chinese medical texts are immeasurable. However, the opinions of experts sometimes require further scrutiny. Given their significant influence and authority, even some views that have not been subjected to further verification can become widely cited by scholars as authoritative sources.

Here's a clear illustration of the issue: The *Categorized Collection of Medical Formulas* (Yī Fāng Lèi Jù, 医方类聚) doesn't list authors next to the titles it cites, leading Taki Mototane to mistakenly attribute Zhang Zhongjing's *Five Viscera Theory* (Wǔ Zàng Lùn, 五藏论) to *Jivaka's Five Viscera Theory* (Qí Pó Wǔ Zàng Lùn, 耆婆五脏论). In his esteemed *Chinese Medicine Bibliography Researched* (Zhōng Guó Yī Jí Kǎo, 中国医籍考),[5] he asserts that the *Jivaka's Five Viscera Theory* (Qí Pó Wǔ Zàng Lùn, 耆婆五脏论), as cataloged in the *Comprehensive Catalogue of Literature During the Song Dynasty* (Chóng Wén Zǒng Mù, 崇文总目), spans one volume and indeed exists. He notes that the initial discussion on gestation theories within the *Five Viscera Theory* (Wǔ Zàng Lùn, 五藏论) found in the *Categorized Collection of Medical Formulas* (Yī Fāng Lèi Jù, 医方类聚) aligns with what is mentioned in Chen's *Great Herbal Formulas for Women* (Fù Rén Liáng Fāng, 妇人良方) . . . as recorded in the *Comprehensive Catalogue of Literature During the Song Dynasty* (Chóng Wén Zǒng Mù, 崇文总目). Taki Mototane highlights that his brother Saitei (Taki Motokata) extracted it from the collection, thus creating a distinct volume. The gestation theories he refers to are those that describe the ten-month fetal development process, featured at the outset of the *Five Viscera Theory* (Wǔ Zàng Lùn, 五藏论) within the Korean version of the *Categorized Collection of Medical Formulas* (Yī Fāng Lèi Jù, 医方类聚).

When it comes to the *Jivaka's Five Viscera Theory* (Qí Pó Wǔ Zàng Lùn, 耆婆五脏论), it's essential to first understand who Jivaka was. Historical accounts paint him as a revered ancient Indian physician, surrounded by numerous legends and mythological tales about his life. Jivaka's expertise in medicine and his therapeutic methods made their way to China as early as the Eastern Han Dynasty, accompanying the translation of Buddhist scriptures.

The *Jivaka's Five Viscera Theory* (Qí Pó Wǔ Zàng Lùn, 耆婆五脏论), a single volume, first appears in the records of the Song Dynasty, specifically in Zheng Qiao's *Comprehensive Records • Monographs on Arts and Literature* (Tōng Zhì • Yì Wén Lüè, 通志•艺文略) and the *Records of Arts and Literature in the History of the Song Dynasty* (Sòng Shǐ Yì Wén Zhì, 宋史艺文志). The *Comprehensive Catalogue of Literature During the Song Dynasty* (Chóng Wén Zǒng Mù, 崇文总目) from that era lists it as "*Jivaka's Five Viscera Theory*, one volume." This indicates that by the Northern Song Dynasty period, there were already multiple versions of this text in circulation. However, after the Southern Song Dynasty, the text was no longer seen in circulation within China.

Since Taki Mototane proposed that the *Five Viscera Theory* (Wǔ Zàng Lùn, 五藏论) cited in the *Categorized Collection of Medical Formulas* (Yī Fāng Lèi Jù, 医方类聚) is indeed the *Jivaka's Five Viscera Theory* (Qí Pó Wǔ Zàng Lùn, 耆婆五脏论), many scholars have referenced Taki Mototane's argument. Fan Xingzhun, in his study of the Dunhuang *Five Viscera Theory* (Wǔ Zàng Lùn, 五藏论), wrote:

> Among the texts like the *Wu Zang Lun*, although there were several as mentioned above, most have not been transmitted to the present. What is generally known seems to be only what is cited in Chen Ziming's *Great Herbal Formulas for Women* (Fù Rén Liáng Fāng, 妇人良方) from the Song dynasty. . . . The *Wu Zang Lun* we know from the Dunhuang collection and the *Wu Zang Lun* cited in the *Categorized Collection of Medical Formulas* (Yī Fāng Lèi Jù, 医方类聚) are indeed the *Jivaka's Five Viscera Theory* (Qí Pó Wǔ Zàng Lùn, 耆婆五脏论). Its content is that of a medical primer. Although it cannot be said that the content of the *Wu Zang Lun* listed in records after the Sui and Tang dynasties is entirely the same as the *Jivaka's Five Viscera Theory* (Qí Pó Wǔ Zàng Lùn, 耆婆五脏论), their content belongs to the same category of simple medical texts, undoubtedly.[6]

It's evident that both Taki Mototane and Fan Xingzhun referenced the famous quote discussed in volume 10 of Chen Ziming's *Great Herbal Formulas for Women* (Fù Rén Liáng Fāng, 妇人良方) from the Southern Song Dynasty, which mentions "Also, the *Wu Zang Lun* attributes to Jivaka" because of the theories on the ten-month fetal development. In fact, Chen Ziming himself was not certain that the *Wu Zang Lun* he referred to was the *Jivaka's Five Viscera Theory* (Qí Pó Wǔ Zàng Lùn, 耆婆五脏论).[7] The original text states:

> Also, in the *Wu Zang Lun*, there is mention by Jivaka discussing from one month like dew drops . . . to the tenth month when the energy received (by the fetus) is complete. There are also those who attribute it to Zhang Zhongjing in the same manner.

From this, it can be inferred that Chen Ziming believed the discussion on the ten-month gestation could also have originated from Zhang Zhongjing. Chen Ziming's final conclusion was "As for the *Wu Zang Lun*, the types are all shallow and not profound, often falsely attributes to other (big) names." That is, he considered that medical books like the *Wu Zang Lun* were more likely written by later individuals claiming to be Jivaka or Zhang Zhongjing. It appears that even Chen Ziming himself was not clear about the origins of the *Wu Zang Lun*.

Furthermore, in the 15th century, when compiling the *Categorized Collection of Medical Formulas* (Yī Fāng Lèi Jù, 医方类聚), the content of the *Five Viscera Theory* (Wǔ Zàng Lùn, 五藏论) was incorporated into volume 4 under the section "The Five-zang Organs." The compilation did not specify whether the *Five Viscera Theory* (Wǔ Zàng Lùn, 五藏论) was the *Jivaka's Five Viscera Theory* (Qí Pó Wǔ Zàng Lùn, 耆婆五脏论) or attributed to another author. By the late 18th century, when Taki Motokata compiled the lost *Five Viscera Theory* (Wǔ Zàng Lùn, 五藏论) from the *Categorized Collection of Medical Formulas* (Yī Fāng Lèi Jù, 医方类聚), he also did not use the title *Jivaka's Five Viscera Theory* (Qí Pó Wǔ Zàng Lùn, 耆婆五脏论).

Let's examine and compare the theory of the ten-month fetal development as cited by Chen Ziming with the theory described in the *Five Viscera Theory* (Wǔ Zàng Lùn, 五藏论) within the *Categorized Collection of Medical Formulas* (Yī Fāng Lèi Jù, 医方类聚) (Table 12.1):

TABLE 12.1
Comparison of the theory of the ten-month fetal development as cited by Chen Ziming with the theory described in the *Five Viscera Theory* (Wǔ Zàng Lùn, 五藏论) within the *Categorized Collection of Medical Formulas* (Yī Fāng Lèi Jù, 医方类聚).

Month	Wu Zang Lun	Great Herbal Formulas for Women
First month	One month pregnant, (the embryo) is like cheese	One month (pregnant), (the embryo) is like a pearl dew
Second month	Two months (pregnant), the embryo formed; it is like a plum	Two months (pregnant), (the embryo) is like a peach blossom
Third month	Three months (pregnant), (the fetus) started to develop appearance	Three months (pregnant), **can tell the sex (of the fetus)**
Fourth month	Four months pregnant, **can tell the sex (of the fetus)**	Four months (pregnant), (the fetus) started to develop appearance
Fifth month	Five months (pregnant), tendons and bones developed	Five months (pregnant), tendons and bones developed
Sixth month	Six months (pregnant), hair grows	Six months (pregnant), hair grows
Seventh month	Seven months (pregnant), the Hun (of the fetus) floats; it can move its **right hand**. Baby boy is on mother's left side; baby girl is on mother's right side.	Seven months (pregnant), the Hun (of the fetus floats). Baby boy can move its **left hand.**
Eighth month	Eight months (pregnant), the Po (of the fetus) floats; it can move its **left hand**	Eight months (pregnant), the Po (of the fetus) floats; it can move its **right hand**
Ninth month	Night months (pregnant), (the fetus) turns three times	Night months (pregnant), (the fetus) turns three times
Tenth month	Ten months is full-term pregnancy; the mother and baby separates	Ten months (fetus) got sufficient qi

As Table 12.1 demonstrates, the descriptions of embryonic development in the first and second months are entirely different between the two texts. There are discrepancies in the months designated for the formation of male and female genders in the third and fourth months, and whether the fetus first moves its left or right hand in the seventh and eighth months is completely opposite. Whether the first movement is with the left or right hand is determined by the sequence of yin and yang initiation and the differences in the positions of male and female fetuses within the womb. From the perspective of TCM's yin-yang and the five elements theory, distinctions between male and female, left and right, and the months cannot be incorrectly ordered or confused. Therefore, although the discussion of the ten-month fetal development in the *Categorized Collection of Medical Formulas* (Yī Fāng Lèi Jù, 医方类聚) appears superficially similar to that in Chen Ziming's *Great Herbal Formulas for Women* (Fù Rén Liáng Fāng, 妇人良方), the differences in understanding of basic TCM theories suggest that the ten-month fetal development discussed in the *Five Viscera Theory* (Wǔ Zàng Lùn, 五藏论) of the *Categorized Collection of Medical Formulas* (Yī Fāng Lèi Jù, 医方类聚) and the theory cited by Chen Ziming do not stem from the same academic source. Thus, even if Chen Ziming cited the *Jivaka's Five Viscera Theory* (Qí Pó Wǔ Zàng Lùn, 耆婆五脏论), it would still be significantly different from the *Five Viscera Theory* (Wǔ Zàng Lùn, 五藏论) in the *Categorized Collection of Medical Formulas* (Yī Fāng Lèi Jù, 医方类聚). Moreover, Chen Ziming himself was not clear whether his citation was from Jivaka or Zhongjing or if it was attributed to them by later generations.

Going back to the origins, in the field of archaeology, tangible artifacts stand as the most persuasive form of evidence. In Turpan, Xinjiang, China, an original scroll of the *Jivaka's Five Viscera Theory* (Qí Pó Wǔ Zàng Lùn, 耆婆五脏论) was unearthed, written on both sides. The front side contains this text, German collection Ch. 3725 (T II, Y49), and the back side contains *Various Medical Formulas Essence* (Zhū Yī Fāng Suí, 诸医方髓), German collection Ch. 3725V (T II, Y49 V).[8] Most of the beginning of the *Jivaka's Five Viscera Theory* (Qí Pó Wǔ Zàng Lùn, 耆婆五脏论) is missing, leaving only a small section at the end with six lines and 73 characters. Japanese scholar Kuroda Genji argued in his *Four Types of Central Asian Medical Texts in the Collection of the Prussian Academy* (普鲁西学士院所藏中央亚细亚出土医书四种) that this fragment should be *Jivaka's Five Viscera Theory* (Qí Pó Wǔ Zàng Lùn, 耆婆五脏论).[9] Aside from discussions on diseases such as five Zang-organ exhaustion, it lacks content on the ten-month fetal development and sections like "Part on Medicine Names" and "The Constitution of the Five Constants" compiled in the *Categorized Collection of Medical Formulas* (Yī Fāng Lèi Jù, 医方类聚). Hence, there's no evidence linking the *Jivaka's Five Viscera Theory* (Qí Pó Wǔ Zàng Lùn, 耆婆五脏论) with the Japanese or Korean versions of the *Five Viscera Theory* (Wǔ Zàng Lùn, 五藏论). It's no wonder Chinese scholar Luo Fuyi stated in the postscript of his *Compilation of Ancient Medical Formula Fragments from the Western Frontier* (Xī Chuí Gǔ Fāng Jì Shū Cán Juàn Huì Biān, 西陲古方技书残卷汇编) in 1953:

> The *Jivaka's Five Viscera Theory* (Qí Pó Wǔ Zàng Lùn, 耆婆五脏论), recorded in volume sixteen of Taki Mototane's *Chinese Medicine Bibliography Researched* (Zhōng

Guó Yī Jí Kǎo, 中国医籍考), was said to have been compiled from the Korean *Categorized Collection of Medical Formulas* (Yī Fāng Lèi Jù, 医方类聚). However, upon examination, the *Five Viscera Theory* (Wǔ Zàng Lùn, 五藏论) cited in the *Categorized Collection of Medical Formulas* (Yī Fāng Lèi Jù, 医方类聚) is actually authored by Zhang Zhongjing, with the Dunhuang fragments as evidence. Taki's attribution of the *Jivaka's Five Viscera Theory* (Qí Pó Wǔ Zàng Lùn, 耆婆五脏论) was a mistake.[10]

It is clear that the *Five Viscera Theory* (Wǔ Zàng Lùn, 五藏论) cited in the *Categorized Collection of Medical Formulas* (Yī Fāng Lèi Jù, 医方类聚) and the Gakkundō wooden-movable type edition *Five Viscera Theory* (Wǔ Zàng Lùn, 五藏论) from Japan bear no resemblance to the *Jivaka's Five Viscera Theory* (Qí Pó Wǔ Zàng Lùn, 耆婆五脏论) unearthed in Turpan, Xinjiang. However, they are strikingly similar to the Zhang Zhongjing *Five Viscera Theory* (Wǔ Zàng Lùn, 五藏论) discovered in Dunhuang. With this, a long-standing question has finally been resolved satisfactorily. The *Five Viscera Theory* (Wǔ Zàng Lùn, 五藏论) referenced in the *Categorized Collection of Medical Formulas* (Yī Fāng Lèi Jù, 医方类聚) is indeed the work of Zhang Zhongjing, not the *Jivaka's Five Viscera Theory* (Qí Pó Wǔ Zàng Lùn, 耆婆五脏论).

Japan is home to a wealth of TCM literature, providing rich resources for comprehensive research. In the 1960s, Iwanami Shoten, a prestigious Japanese publisher, released the *General Catalog of National Books* (Kokusho Sōmokuroku, 国书总目录), which cataloged an impressive array of 14,500 titles of ancient TCM and Japanese Kampo books, amounting to over 1 million volumes across 42 libraries, many are considered rare and esteemed editions, showcasing a collection that competes in both volume and quality with those in China. The Gakkundō wooden-movable type edition of *Five Viscera Theory* (Wǔ Zàng Lùn, 五藏论), among this vast collection of 14,500 ancient Japanese Kampo texts, is meticulously preserved at Waseda University Library in Japan. This edition is also accessible online in high-definition digital format, freely available to all. In today's world, where Western medicine is rapidly evolving, the question of whether this text is a work by the Indian sage Jivaka or a manuscript by the Chinese medical saint Zhang Zhongjing might seem obscure to many. Chinese scholar Ma Jixing, in his work *Annotations on the Ancient Medical Texts from the Dunhuang Cave Library* (Dūn Huáng Gǔ Yī Jí Kǎo Shì, 敦煌古医籍考释), noted:

> By the end of the 18th century, Taki Saitei (Taki Motokata) had compiled and published this book (*Wu Zang Lun*) from the *Categorized Collection of Medical Formulas* (Yī Fāng Lèi Jù, 医方类聚) using movable type, but the original manuscript has since vanished.[11]

Furthermore, Chinese scholar Li Qian, in her master's thesis, Research on Ancient Chinese Medical Texts Cited in the "Categorized Collection of Medical Formulas," suggests that the *Five Viscera Theory* (Wǔ Zàng Lùn, 五藏论) cited from the *Categorized Collection of Medical Formulas* (Yī Fāng Lèi Jù, 医方类聚) and its compilation exist in Japan, but the status of the copied volume – whether it has survived or not – is difficult to ascertain and needs further investigation.[12] Essentially, it was believed that this particular version of *Five Viscera Theory* (Wǔ Zàng Lùn, 五藏论), once cataloged in Japan, had been lost. Yet after extensive research, it was found that the edition of *Five Viscera Theory* (Wǔ Zàng Lùn, 五藏论) kept at Waseda University Library is precisely the *Five Viscera Theory* (Wǔ Zàng Lùn, 五藏论) manuscript Ma Jixing and Li Qian had mentioned in their works.

Zhang Zhongjing's *Five Viscera Theory* (Wǔ Zàng Lùn, 五藏论) has not been forgotten by history. Today, in addition to the five handwritten copies discovered in Dunhuang, the academic community recognizes several other versions of Zhang Zhongjing's *Five Viscera Theory* (Wǔ Zàng Lùn, 五藏论): one included in the Korean *Categorized Collection of Medical Formulas* (Yī Fāng Lèi Jù, 医方类聚), a copied manuscript by the renowned Zhejiang physician Zhang Yicheng, and the Gakkundō wooden-movable type edition preserved in the Waseda University Library in Japan. In total, there are eight known versions of this work in existence.

The following is a direct translation of the entire text of Zhang Zhongjing's *Five Viscera Theory* (Wǔ Zàng Lùn, 五藏论) from the Japanese Gakkundō wooden-movable type edition. The translation process was strictly adherent to the original text, translating word by word, sentence by sentence, to ensure that every character and every sentence remains faithful to the original manuscript:

題言

Preface

五藏論不著人名氏。考舊唐經籍志五藏論一卷，新唐藝文志同。則其書基系於唐代編輯，原本久佚。待醫劉君茝庭從朝鮮國醫方類聚錄出，衰然還舊，洵為希觀之秘笈矣。予近以活字印鄙著，僚友山崎次聞之，寄字子一櫃。曰是先人所銅也，未及裨事，而捐館徒委塵土。如有被藏於吾子，先人之誌或可少賞也。予得之驚喜，然與印鄙著字格不同，於是命工補刻若干字，又將有所刷，因謂此編卷頁短少，易於下手。乃請劉君本倣武殿聚珍式，依近人說，鎔化松脂填著版底，其法甚便，因印數十部，以貽同好。顧此小冊子僅為開雕嚆矢，自是以往津逮捕鄉嬛，每遇奇編，輒為擺刷，以資醫林欣賞。庶其字子不致淪墜。謂之活續次圭先人之志，於不朽可也，聊記此為弁首。

The book *Wu Zang Lun* lacks an author's name. In the *Old Tang Dynasty Records of Classics and Books* (Jiù Táng Jīng Jí Zhì, 旧唐经籍志), there's a record of a single volume titled "Wu Zang Lun." It's also mentioned in the *New Tang Dynasty Records of Arts and Literature* (Xīn Táng Yì Wén Zhì, 新唐艺文志), indicating that the book was edited during the Tang Dynasty, but the original version has been lost for a long time. When the royal physician Saitei brought back excerpts from *Categorized Collection of Medical Formulas* (Yī Fāng Lèi Jù, 医方类聚) from Korea, he restored the lost *Wu Zang Lun*, making it a very precious and valuable secret text. I recently printed this work using movable type, and upon hearing this, my friend Yamazaki sent me a cabinet of types. He said these were carved by his predecessors and, having not been put to significant use, they were just left gathering dust in a corner. If these types could help solve some of the difficulties in printing this book, it would also serve to fulfill or inspire the ambitions of my ancestors, which would be somewhat comforting. I was surprised to receive these items, as they were slightly different from the format of my printed work. So I had the craftsmen carve some characters and considered reprinting, as the volume of this compilation is not too large, making it easy to produce. I then requested Saitei to follow the format of the *Categorized Collection of Medical Formulas* (Yī Fāng Lèi Jù, 医方类聚) edition and, based on other experts' advice, melted rosin to fill the bottom of the printing plates, a convenient method. I plan to print several dozen more copies to give to those who appreciate such books. However, printing this booklet is just the beginning, merely an initial effort to lead and guide. Many medical books accumulated over time are printed whenever a new and interesting compilation arises, to be appreciated by the medical community and prevent these texts from being lost. In doing so, we continue the aspirations of our predecessors, ensuring the immortality of this cultural heritage. For now, I record this experience as a preface.

嘉永辛亥初冬既望江戶喜多村直寬士栗志

Kaei XinHai (the year 1851) early winter, after the full moon, in Edo (Tokyo), Chokukan Kitamura, styled Shi Li.

五藏論

Wu Zang Lun

夫天地之精氣，化萬物之形。父之精氣為魂，魂則黑；母之精氣為魄，魄則白也。以分晝夜。一月懷其胎，如酪。二月成其果，而果李相似。三月有形象。四月男女分。五月筋骨成。六月髮鬢俱生。七月遊其魂而能動右手，是男於母左，是女於母右。八月遊其魄能動左手。九月二轉身。十月滿足，母子分解祷。其中亦有延月者，有相富貴；而有月不足者，下賤而貧窮。子生經六十日，瞳子成，能喜笑。二百一十日，掌骨成而能匍匐。三百日，髀骨成而能獨立。三百六十日為一歲，膝骨成而能行動。若不能依此者，男女不安，必有疾病。又兒女三十二日為一變，六十四日為再變。父母三年之中，迴乾就濕，嚥苦吐甘，始得離父母之懷抱，割損母之形像，毀傷母之筋骨，以成其身。夫內有五藏，外應五行，頭圓像天，足方像地，因緣而生。

The essence of heaven and earth has transformed the shape of everything. The Jing Qi from father is called Hun, and the Hun is black; the Jing Qi from mother is called Po, and the Po is white. Like day and night, (Jing Qi can be divided into yin and yang). The first month of pregnancy, (the embryo) is like cheese. The second month of pregnancy, (embryo) begins to take shape, and it looks like a plum. Into the third month, (the fetus) began to form humanoid. The fourth month, the gender of the baby can be revealed. Into the fifth month, tendons, ligaments and bones of the fetus begin to form. Hair grows in the sixth month. Into the seventh month, Hun awakes, the fetus is able to move the right hand; boy situated in the left side of mother's womb, while girl lies on the right side of mother's womb. During the eighth month, Po awakes, and the fetus can move the left hand. The 9-month-old fetus starts to be very active, turning the body many times. After ten months of pregnancy, the fetus is separated from the mother. If the child is born beyond the gestation period, there are signs of wealth; if it is a premature baby, there are signs of poverty. 60 days after the child is born, the child's pupils form. He/she can see, can feel joy, and can laugh. 210 days after the birth (about seven months), metacarpal bones are formed, and the baby can crawl. After 300 days, the femur is formed, and the baby can stand alone. 360 days after the birth marked 1 year old, the child's knee bone is formed, and he/she can walk. If the baby does not develop according to this progress, no matter it's a boy or girl, it must have illnesses. An infant has the initial growth spurt around 32 days after birth, then another one around 64 days. In the first three years since the child born, the parents (take care of the baby in every possible way). They let the child live in a dry place while they are bearing the pain from living in a damp place; the parents eat simple foods themselves but feed the baby with nutritious foods. To helping the child to grow so that he/she can walk independently, the mother's appearance was deteriorated; her muscles and bones were damaged. In human body, there are five internal organs, which corresponds to the five elements on earth. The head is round, which symbolizes the sky. The foot is rectangular, which symbolizes the ground. (The existence of all things) is produced by the union of destiny.

因依足根，以拄著踝骨，以拄脛骨。因依脛骨，以拄膝骨，拄腿骨。因依腿骨，以拄髀骨、胯骨、腰脊骨、胷骨、項骨、頭骨、髑髏骨、肩骨、臂骨、肘骨、腕骨、掌骨、指骨。

The heel is the base point to support the ankle bone, and the ankle bone supports the tibia. The tibia is the base point to support the knee bone, and the knee bone supports the leg bone. The leg bone is the base point to support the femur, hip joint, lumbar spine, thoracic spine, cervical spine, skull, scapula, humerus, ulna and radius, wrist bones, metacarpal bones, and finger bones.

已上指骨，都共有三百六十五骨節，以應天三百六十五度。身上有五百筋脉，復有八萬毛孔，復有八萬戶此户字合是尸虫，虫戶八萬種，譬如窟中無所不成，名字各異。

Including the phalanges, the human body has 365 joints, corresponding to 365 days in a year. The human body has 500 veins, plus 80,000 pores, and 80,000 insects. And the insects have 80,000 species. It seems that all kinds of insects can grow in the "cave" and all have different names.

五藏者：心 肝 脾 肺 腎上是陰陽也。

The five Zang-organs refers to the heart, liver, spleen, lung, and kidney. (Kidney has kidney Yin and kidney Yang.)

六府者：大腸 小腸 膽 胃 膀胱是三焦也。

The six Fu-organs refers to the large intestine, small intestine, gallbladder, stomach, and bladder (the bladder has the function of triple burner).

肝合於膽，膽者中精之腑。
心合於小腸，腸受盛之腑。
脾合於胃，胃者水穀之腑。
肺合於大腸，大腸者傳導之腑。
腎合於膀胱，膀胱者津液之腑。

The liver and gallbladder are connected, and the gallbladder is the Fu-organ that stores pure essence (bile). The heart is connected to the small intestine; the small intestines is the Fu-organ to digest and absorb nutrients. The spleen is connected to the stomach; the stomach is the Fu-organ to receive food and water. The lung is connected to the large intestine; the large intestine is the Fu-organ to transport the waste. The kidney is connected to the bladder; the bladder is the Fu-organ to excrete water.

三焦者，中腑水道出於膀胱，膀胱者為三焦之腑。血氣之津液皆出於血，血海有餘，自然無疾；血海不足，身少顏色，面無精光。氣海有餘，胷面具赤；氣海不足，少氣力，不多言。水穀之海有餘，則消食腸滿；水穀之海不足，則多飢，不消食。髓海有餘，輕便多力；髓海不足，則肝轉耳鳴。

The triple burner is in charge of the internal water metabolism, and the fluids end up in the bladder, so the bladder is the fu of the triple burner. The fluid of blood and Qi both come from blood. If the sea of blood is full, there will be no sickness. If the sea of blood is insufficient, the body will have little color, and the face will be pale and dull. If there is too much in the sea of Qi, the excess qi accumulates in the upper part of the body, resulting in a red face and chest. If the sea of Qi is deficient, the person may have no strength, and unwilling to speak. If the sea of grain is sufficient, one will be able to digest food while also can feel full. If the sea of grain is weak, one will often be hungry but unable to digest food. If the sea of marrow is sufficient, the body feels light and energetic; if the sea of marrow is deficient, one will feel dizzy and tinnitus may occur.

肝屬東方甲乙木，外應於眼。
心屬南方丙丁火，外應於舌。
肺屬西方庚辛金，外應於鼻。
腎屬北方壬癸水，外應於耳。
脾屬中央戊巳土，外應於唇。

Liver corresponds to the direction of east, the first and second of heavenly stem, and the five elements of wood, and connected to the eyes on the outside. Heart corresponds to the direction of south, the third and fourth of heavenly stem, and the five elements of fire, and connected to the tongue on the outside. Lung corresponds to the direction of west, the seventh and eighth of heavenly stem, and the five elements of gold, and connected to the nose on the outside. Kidney corresponds to the direction of north, the ninth and tenth of heavenly stem, and the five elements of water, and connected to the ears on the outside. Spleen corresponds to the direction of middle, the fifth and sixth of heavenly stem, and the five elements of earth, and connected to the lips on the outside.

六神配五藏

Six Shen and five zang relations

胆為滕蛇。心為帝王监领四方。肺為將軍應四方。肝為尚书有流淚。腎為列女命主之門。脾為大夫王在四時。

The gallbladder is like a flying snake. The heart is the emperor, who supervises and controls all four directions. The lung is the general, who manages far and near. The liver is the minister, who weep sometimes. The kidney is like an upright woman with moral integrity, and it is the entrance to life. The spleen is a senior official, who is in charge of the end of four seasons.

夫五藏象天，六腑象地，上下相對，以合陰陽之氣，外有耳、鼻、舌、口、眼，內有五藏六腑。

The five Zang-orans corresponds to the heaven, and the six Fu-organs corresponds to the earth. The heaven and the earth are facing each other, and the Yin and Yang energy integrates. There are ears, nose, tongue, mouth, and eyes on the outside of human body, while inside, there are five Zang-organs and six Fu-organs.

心病則口焦，肝病則目暗，脾病嘔逆不下食，肝病則鼻塞不通，腎病則耳聾。心主於血，肺主於涕，肝生於淚，腎生於津液，脾生於涎。心是神，肺是魄，肝是魂，腎是志，脾是意。色脉為心，毛髮為肺，爪甲為肝，脂肉為腎，化食為脾。心逆則憂，肺逆則滿，肝逆則怒，腎逆則蹇，脾逆則嘔。心順面赤，肺順面白，肝順目明，腎順耳目精明，脾順則變化飲食。久坐濕地，強力入水，傷腎；愁憂必慮，傷心；形寒飲冷，傷肺；恚怒逆不可食，傷肝；飲食勞倦，傷脾。

Heart disease manifests as dry mouth; liver disease manifests as diminished vision; spleen disease manifests as vomiting, hiccups, and inability to take food; liver (pulmonary) disease manifests as nasal congestion; and kidney disease manifests as deafness. Heart dominates blood, lung dominates nasal mucus, liver dominates tears, kidney dominates fluid, and spleen dominates saliva. Heart houses Shen (mind), lung houses Po (the corporeal soul), liver houses Hun (the ethereal soul), kidney houses Zhi (the will-power), and spleen houses Yi (the intellect). The health of heart reflects through complexion and blood vessels. The health of lung reflects through hair. The health of liver reflects through nails. The health of kidney reflects through adipose tissues and muscles. And the health of spleen reflects through the ability of digesting food. Imbalance in the heart will cause depression, imbalance in the lung will cause chest tightness, imbalance in the liver will cause irritability, imbalance in the kidney will cause blockage of urination, and imbalance in the spleen will cause vomit. Heart being healthy makes the skin rosy, lung being healthy makes the skin pale, liver being healthy makes the eyes clear, kidney being healthy makes the ears and eyes sharp, and spleen being healthy makes the body digest and absorb food. Sitting in a humid place for a long time, or entering the water after overwork, will hurt the kidney; depressed and worried about everything will hurt heart; the body catching cold or eating cold food will hurt the lung; being angry to an extend that one does not want to eat, this will hurt liver; and intemperate diet, or overwork, can hurt the spleen.

夫五勞、七傷、六極、五藏敗、九候、十絕及婦人產後餘疾，悉緣內積風冷所致。

Five strains, seven impairments, six exhaustions, five Zang-organ damages, nine dangerous symptoms, ten critical conditions, and diseases caused by childbirth are all caused by the accumulation of wind and coldness in the body.

五勞者

The five kinds of strains are:

一、忽喜怒，大便苦難，口內生瘡，此為心勞；二、短氣面腫，鼻不聞香，咳嗽餘痰，兩脇脹痛，喘息不定，此為肺勞；三、面目乾黑，口中復苦，精神不定，不能獨臥，目視不明，如隔羅幕，頻頻下淚，此為肝勞；四、口苦，舌卷強直，不得嘔逆，醋心氣脹，脣焦，此為脾勞；五、小便黃赤，兼有餘瀝，腰痛耳鳴，夜間多夢，此為腎勞。

1. Sudden mood change, constipation, and sore in the mouth, these are the manifestations of heart strain; 2. shortness of breath, puffy face, loss of smell, cough out phlegm, intercostal tightness and pain, and breathlessness, these are the manifestations of lung strain; 3. dark complexion, dry eyes, bitter taste in mouth, restlessness, can't sleep alone, eyes can't see clearly like there is curtain in front, and tears often, these are the manifestations of liver strain; 4. bitter taste in mouth, tongue stiffness, often vomiting, heartburn, flatulence, and dry lips, these are the manifestations of spleen strain; and 5. yellow or dark urine, dribbling urination, back pain, tinnitus, insomnia and dreaminess, these are the manifestations of kidney strain.

七伤者

The seven types of impairments are as follows:

一陰汗；二精寒；三精清；四精少；五囊下濕癢；六小便數；七夜夢陰。

1. sweaty in male's genital area; 2. cold semen; 3. thin seminal plasma; 4. sparse semen; 5. wet and itchy scrotum; 6. frequent urination; and 7. nocturnal emission.

六極者 筋、骨、血、肉、精、氣。

The six exhaustions are (the overstrain of) tendons, bones, blood, muscles, essence, and Qi.

筋極則數轉筋，十指爪甲皆痛；骨極則牙齒痛，手足疼，不能久立；血極則令人面元顏色，頭髮墮悲；肉極則令人身上往往如鼠走，體上乾黑；精極則令人氣少無力，漸漸內虛，身上無潤澤，翕翕羸瘦，眼元精光，立不能定，身中若癢，瘙之生瘡；氣極則令人胷脇逆滿，邪氣沖胷，恒欲大怒，氣少不能言。此為六極。

The tendon exhaustion will cause frequent cramps, and the fingers and nails will be painful; the bone exhaustion will cause toothache; the hands and feet are also painful so that one cannot stand for long; the blood exhaustion will cause pale complexion and the thinning of hair; the muscle exhaustion will make one feel foreign objects crawling on the body, and the body is dry and dark; the essence exhaustion will cause fatigue, then gradually feels weak inside, and the skin is not shiny; the body emaciated like an old person, dull eyes, unstable posture or tremor, itching, and sores may develop after scratching; the qi exhaustion will cause chest fullness, rebellious Qi in the chest, easily burst in anger to an extend that one cannot even speak. These are the six exhaustions.

九候者

The nine dangerous symptoms are as follows:

一手足青；二手足久腫；三脉枯齒禁；四語聲散，鼻虛張聲勢；五脣寒冷宣露；六脣腫齒焦；七手順衣縫；八汗出不流；九舌捲卵縮。

1. The hands and feet are blue; 2. chronic edema on the hands and feet; 3. the blood vessels dry up and the teeth are clenched; 4. the voice is scattered and the nose flaps; 5. the lips are cold, and the gums are atrophied; 6. the lips are swollen, and the teeth are black; 7. the hands unconsciously smooth out the corner of clothes; 8. the sweat stays on the skin, does not drip; and 9. the tongue curls and the scrotum retracts.

五敗者

The five (Zang-organ) damages are as follows:

手足腫，無交文，心敗；唇反黑無文，肺敗；面黑有瘡，肝敗；陰腫囊縮，腎敗；臍腫滿，脾敗。

Edema on hands and feet. The edema is so severe that there is no wrinkle on skin, this is heart damage; darkened lips with no luster, this is lung damage; darkened complexion with sores outbreak, this is liver damage; swollen or contracted scrotum, this is kidney damage; full and swollen belly button, this is spleen damage.

十絕者

The ten critical conditions are as follows:

氣短，目視亭亭無精光，心絕；口鼻虛張聲勢，氣復短，肺絕；面青，眼視人不具數出淚，肝絕；面黑，眼睛黃，素汁流，腎絕；泄涎唾不覺，時時忘語，脾絕；手上爪甲青黑，惡罵不休，筋絕；背脊酸疼，腰中復重，骨絕；面無精光，頭髮自落，血絕；舌捲卵縮如紅丹，嚥唾不得，足踝小腫，肉絕；髮直如竿，汗出不止，腸絕。

Shortness of breath, straight and dull look in the eyes, this is heart failure; mouth and nose are feebly open with shortness of breath, this is lung failure; a bluish color to the skin, eyes are not focused and watery, this is liver failure; face is dark, eyes are yellow, spontaneous sweat, this is kidney failure; unconsciously drooling and often forget words, this is spleen failure; the nails on the hands are blue and black, constantly cursing, this is tendon failure; the back is sore, there is heavy sensation around the waist, this is bone failure; dull complexion with eyes lacking in luster, hair loss, this is blood failure; the tongue is curled, the scrotum is retracted like a red pellet, having trouble of swallowing saliva, and the ankle is swollen, this is muscle failure; hair is stiff like a bamboo pole, sweat continuously, this is intestine failure.

五氣不足歌 五言

Song of the Five Qi Insufficiencies (five characters to a line)

心氣若不足，衄血眼中黃。悲愁及喜怒，煩悶即荒忙。夢寤不自覺，心熱須水漿。喉嚨中滿痛，舌強口誇張。冷汗出不止，忘語忽驚忙。此為損心氣，不療轉加傷。

If heart Qi is deficient, will have nose bleeding and eyes will turn yellow. Sometimes sad, sometimes worried, sometimes happy, and sometimes angry. One moment being bothered, and in a flurry the next. Dreamful sleep but does not remember the dreams, dysphoria with thirst. Pain in the throat, stiff tongue, mouth wide open. Continuous cold sweat, forgetful and has sudden panic. This is the deficiency of the heart and will be more serious if left untreated.

肺氣若不足，肚脹不能安。嘔逆及上氣，悲思數多端。形寒似飲冷，肺損唾痰涎。皮毛不覺起，恚怒數千般。肩脊背強痛，夢裏鬼相牽。鼻中不覺氣，尋常骨膈乾。此為肺不足，不療病成難。

If lung Qi is deficient, there will be fullness in the stomach so that it is hard to feel comfortable. Nauseous, vomiting, and belching, often feels sad and worried. Body feels chilly like drinking cold water. Because the lung is damaged, which leads to excessive amount of sputum and saliva. The hair on the skin erected unconsciously and often gets angry. The shoulders, spine, and back are stiff and painful. There are ghosts in the dream. Nasal obstruction and dryness. This is the deficiency of the lung. If it is not treated, the disease will be more difficult to treat.

肝氣若不足，遠視目失力。兩脇氣脹滿，上下連胷臆。四肢熱復冷，肚痛不能食。眼前見火生，冷淚頻頻拭。不療恐失明，此為肝不足。

If liver Qi is deficient, it is difficult to see from a distance. The hypochondriac area feels full, and the chest is also affected by the tightness of the surrounding areas. The limbs are one moment hot and cold right after. Pain in the abdomen is so severe that one cannot eat. Seeing the hot fire in front the eyes but has to constantly wipe off the cold tears. If leave it untreated, one may be blind. This is liver deficiency.

腎氣若不足，腰胯收攝難。恍惚心少力，重聽不聞言。眼前如艷水，冷氣在腰間。身中悉皆癢，骨痛不能安。坐復身拘急，氣乏咽喉乾。狀似洋膠汁，腰胯強如寒。此為腎不足，於身不自安。

If kidney Qi is deficient, it is difficult to stretch the back and hips. One may feel uneasy and powerless, may have tinnitus or hearing loss. Sparkles dance before the eyes, and there is chilliness in the back. Itchy everywhere, pain in the bone so that one cannot find a comfortable position. The body contracts as soon as one sat down, shortness of breath with dry throat. Body is so weak, soft like gel; but the back and the hips are stiff and cold. This is the kidney deficiency. With this disease, one cannot be at ease.

脾氣若不足，令人面目黃。食即欲嘔逆，脣乾復口瘡。氣脹四支重，意相竝慞惶。不欲聞人語，脾渴即須漿。此為脾臟不足，急療可為良。醫人。

If the spleen Qi is deficient, it will cause yellow eyes and sallow complexion. Feels nauseous right after eating. Lips are dry and sores in the mouth. Bloated with heavy limbs, easy to get worried and terrified. Doesn't want to hear other people's voice, wants to drink as soon as the spleen is thirsty. This is spleen deficiency. The prognosis will be good if treated as soon as possible. The healer.

藥名之部，所出醫王。黃帝造針經曆有千卷。藥姓名品，若匪神仙，何能備著？且神農本草，辯土地而顯君臣，岐伯經方，說酸鹹而陳冷熱。雷公妙典，略述炮炙之宜，弘景奇方，備說根莖之用。

Medicine is contributed by the works of (later) various kings of medicine. The Yellow Emperor wrote "The Canon of Acupuncture" that consists of one thousand volumes. The medicines did not only have their names but also the functions. If this were not a celestial being, how could anyone write such a great book? Meanwhile, the *Shennong's Classic of Materia Medica* (Shén Nóng Běn Cǎo Jīng, 神农本草经) did not only tell the region/place that produces the medicine/herb but also classified each medicine. The classics written by Qi Bo explained medicine's (properties like) sour and salty and cold or hot nature. Lei Gong's marvelous classic talked in detail about herbal processing. Tao HongJing's miraculous formulas tirelessly discussed the use of stems and roots.

只如犀角觝觸之義，故能逐汪驅邪。牛黃壞鴆之功，是以安魂，藍田玉屑，可以鎮壓精神，中條麝香，堪將辟邪除鬼。河內牛膝，去腠冷而止腰疼。防風除頭風而抽脇痛。半夏有消痰之力，制毒要用生薑；當歸有止痛之能，會須白芷。晉地龍齒偏差顛癎，太山茯苓延年却老。仁參、薯蕷能令耳目聰明，遠志、菖蒲妙能開心益智。甘草安和諸藥，遂得國老之名；大黃宣引眾功，乃得將軍之号。秦膠結羅紋之狀，乾漆作蜂巢之形。丹砂會取光明，升麻破求青綠。秦椒須汗，樸硝、礬石須熬。杜仲削去麄皮，桂心還求肉味。石英須研似麵，杏仁別擣如膏。兔絲得酒乃良，礬石燒之力好。防葵唯輕唯上，狼毒唯重彌佳。黃芩以腐爛為精，閭茹蚛頭為上。石南採葉，甘菊收花。五茄剝取其皮，牡丹要須去骨。鬼箭破血，乃有射鬼之靈，神屋除瘟，非無保神之驗。嘔吐湯煎乾葛，轉筋酒煮木瓜。目赤宜點黃連，口瘡宜含石膽。木蘭皮能除點䵟，流黃妙去死痺。茵草殺齒內之虫，藜蘆爛鼻中宿肉。赤油宜塗雞子，白癲偏衣越挑。火燒多佔水萍，杖打須加松實。琥珀拾芥乃辯其真，磁石引針將知不謬。石得鴆糞乃爛如泥，漆遇蟹黃便化為水。三稜破癖，本出行從，劉寄奴療瘡起於田獵。牡蠣助栢仁之力，地黃益天門冬之功。斂及反烏頭之精，梔子解躑躅之毒。苦參、酸棗以味為名，白术、黃連，將色為號。蜈蚣、蜀漆，陸地標名，狗脊、狼牙，因形為記。只如八味腎氣，補六極而差五勞；四色神丹，蕩千痾而除萬病。檳榔下蟲除氣，玉壺丸去積冷消堅。李子預有殺鬼之方，劉涓有遣鬼之錄。耆婆童子，妙述千端，喻父醫王，神方萬品。是以有命者必差，虢太子死而更甦；無命者難理，晉公生而致死。此之養病，如積薪投火而薪存，人若有病，去病而人活，不去火而薪被焚，病不除而徒喪命。是以神方千卷，藥名八百。中黃丸能差千痾，底野迦善除萬病。扁鵲秘論乃揔君臣，冷熱不調，酸鹹各異。

Xi Jiao (犀角, rhinoceros horn) has the power to fight against illness, so it can eliminate chronic infectious disease and disperse evil. Niu Huang (牛黃, cattle gallstone) has the function to damage Zhen (a legendary bird with poisonous feathers) so that it can calm the soul (hun). Yu Xie (玉屑, Jade Chips) from Lan Tian can tranquilize the mind. She Xiang (麝香, musk) from Zhong Tiao can drive out evil.

Niu Xi (牛膝, twotoothed achyranthes root) from He Nei treats cold knee and relieves lower back pain. Fang Feng (防風, siler root, or divaricate saposhnikovia root) heals the head wind, also relieves the hypochondriac pain. Ban Xia (半夏, pinellia tuber) dissolves phlegm; Sheng Jiang (生薑, fresh ginger) can counteract its toxicity. Dang Gui (當歸, Chinese angelica root) can stop pain, but it must be combined with Bai Zhi (白芷, Dahurian angelica root). Long Chi (龍齒, fossilized animal teeth) from Shanxi can treat epilepsy; Fu Ling (茯苓, Indian bread, or poria*) from* Taishan can prolong life. Ren Shen (仁參 or 人参, ginseng root) and Shu Yu (薯蕷 or "Shan Yao" 山药, dioscrea rhizome) can make your eyes bright and ears sharp. Yuan Zhi (遠志, Thinleaf milkwort root) and Chang Pu (菖蒲 or "Shi Chang Pu" 石菖蒲, grass-leaf sweetflag rhizome) can clear the brain and improve the intelligence. Gan Cao (甘草, licorice root) has the function of harmonizing; thus, it has been called the "Guo Lao," a respected elder in the kingdom. Da Huang (大黄, rhubarb root) has the function of opening and inducing the elimination. That's why it was called the "Marshall General." Qin Jiao (秦膠or 秦艽, largeleaf gentian root) pertains spiral shape; Gan Qi 乾漆, dried lacquer) looks like honeycomb. Dan Sha (丹砂 or "Zhu Sha" 朱砂, cinnabar) should be shiny; Shen Ma (升麻, largetrifoliolious bugbane Rhizome) should be blue and green. Qin Jiao (秦椒, prickly ash peel) needs to be steamed; Pu Xiao (樸硝, a crude form of sodium sulfate) and Fan Shi (礬石 or "Ming Fan" 明矾, a sulfate of alum-stone, or white alum-stone) should be roasted; Du Zhong (杜仲, eucommia bark) must peel off the outer skin; Gui Xin (桂心 or "Rou Gui" 肉桂, cinnamon bark) must have meaty fragrance. Shi Ying (石英, Cristobalite) must be powdered; Xing Ren (杏仁, apricot seed) should be grinded until gets creamy. Tu Si (菟丝, Chinese dodder seed) must be soaked with alcohol; Fan Shi (礬石 or "Ming Fan" 明矾, a sulfate of alum-stone, or white alum-stone) must be calcinated. Fang Kui (防葵, white flower hog fennel root) the lighter the better; Lang Du (狼毒, Bracteole-lacked Euphorbia root) the heavier the better. Good Huang Qin (黄芩, Baical skullcap root) looks like rotten intestine; only use Lin Ru's (閭茹, Euphorbia Lanru root) top part. Shi Nan (石南, Chinese photinia Leaf) should pick its leaves; Gan Jü (甘菊, sweet chrysanthemum flower) uses its flower. Wu Jia (五茄, slenderstyle acanthopanax Bark) only uses the bark; Mu Dan (牡丹, tree peony bark), need to take the bone out. Gui Jian (鬼箭 or "Gui Jian Yu" 鬼箭羽, winged branches) can break up the blood stasis thus to kill ghost toxins. Shen Wu (神屋 or 龟板, tortoise carapace and plastron) clears the heat and has magical effect. Decoct Ge Gen (乾葛 or "Ge Geng" 葛根, dried pueraria root) to treat vomiting; use alcohol to decoct Mu Gua (木瓜, Chinese quince fruit) for muscle spasm. Use Huang Lian (黄連, yellow coptis root) to make eye drops for red eyes. Hold Shi Dan (石膽 or "Dan Fan" 膽矾, chalcanthite) in the mouth for mouth ulcer. Mu Lan (木蘭, lily magnolia bark) can remove dead skin; Liu Huang (流黄 or 硫磺, yellow Sulfur) is to treat gangrene. Wang Cao (莔草, leaf of poisonous eightangle tree) treats cavity inside the teeth; Li Lu (藜蘆, veratrum root and rhizome) can dissolve polyps in the nose. Red ulcer should apply Ji Zi (雞子, chicken eggs); tuberculoid leprosy needs to use Yue Tao (越桃 or "Zhi Zi" 栀子, gardenia fruit); burns to be treated by applying Shui Ping (水萍 or "Fu Ping" 浮萍, floating duckweed) topically; wounds from caning can use Song Shi (松實or "Song Zhi" 松脂, pine resin). Real Hu Po (琥珀, amber) can pick up tiny things; if the Ci Shi (磁石, magnetite) can attract needles, which means it is not fake. Zhen Fen (鴆糞, the excrement of a legendary poisonous bird) can make stones melt like mud; Xie Huang (蟹黄, crab yolk) can make paint melt like water. San Leng (三棱, common burred tuber) can break the nodule; this comes from Xing Cong's story; Liu Ji Nu (劉寄奴, diverse wormwood herb) heals the wound. This function was discovered from field hunting. Mu Li (牡蠣, oyster shell) can help the function of Bo Ren (柏仁, Oriental arborvitae seed kernel); Di Huang (地黄, rehmannia root) can benefit the function of Tian Men Dong (天門冬, Cochinchinese asparagus root). Bai Lian (白蔹, Japanese ampelopsis root) is incompatible with Wu Tou (烏頭, Sichuan aconite root); Zhi Zi (栀子, gardenia fruit) is the antidote of Zhi Zhu (躑躅, Chinese azalea flower). Ku Shen (苦参, light-yellow sophora root) and Suan Zao (酸棗, Chinese sour jujube) are named after their taste; Bai Zhu (白术, white atractylodes tuber) and Huang Lian (黄連, yellow coptis root) are named after their colors; Wu Gong (蜈蚣, centipede) and Shu Qi (蜀漆, Sichuan dichroa leaf) are named after their place of origin; Gou Ji (狗脊, cibot rhizome) and Lang Ya (狼牙, the underground winter bud of Agrimonia root) are named after their shapes. Just like Ba Wei Shen Qi (八味腎氣, Eight-Ingredient Kidney Qi Pills), it nourishes the six exhaustions and cures the five strains; Si Se Shen Dan (四色神丹, Four-Color Magic Pills) eliminates thousands of diseases and cures 10,000 illnesses. Bing Lang (檳榔, betel nut) eliminates parasites and relieve bloating; Yu Hu Wan (玉壺丸, Jade Pot Pills) expels coldness and dissolves hardness. Li Ziyu was known to kill ghosts; Liu Juan has a record of expelling ghosts. Jivaka understood medical theory profoundly. He was known as the king of medicine; he had many magical formulas. Those destined to live will recover from illness. Like the Prince of Guo ("Guo" is one of the ancient feudal states), he was resurrected, even though he was considered dead already. Those destined to die are difficult to save. Like the death of the Duke of Jin. Treating an illness is like a fire within a pile of firewood; removing the fire keeps the firewood intact, removing the illness allows the person to live. If the firewood is not removed from the fire, it will be burned in vain; if a person's illness is not treated, they will lose their life in vain. There are thousands of good formulas and 800 names of medicines in the world. Zhong Huang Wan (中黄丸, Central Yellow Pills) can treat thousands of illnesses, and Di Ye Jia (底野迦, Theriac) can cure tens of thousands of diseases. The secret in Bian Que's talk about medicine is that the medicines are categorized into Kings and Ministers. They have cold or hot natures. Their tastes are different as well.

夫五常之體，因暑濕而結百疾。頭風目眩須好菊花，脚弱行遲多添石斛。卒中霍亂宜服茅香之湯，久患脊痾急內蚺蛇之膽。痺濕攣痛須用茵芋，皮膚瘙癢宜加蒴藋。傷寒發汗要用麻黃，壯熱不調宜加竹葉。恒山、鱉甲療瘧之功，枳實、芎藭善除心家之悶。卒患鬼注須用雄黃，忽爾驚邪時須龍齒。當歸、芍藥去肚痛之痾，款冬、紫菀除穎嗽之疾。檳榔、白术理宿食不消，硇硝、大黃瀉癥瘕之病。黃連、阿膠善能止痢，通草有發聲之能。水蛭、虻虫善能破血。蕤仁明目，秦皮、決明去瞖，牛膝止膝痛風冷，鵝脂善治耳聾，蜂房能消毒腫，蟹黃善去漆瘡，蕪夷、狼牙殺白虫，桔梗、蘘荷善除蠱毒，亂髮灰能止血汗，滑石通淋瀝之疾。莨草定其牙疼，海藻能除癭氣。知母、栝樓止渴，麥門冬、石膏除溫。署預補骨，澤瀉能治膀胱，遠志、菖蒲聰明益智。脇中乏痛宜用防風、當歸。艾葉、阿膠善治動，連翹止癧，礬石療耳內之膿，小便不利宜服亭歷，杏人益氣身體輕肥。婦人產後羸弱宜服黃精、酸棗、紫花、白微、生葛。人參治五藏虛熱，麥門、鍾乳補肺安心，紫苑、柴胡療人上氣，雄黃、薤白能止狂風，犀角、升麻、烏梅偏醫熱腫，獨活理人面上游風，茵芋、閭茹治人髭落。天行溫病宜服芍藥、生薑，壯熱口乾宜下大青、知母。甘草宜補五藏，人參好定精神。丹參養魂安魄，地黃能通血脉，黃精定長肌膚。

Human beings as an integral part of nature will get hundreds of diseases due to heat and dampness. Head wind with dizziness must use Ju Hua (菊花, chrysanthemum flower). Weakness of limbs caused difficult walking will be benefit from Shi Hu (石斛, dendrobium stem). Suffering from acute gastroenteritis should take Mao Xiang (茅香 or "Mao Gen" 茅根, imperata rhizome) decoction. Long-term suffering from spinal disease requires immediate use of Ran She Dan (蚺蛇膽, python gallbladder). Painful arthritis uses Yin Yu (茵芋, Japanese skimmia stem and leaf); severe skin itch uses Shuo Huo (蒴藋, Chinese elder). Promote sweat during Shang Han, exogenous pathogenic cold-induced diseases, uses Ma Huang (麻黄, ephedra stem). Constant high fever can benefit from Zhu Ye (竹葉, bamboo leaves). Heng Shan (恒山 or "Chang Shan" 常山, dichroa root) and Bie Jia (鱉甲, Chinese soft-shelled turtle shell) have great function to relieve malaria. Zhi Shi (枳實, immature range fruit) and Xiong Qiong (芎藭 or "Chuan Xiong" 川芎, Sichuan lovage rhizome) are good at treating oppression in the heart. Pestilential illness uses Xiong Huang (雄黄, realgar) immediately. Sudden frightening should ask for Long Chi (龍齒, fossilized animal teeth) in no time. Dang Gui (當歸, Chinese angelica root) and Shao Yao (芍藥, white peony root) can heal the disease in the abdomen; Kuan Dong (款冬, Common coltsfoot flower) and Zi Wan (紫苑, Tatarian aster root) are good to eliminate cough. Bing Lang (檳榔, betel nut) and Bai Zhu (白术, white atractylodes tuber) can treat food stagnation; Nao Xiao (硇硝 or "Mang Xiao" 芒硝, Nitrate from saline alkali land) and Da Huang (大黄, rhubarb root) can eliminate abdominal mass. Huang Lian (黄連, yellow coptis root) and E Jiao (阿膠, donkey-hide glue) are good at stopping dysentery disease; Tong Cao (通草, rice paper plant pith) helps to open up voice. Shui Zhi (水蛭, leech) and Mang Chong (虻虫, horse fly) are to break blood stasis; Rui Ren (蕤仁, hedge prinsepia nut) can brighten the eyes; Qin Pi (秦皮, fraxinus bark) and Jue Ming (决明, cassia seeds) can treat cataract. Niu Xi (牛膝, twotoothed achyranthes root) stops knee pains due to wind cold; E Zhi (鹅脂, goose fat) treats deafness; Feng Fang (蜂房, honeycomb) reduces swelling due to toxin; Xie Huang (蟹黄, crab yolk) can heal lacquer dermatitis; Wu Yi (蕪夷, large-fruited elm seed) and Lang Ya (狼牙, the underground winter bud of Agrimonia root) can kill parasites; Jie Geng (桔梗, platycodon root) and Rang He (蘘荷, Mioga ginger rhizome) can treat insect poison; Luan Fa Hui (亂髮灰, human hair ash) can stop bleeding. Hua Shi (滑石, talc) can treat Lin syndrome. Wang Cao (茵草, leaf of poisonous eightangle tree) stops toothache; Hai Zao (海藻, seaweed) reduces goiter. Zhi Mu (知母, common anemarrhena rhizome) and Gua Lou (栝樓 or "Tian Hua Fen" 天花粉, trichosanthes root) quenches thirst; Mai Men Dong (麦門冬, dwarf lilyturf tuber) and Shi Gao (石膏, gypsum) clears heat. Shu Yu (署預 or "Shan Yao" 山药, dioscrea rhizome) can strengthen bones; Ze Xie (澤瀉, alisma tuber) can regulate the bladder function. Yuan Zhi (遠志, Thinleaf milkwort root) and Chang Pu (菖蒲 or "Shi Chang Pu" 石菖蒲, grassleaf sweetflag rhizome) can improve a person's intelligence. Fang Feng (防風, siler root) can treat hypochondriac pain; Dang Gui (當歸, Chinese angelica root);

Ai Ye (艾葉, argy wormwood leaf) and E Jiao (阿膠, donkey-hide glue) can calm the fetus; Lian Qiao (连翹, weeping forsythia Capsule) can eliminate scrofula; Fan Shi (礬石, "Ming Fan" 明矾, a sulfate of alum-stone) can treat pus in the ear; difficult urination should take Ting Li (葶歷 or "Ting Li Zi" 葶歷子, tansymustard seed). Xing Ren (杏人 or 杏仁, apricot seed) can supplement qi and help to lose weight. Postpartum women should take Huang Jing (黄精, solomonseal Rhizome) for weakness after childbirth. Suan Zao (酸棗, Chinese sour jujube seed), Zi Hua (紫花 or "Zi Hua Di Ding" 紫花地丁, Tokyo violet herb), Bai Wei (白薇, blackened white swallowwort root), Sheng Ge (生葛 or "Ge Gen" 葛根, dried pueraria root), and Ren Shen (人参, ginseng root) can treat deficiency heat in five zang. Mai Men (麥門 or "Mai Men Dong" 麥門冬, dwarf lilyturf tuber) and Zhong Ru (鍾乳 or "Zhong Ru Shi" 鍾乳石, stalactite) can tonify lung and calm the mind; Zi Wan (紫苑, tatarian aster root) and Chai Hu (柴胡, Chinese thorowax root) can treat rebellious qi; Xiong Huang (雄黄, realgar) and Xie Bai (薤白, long-stamen onion bulb) can stop maniac; Xi Jiao (犀角, rhinoceros horn), Sheng Ma (升麻, largetrifoliolious bugbane Rhizome), and Wu Mei (烏梅, smoked plum) tend to treat swelling and pain due to heat toxin; Du Huo (獨活, doubleteeth pubescent angelica root) can take care of wandering wind on face; Yin Yu (茵芋, Japanese skimmia stem and leaf) and Lü Ru (閭茹, Euphorbia Lanru root) can treat hair loss. If there is a contagious warm disease, take Shao Yao (芍藥, white peony root) and Sheng Jiang (生薑, fresh ginger); if there is high fever and dry mouth, take Da Qing (大青 or "Da Qing Ye", 大青叶, Isatis leaf) and Zhi Mu (知母, common anemarrhena rhizome). Gan Cao (甘草, licorice root) nourishes five Zang-organs; Ren Shen (人参, ginseng root) replenishes the vital energy. Dan Shen (丹参, salvia root) calms the Hun and Po; Di Huang (地黄, rehmannia root) unblocks the blood vessels. Huang Jing (黄精, solomonseal Rhizome) helps to grow muscles and skin.

夫以三焦為性，處用不同；五昧酸鹹，其根各異。只如天有五星，地有五岳，而運五藏。所以肺為丞相，肝為尚書，心為帝王，脾為大夫，腎為列女。肝與膽合，脾與胃通，小腸連心，大腸連肺，膀胱合腎。是以肝藏盛則目赤，心熱即舌乾，腎虛即耳鳴，肺風即鼻塞。目是肝候，舌是心官，耳作腎司，鼻為肺應。心主血，肺主皮膚，肝主於筋，腎主於骨。骨假筋立，筋籍肉行，肉假皮存，皮因骨長。故骨患從腎，筋患出肝，肉患傷脾，皮患由肺。只如十二經脉，上下巡還；八八脉冀傾，內外流轉。三焦六腑，四海七神，胷膈咽喉，唇齒臂肋，股肱胦胯，指腕爪甲，九竅八扇，三陰五會，小腸胃口，臍脇脊膂，項頰曲鬢，頷額鼻柱，唇齗牙齒，掌腋髮，已上但有患處，皆有所因，莫不內積虛勞，外緣風濕。察其顏色，即辯寒溫；聽聲音，便知損益。只如戲驚者心疾，多笑者腎邪，呻吟者患脾，啼哭者損肺。聲細者是冷，聲絕者患風，聲輕者患虛，聲麁者患熱。膚白是冷，皮青是風，顏黑者是溫，面黃即熱。心虛忘，脾虛患飢，腎冷腰疼，肝實多怒。視毛知血，見瓜知筋，看目知肝，舉齒知骨。骨傷齒黑，損燋筋絕爪乾，氣少聲短，聲聲氣促。髮是血餘，是患之意，原見之可作醫療，即如此委細，乃是良醫。又須用醫方，妙閑藥性，應病與藥性，不羌者是以代無良醫，枉死者半。天地之內，以人為貴，頭圓象天，足方象地。天有四時，人有四支；天有五行，人有五藏；天有六律，人有六腑；天有九星，人有九竅；天有八風，人有八節；天有十 二時，人有十二經脉；天有二十四氣，人有二十四俞；天有三百六十五度，人有三百六十五骨；天有日月，人有眼目；天有晝夜，人有寐寤；天有雷電，人有喜怒；天有雨露，人有啼泣；天有陰陽，人有寒暑。地有九州，人有九竅；地有泉水，人有血脉；地有草木，人有毛髮；地有金石，人有牙齒。是以經云皆禀四大五常，假合成身。夫陰陽之氣，情有喜怒哀樂之性，人有禮義智信。故天圓地方，四時八節，五藏六腑，榮衛之氣，九竅呼吸，寒暑皮毛骨齒，經脉表裏虛實。男子陰陽相繫，為之五勞；冷熱相衝，遂為七傷之疾。厥氣入膀胱，夢遊走。陰氣沉而夢大水，兼之恐懼；陽氣發上，夢見大火而煩。上盛則夢飛空，下盛夢見沉水。中渴，渴即是熱也。

San Jiao (triple burner) has different functions based on the locations. Foods have different tastes because they grow up from different plants and places. The heaven has five stars, the earth has five mountains, and the human body has five Zang-organs. So that the lung is like the Cheng Xiang (prime minister), the liver is like the Shang Shu (minister), the heart is like the Emperor, the spleen is like a senior official, and the kidney is like a woman with moral integrity. The liver works with the gallbladder, the spleen connects the stomach, the small intestine links to the heart, the large intestine coordinates with the lung, and the urinary bladder connects the kidney. Therefore, liver excess causes red eyes, heart heat causes dry mouth, kidney deficiency causes tinnitus, and lung wind causes sinus blockage. The liver manifests on eyes, heart manifests on the tongue, kidney manifests on ears, and lung manifests on the nose. The heart rules the blood vessels, the lung rules the skin, the liver rules the tendons, and the kidney rules the bones. Bones depend on tendons to stand straight, tendons make use of muscles so that one can walk, muscle depends on skin to exist, and skin depends on bones to grow. Therefore, the bone disorders are related to the kidney, the tendon disorders are related to the liver, the muscle disorders will damage the spleen, and the skin disorders are related to the lung. There are 12 meridians that circulate upward and downward and eight extraordinary meridians that flow in the human body internally and externally. There are also triple burners and six Fu-organs; four seas and seven spirits; chest, diaphragm, pharynx, and throat; lips, teeth, arms, and ribs; thighs, forearms, and pelvis; fingers, wrists, and fingernails; nine orifices (for human) and eight holes (for animals other than human), three Yin (channels) and five (Zang-organs and six Fu-organs) meeting points, and small intestine and stomach; navel, hypochondriac area, and spine; neck, cheeks, and mustache (bended knees); chin, forehead, and nose; lips cover the teeth; palms, armpit, and hair, all the aforementioned places could suffer from illness, and the illness must have their causes, which are either internal deficiency and impairment or externally caught wind damp. By looking at the facial color, you will be able to tell if it is cold syndrome or warm syndrome. By listening to the voice, you will know if the person has excess or deficiency. Someone easy to be frightened could have heart sickness; laughing too much means there is evil in the kidney; moaning and groaning are because of the illnesses of the spleen; and crying and sobbing are due to the illnesses of the lung. A soft voice indicates suffering from cold, no voice indicates suffering from wind, a weak voice indicates suffering from deficiency, and a rough voice indicates suffering from heat. Pale skin indicates cold in the body, blue skin tone indicates wind invasion, dark facial color indicates warmth in the body, and sallow face indicates the heat in the body. Heart deficiency causes forgetfulness, spleen deficiency causes hunger, kidney cold causes the lumbar pain, and liver excess causes anger. Looking at hair can know about the blood, looking at nails can know about tendons, looking at eyes can know about the liver, and looking at the teeth can know about bones. The bone injury causes the teeth to turn into a dark color, the blood injury causes the hair to look burned, the tendon damage causes the nail to be dried, and deficient qi causes shortness of breath and shallow breathing. Hair is the residual of blood. According to the clinical manifestations of these diseases to determine the root cause for treatment. If it can be investigated in such detail, this is a good doctor. When prescribing herbal formulas, (a good doctor) needs to know each medicine well and prescribe the medicine according to the illness. (If do so), no disease cannot be cured! But there is no good doctor now. Half of the patients died due to improper treatments. Between the heaven and earth, the human being is the most valued. The head is round shaped that imitates the heaven; the feet are square shaped that imitates the earth. (On the analogy concept), the heaven has four seasons, correspondingly, human has four limbs; the heaven has five elements, so does human has five Zang-organs; the heaven has six rhyms, so does human has six Fu-organs; the heaven has nine stars, so does human has nine orifices; the heaven has eight kinds of winds, so does human has eight (big) joints; the heaven has 12 two-hour periods, so does human has 12 meridians; the heaven has 24 divisions of the solar year, so does human has 24 acupuncture shu points. The heaven has 365 days, so does human has 365 bones; the heaven has sun and moon, so does human has eyes; the heaven has days and nights, so does human knows when to sleep; the heaven has thunder and lightning, so does human has joy and anger; the heaven has rains and dews, so does human has cry and weep; the heaven has Yin and Yang, so does human has cold and heat; the earth has nine states, so does human has nine orifices. The earth has spring water, so does human has blood vessels. The earth has trees and grass, so does human has hair. The earth has metals and rocks, so does human has teeth. So theoretically speaking, it is all the human body formed by the aforementioned reasons due to the "four major and five constants." Qi has Yin and Yang temperament has happiness, anger, sorrow, and joy; and people have (constant virtues of) propriety, righteousness, wisdom, and fidelity. So the sky is round; the earth is square; four seasons and eight solar terms; five Zang-organs and six Fu-organs; Ying Qi and Wei Qi; nine orifices to breathe; skin and hair, bones and teeth to withstand the cold and heat; through the meridian pulse to indicate whether the disease is internal or external and deficiency or excess. Too much sex for men will cause five strains; the imbalance between heat and cold will cause seven impairments. Rebellious Qi that enters the urinary bladder will cause sleepwalks. When Yin-Qi is sinking, one will dream of flooding and having nightmares. If Yang-Qi rises upward, one will dream of catching fire and get irritated. When the upper part of the body is full, one will dream of flying in the sky, and when the lower part of the body is full, one will dream of sinking into the water. Feeling thirsty is caused by heat.

夫五藏重斤两

The weight of five Zang-organs

心為帝王，監領四方，重十二兩，中有七孔，孔有三毛，盛精汁三合，主藏神。肝為尚書，有五葉，應五常，重三斤十兩。膽為將軍決曹吏，在肝短葉下，重九兩，精汁四合。脾為諫議大夫，重二斤三兩，闊三寸，長五寸，有膏半斤，主囊濕血溫，主藏意，在胃下，助胃氣，主化穀食也。胃重二斤十四兩，盛穀三斗五升。肺為丞相，有四葉，應四時，重二斤十二兩，主藏魄，出音聲。腎臟為列女，在後宮，有兩枚，重二斤一兩。主藏末，灌注諸脉也。

The heart is like an emperor, who monitors and controls all four directions. (The heart) weighs 12 liang (a unit of weight). There are seven holes inside the heart. The hole has three hairs. (The heart) contains 3 he of essence liquid ["he" is a unit of dry measure for grain (=1 decilitre)] and houses Shen (mind). The liver is like a minister, who has five leaves, corresponding to the five elements, and the weight is 3 jin [a catty (approximately 500 g)] and 10 liang. The gallbladder is like a general or a clerk in the Bureau of Decision. Below the short lobe of the liver, which weighs 9 liang, contains 4 he of essence liquid. The spleen is like an imperial advisor. It weighs 2 jin and 3 liang. It is 3 inches wide, 5 inches long, with a half a catty gao ("gao" is a kind of tissue has the texture of fat). It mainly stores warm blood. It houses Yi (will). It is located under the stomach and helps the stomach to digest food. The stomach weighs 2 jin and 14 liang. It can hold 3 buckets and 5 liters of grain. The lung is like a prime minister, with four leaves, corresponding to four seasons, weighing 2 jin and 12 liang. It houses Po (the corporeal soul) and is in charge of making voices. The kidney is like an upright woman with moral integrity and lives in the harem. It has 2 pieces, weighing 2 jin and 1 liang, and mainly collects the essence, then infuses the essence into the blood vessels.

五藏論 終

Wu Zang Lun (the end)

是摘錄古醫書中關於藏象之說，以成編者，藥名之部及五常之體，其文理殆類雷公炮論序，看體製古樸實，非唐以後之書也。陳自明婦人良方引卷首生育說五藏論有稱耆婆者，今推其說類皆淺鄙，不經妄託其名於三藏佛者，語涉怪誕。考崇文總目載耆婆五藏論一卷，今檢書中有黃帝為醫王，耆婆童子妙述千端，又稟四大五常，假合成身等語，則所謂訥於耆婆三藏者，則　是書也，是亦醫方類聚採輯本，弟亦柔嘗所鈔出也。

This is a compilation based on excerpts from ancient medical texts concerning the theory of the Zang-organs. The sections on medicinal names and the essence of the Five Constants. Its logic and structure are very similar to the preface of *Master Lei's Discourse on Medicinal Processing* (Léi Gōng Pào Zhì Lùn, 雷公炮炙论), embodying an ancient and straightforward composition, not a book from after the Tang Dynasty. In Chen Ziming's *Great Herbal Formulas for Women* (Fù Rén Liáng Fāng, 妇人良方), he mentions someone attributing the *Five Viscera Theory* (Wǔ Zàng Lùn, 五藏论) to Jivaka. However, upon examination, their theories are shallow and contemptible, just like attributing the author to Tripitaka, with bizarre and strange language. I examined the *Comprehensive Catalogue of Literature During the Song Dynasty* (Chóng Wén Zǒng Mù, 崇文总目) listed one volume of *Jivaka's Five Viscera Theory* (Qí Pó Wǔ Zàng Lùn, 耆婆五脏论). In this book, the Yellow Emperor is named the King of Medicine, and Jivaka, described as a youth of extraordinary erudition, elaborately discusses various aspects, also incorporating the Four Major Principles and the Five Constants, and theories on the composition of the body. Thus, what is falsely attributed to Jivaka or Tripitaka is actually this book, which is also a compilation included in *Categorized Collection of Medical Formulas* (Yī Fāng Lèi Jù, 医方类聚), previously copied by my younger brother Saitei.

文政庚辰霜月初六日識於柳沜精盧

Written on the sixth day of the frost month during the "Wenzheng" period, in the "Gengchen" year, at the place called Liu He Jinglu.

東都丹波元胤紹翁

Taki Mototane of the Eastern Capital, styled Shaoweng.

REFERENCES

1. 多紀元胤, 五藏論/丹波元胤 ［編］ (江户: 学训堂, 1851). www.wul.waseda.ac.jp/kotenseki/html/ya09/ya09_00406/index.html
2. 梁永宣，“朝鲜《医方类聚》的版本流传[J].” *江西中医院学报*, Vol. 19, No. 5 (1964): 47–50.
3. 金秀梅，“丹波父子与《伤寒论》研究[D].” 硕士论文 山东中医药大学 (2001), 3.
4. 曹丹，“《金匮要略疏义》文献研究[D].” 硕士论文 山东中医药大学 (2022), 3.
5. 丹波元胤，*中国医籍考*[M] (北京：人民卫生出版社, 1956), 232.
6. 范行准，*医家训蒙书-五脏论的研究[A]*. 见：王咪咪.，*范行准医学论文集[M]* (北京:学苑出版社, 2011), 27.
7. 陈自明，*妇人大全良方[M]* (北京：人民卫生出版社, 1985), 304.
8. 陈明，“俄藏敦煌文书中一组吐鲁番医学残卷[J].” *敦煌研究*, No. 3 (2002): 102.
9. 黑田源次，“普鲁西学士院所藏中央亚细亚出土医书四种[J].” *支那学*(京都：Vol. 7, No. 4, 1925): 91–124.
10. 罗福颐，“西陲古方技书残卷汇编[J].” *中华医史杂志*, Vol. 4, No. 1 (1953): 27–30.
11. 马继兴，*敦煌古医籍考释[M]* (南昌：江西科学技术出版社, 1988), 37.
12. 李倩，“《医方类聚》所引中国古代医籍研究[D].” 硕士论文，*北京中医药大学* (2006), 30.

Appendix

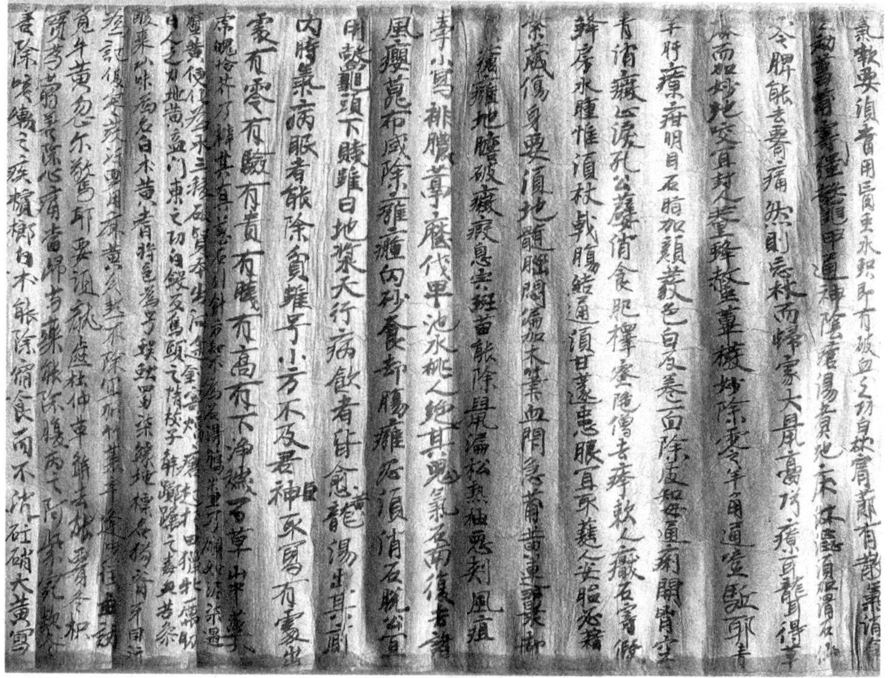

The central section of Pelliot's Dunhuang collection P.2755V scroll, housed at the National Library of France. (Used with permission.) This manuscript focuses on Chinese medicinal herbs and their clinical applications. The content is very similar to the other *Five Viscera Theory* (Wǔ Zàng Lùn, 五藏论), yet remains untitled and lacks an attributed author. (see Chapter 5 for details)

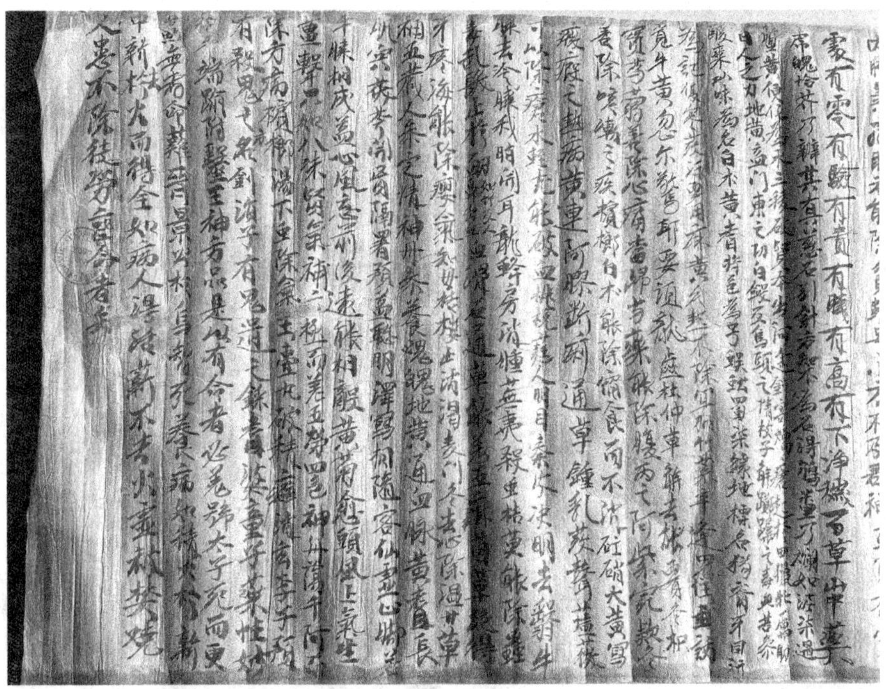

The last section of Pelliot's Dunhuang collection P.2755V scroll, housed at the National Library of France. (Used with permission.) This manuscript focuses on Chinese medicinal herbs and their clinical applications. The content is very similar to the other *Five Viscera Theory* (Wǔ Zàng Lùn, 五藏论), yet remains untitled and lacks an attributed author. (see Chapter 5 for details)

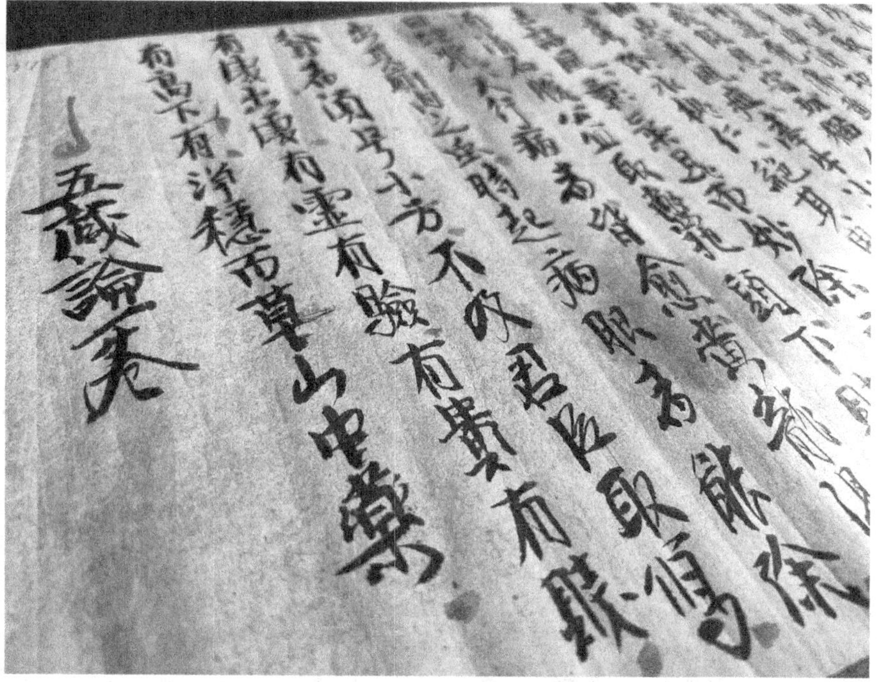

The final section of Pelliot's Dunhuang collection P.2378 scroll at the National Library of France. (Used with permission.) The last section is inscribed with "Wu Zang Lun, one volume" in deep-black ink, lacking the author's name. (See Chapter 6 for details.)

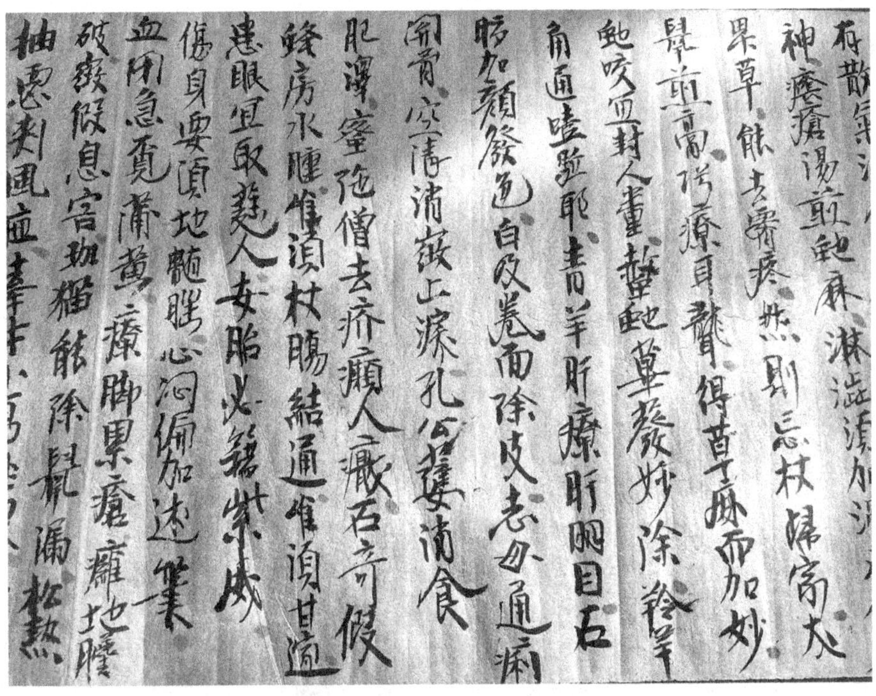

Pelliot's Dunhuang collection P.2378 scroll at the National Library of France. (Used with permission.) This section focuses on Chinese medicinal herbs and their clinical applications. The content is very similar to the other *Five Viscera Theory* (Wǔ Zàng Lùn, 五藏论). (See Chapter 6 for details.)

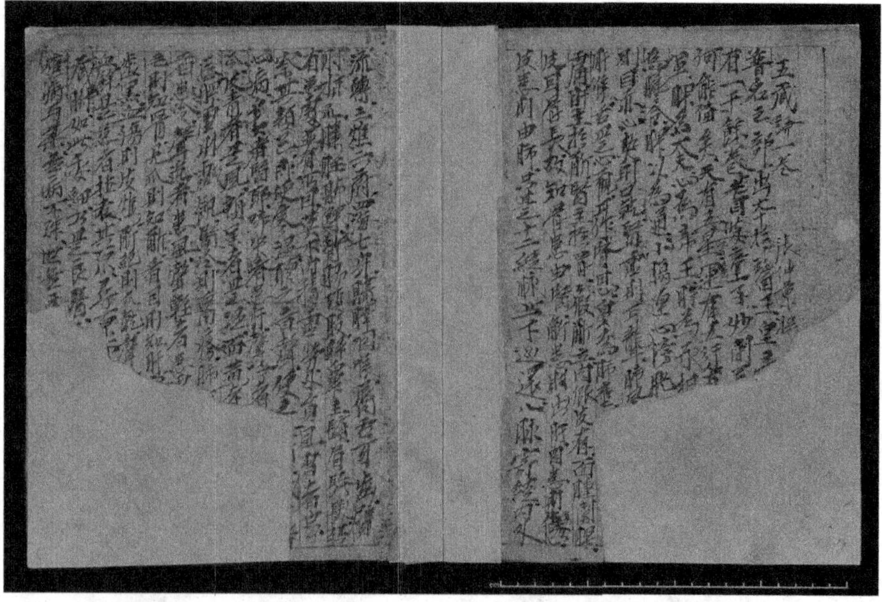

First page of the *Five Viscera Theory* (Wǔ Zàng Lùn, 五藏论) from Stein's Dunhuang collection S. 5614 booklet at the British Library. (Used with permission.) The torn bottom corners give it a butterfly-like appearance. The content resembles other *Five Viscera Theory*. (See Chapter 7 for details.)

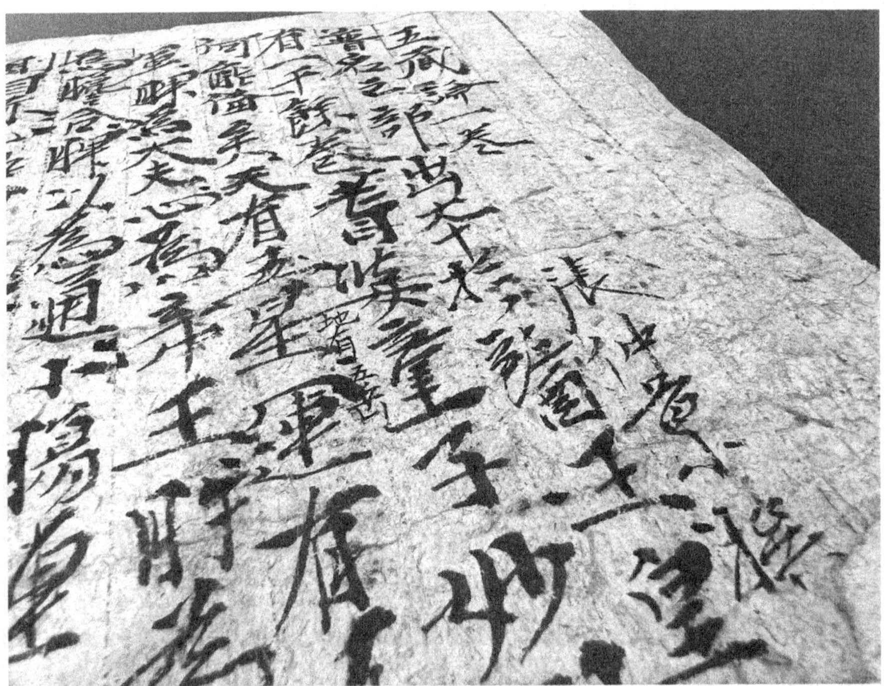

First page of the *Five Viscera Theory* (Wǔ Zàng Lùn, 五藏论) from Stein's Dunhuang collection S. 5614 booklet at the British Library, titled "Wu Zang Lun, One Volume, written by Zhang Zhongjing". (Used with permission.) (See Chapter 7 for details.)

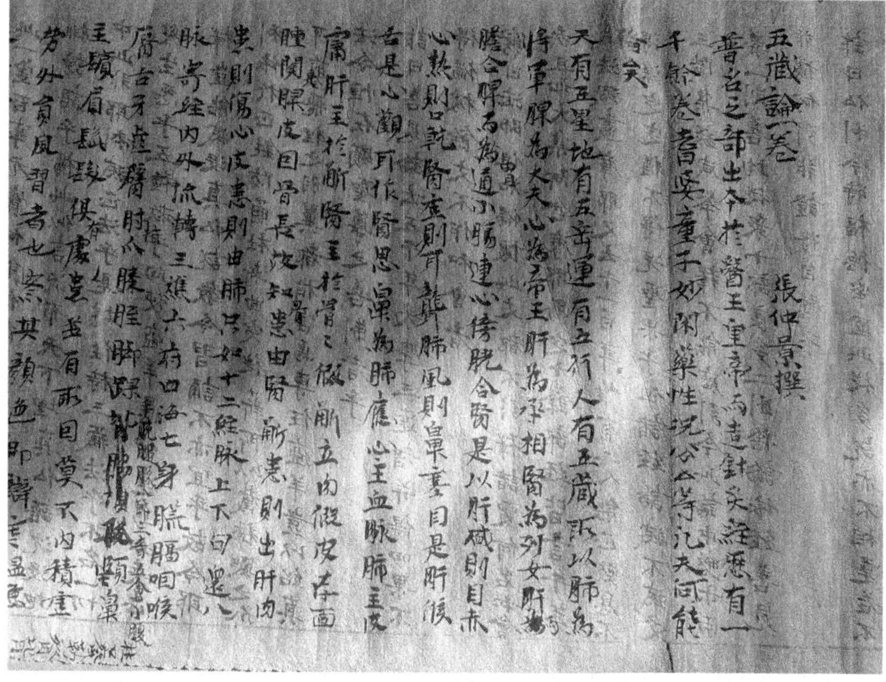

五藏論一卷 張仲景撰

Beginning of the Pelliot Dunhuang collection P.2115V scroll at the National Library of France, titled "Wu Zang Lun, One Volume, written by Zhang Zhongjing". (Used with permission.) The content resembles other *Five Viscera Theory* manuscripts. (See Chapter 9 for details.)

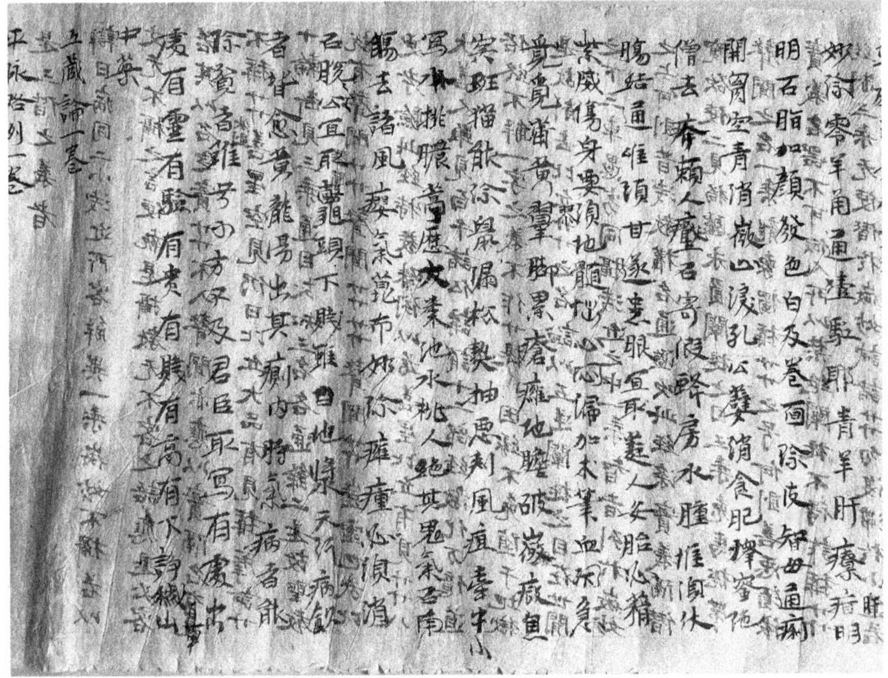

End section of the Pelliot Dunhuang collection P.2115V at the National Library of France. (Used with permission.) Like the P.2378 scroll, it ends with the title "Wu Zang Lun, One Volume". (See Chapter 9 for details.)

Index

C

D

E

F

G

H

I

M

N

Q

R

T

U

V

W

X

Y

Z

Printed in the United States
by Baker & Taylor Publisher Services